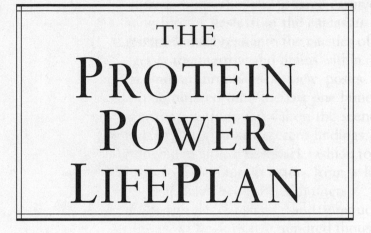

THE
PROTEIN
POWER
LIFEPLAN

THE
PROTEIN
POWER
LIFEPLAN

MICHAEL R. EADES, M.D.
MARY DAN EADES, M.D.

WARNER BOOKS

A Time Warner Company

The authors do not intend this book to be a substitute for advice from your own medical or health professional who should be consulted before you proceed with any recommendations in *The Protein Power Lifeplan*. Anyone with a known disease or serious health condition or who is taking prescription or non-prescription medications should especially seek professional medical advice before beginning *The Protein Power Lifeplan* or following specific recommendations as to types and dosages of medications, supplements, or products. In any case, you should discuss all aspects of *The Protein Power Lifeplan* with your doctor or health professional as he or she may wish to tailor the program to your specific needs. The authors and the publishers expressly disclaim responsibility for any adverse effects arising from the use or application of the information contained in this book.

Warner Books, Inc., 1271 Avenue of the Americas,
New York, NY 10020

Visit our Web site at www.twbookmark.com

W A Time Warner Company

Printed in the United States of America
First Warner Books Printing: January 2000
10   9   8   7   6   5   4   3

Library of Congress Cataloging-in-Publication Data

Eades, Michael R.
The protein power lifeplan / Michael R. Eades and Mary Dan Eades.
p.   cm.
Includes index.
ISBN 0-446-52576-6
1. Low-carbohydrate diet.   2. High-protein diet.   I. Title.   II. Eades, Mary Dan.
RM237.73.E229   2000
613.2'821—dc21   99-043052

Text design by Stanley S. Drate/Folio Graphics Co. Inc.
Illustrations in chapter 10 by Scott Eades.

To our parents:
Larry and Edith Mary Crane
and
Jerald and Virginia Eades

ACKNOWLEDGMENTS

Every book is more than just the written product of its authors; this one is certainly no different. We wish to gratefully acknowledge some of the people who helped us to bring this book to you.

First, to Larry Kirshbaum, Maureen Egen, and Diana Baroni, who believed in the project strongly enough to throw the considerable power of Warner Books behind it, our heartfelt gratitude—we hope we've justified your faith in us. Thanks as well to both our hardworking and loyal agents, Carol Mann and Channa Taub, who helped us to find this new and congenial publishing home. A special additional thanks must go to Channa, who throughout this project (as always) stood ready with her sharpened pencil and whip to keep our noses to the grindstone.

A bow to our copyeditor, Pamela Marshall, who didn't let a thing slip by and, along with Bob Castillo and the other Warner editorial staff, did her best to keep us honest.

To all our own staff, especially Michelle Hegwood (who has put up with us for a dozen years) and Debbie Nelson and Kristi McAfee (who are just learning to put up with us), thanks for holding the fort.

For always being ready to read and discuss the finer points of metabolic medicine and Paleolithic nutrition, thanks especially to Ron Rosedale, Larry McCleary, Loren Cordain, and Robert Crayhon.

And, as always, thanks to our children, Ted (and wife, Jamye), Dan, and Scott, for enduring the lack of our usual fawning attention during the writing of this book. We love you.

CONTENTS

x   *Contents*

INTRODUCTION

S ince the publication of our previous book *Protein Power* in early 1996, readers have sent us tens of thousands of letters and e-mails, telling us of their successes, not just with losing weight, but in solving many serious health problems with which they'd struggled. And while we're always delighted to hear that our plan has helped, these beneficial effects didn't surprise us at all—we'd seen them many times before. Although our previous publisher chose to feature weight loss as the primary benefit of our plan—and as a result many people mistakenly categorized our book as simply a diet book—we have always emphasized the effectiveness of the *Protein Power* nutritional program in treating diabetes and cholesterol and triglyceride disorders. It still remains the most effective tool we've ever seen to stabilize blood sugar and improve lipid profiles—as evidenced by the success of the many thousands of our own patients on whom we've used it and as the many thousands more of readers who have written to us attest. But over the dozen-plus years we've prescribed this nutritional regimen, we've seen its therapeutic power in other areas of health as well, such as in reducing the inflammatory symptoms of such autoimmune disorders as ulcerative colitis, rheumatoid arthritis, and Crohn's disease. We didn't have space in our first book to fully explore the range of health benefits that readers might experience using the plan, and when they got relief from symptoms of such diverse disorders as gastroesophageal reflux, or severe heartburn (which virtually always improves), and chronic inflammatory bowel disorders, they wrote by the thousands to tell us. Over the years, we've seen these kinds of dramatic results time and again. This second book gives us the opportunity to answer readers' queries, to include information on the many far-ranging benefits of the regimen, and to offer, at last, a comprehensive plan for living what we think of as a *Protein Power*ed life.

You see, our premise—the one we've lived by now for over a decade—is that humans are born to be well, but they spend the greater part of their lives mortgaging that birthright and squandering their health potential. We like to examine ideas, not against the limited experience of nutritional and scientific information gathered over the last five, ten, twenty, or even hundred years, but against the hundred thousand or so generations of human experience that have come before to see what's valid and what's not. Examining nutrition and lifestyle through that "Paleolithic lens" points up a number of major shifts in the way we live, work, eat, and play today compared to the optimal design molded over the millennia by the forces of nature. Our physiologies are the same as they were fifty thousand years ago—truly, we're cavemen in designer suits with cell phones. What we've come to understand—and what we lay out in this book—is that if we can identify and correct these major differences in nutrition and lifestyle, we can return to the state of natural health that we were born to enjoy. Our goal here is to acquaint you with these differences and to teach you how to best resolve them in a twenty-first-century world.

We'll begin by reintroducing you to your hunting past and by making the strong case for eating meat (that's not to say it's impossible to stick to a *Protein Power LifePlan* if you're a vegetarian—it's not; it just takes more effort). Then, in chapter 2, "The Insulin Connection," we'll review the Diseases of Civilization—the diabetes, heart disease, lipid disorders, hypertension, and obesity that resulted from our adoption of agriculture some ten thousand years ago when we opted out of hunting and gathering in favor of grains. In the four plus years since we completed the manuscript for *Protein Power* many new disorders, such as metabolic iron-storage disease, clotting disorders, sleep apnea, polycystic ovary disease, and even colon cancer, have entered as possible competitors in the insulin-resistance sweepstakes. As far as we are able, we'll cover these disorders here. But bear in mind: new ones are being added almost faster than we can write about them.

We've devoted separate chapters to covering much of this new information. We'll examine the dangers of excess iron storage and make recommendations on how to determine your level of risk and to reduce that risk. We'll weigh in on the dangers of artificial sweeteners with critical new information that, in some cases, has changed our position on their safety. We'll explore the science behind the damage that cereal grains can do to your gut and their possible connection to the development of autoimmune disorders. We'll look at the addictive nature of grains. We'll cover the issue of dietary fats and help you to better understand their essential nature, including those kinds of fat you should eat for health and those you should avoid. We'll look at the crucial protective role of antioxidants, showing you how and where they help as well as which foods provide the best sources and how best to supplement their levels.

We've refined our nutritional plan, presenting it here on three levels that we call Hedonist, Dilettante, and Purist. While the general biochemical principle remains the same for all three groups—namely, that restricting carbohydrate intake lowers insulin and ultimately leads to health benefits—the level of restriction of specific foods or groups of foods that research has shown can cause health problems for some people varies. The Hedonist plan, the least restrictive of all, offers the most health benefits possible for the least nutritional change. It picks up where the original *Protein Power* strategy left off with three new and important caveats: no trans fats (i.e., partially hydrogenated), no aspartame as a sweetener, and no added fructose.

For people who will accept slightly more restriction for better health, we designed the Dilettante plan, in which we eliminate a few of the more troublesome foods—primarily certain grains associated with gut damage and arthritic disorders—and aim toward purging the diet of potentially toxic additives, such as the hormones, antibiotics, and pesticides found in some products. (It is, in fact, the version we stick to ourselves most of the time.)

And finally, for those people who wish to wring the most health benefits possible from their nutrition and lifestyle, who want to hew more nearly to a truly Paleolithic diet, we've designed that which comes closest, the Purist plan, in which we eliminate virtually everything not available to early humans—all grains, all dairy, all sources of added hormones, antibiotics, pesticides, alchol, and caffeine—in short, coming as close as is possible in a modern world to eating the diet that nature designed for us to eat.

But our modern lifestyle has deviated from our ancestral one in more ways than simply nutrition, and we'll examine those as well, covering such areas as the modern widespread magnesium deficiency and how best to treat it, the consequences of sunlight deprivation, and the benefits of high-intensity exercise. In these chapters, we'll show you how to return to a more natural lifestyle even in this modern and fast-paced world. We've also included some information on how you can keep your brain as sharp as your body—both through proper nutrition and regular use.

We've endeavored to answer the questions that have regularly come up over the last several years, to include the benefits of our plan that space didn't permit in the previous book, to fill in some gaps that needed filling, and to showcase the new, cutting-edge information that's come to light since we turned in the previous manuscript to our editor in the summer of 1995. Our purpose is to provide you with a comprehensive blueprint—a complete life plan—that will enable you to be as well as you can possibly be.

Throughout the book, we've tried to present scientific information in a way that makes it accessible to anyone interested in finding out more. For those readers who have a scientific bent we've tried to explain the science fully without resorting to medical or scientific jargon. But we feel the new information is critical to all readers—even those who don't have the inclination to wade through all the scientific underpinnings. For this group, as we did in *Protein Power*, we've provided a short summary of each chapter that gives the high points without all the detail. We understand that time is often a precious commodity and that you may want to get to the "meat" of the plan quickly and perhaps go back later to those particular chapters that intrigue you or pique your interest to know more. If that's the case, we ask that you at least read the Bottom Line summaries (only a couple of pages at the end of each chapter) before diving into the workings of the plans. The Bottom Line summaries also work well to provide a quick overview; they're a good way to breeze through the entire book on a superficial level and get the gist of things before you go back at your leisure to read in more depth.

In the past four years—often in the face of their patients' successes on our *Protein Power* plan—more and more doctors and nutritionists have begun to question the low-fat, high-carb diet and acknowledge that a diet that limits carbohydrates while ensuring adequate amounts of the protein and fat that is essential for the body's health makes sense. Four years ago, an individual seeing a nutritionist because he or she was overweight or in poor health or fit but feeling tired would have been told to cut fat and get plenty of complex carbs. Now, many will be told instead to make sure they're getting enough protein and watch those carbs. Four years ago, "power bars" had 40+ grams of carbs and 7 grams of protein; now more and more the ratio is reversed. So the landscape has indeed changed for the better, and in that regard we couldn't be happier. Nonetheless, many people still view fat as a dirty word and are afraid to eat those foods that have been forbidden for so long. So we'll take a few moments here to explain once again why the low-fat diet has led most of us astray, setting us as a nation on the most direct path to obesity and the ailments that accompany it.

Tell Me Again Why the Low-Fat, High-Carb Diet Undermines My Health

Many of the letters we've received have expressed some skepticism about our advocacy of a protein-rich, moderate-fat, carbohydrate-restricted diet in the face of the "certain truth" that the low-fat food pyramid diet is the way to health. In many of these missives, the recurring theme includes some reference to the health of the Chinese. Most people assume that the Chinese eat little protein and a lot of rice and vegetables and don't have heart disease; therefore, they conclude, eating a high-carb diet must be healthier.

The idea that the Chinese don't have cardiovascular disease is firmly implanted in the minds of just about everyone. However, the truth of the matter is that the Chinese do indeed have cardio-vascular disease, and lots of it. According to the *1999 Heart and Stroke Statistical Update* published annually by the American Heart Association, the rates of death from cardiovascular disease suffered by both rural and urban Chinese males is almost indistin-guishable from the rate experienced by American males, while the rates of cardiovascular deaths for both rural and urban Chinese women is significantly higher than those suffered by American fe-males.[1] And bear in mind that cardiovascular disease is the num-ber one killer of Americans. The notion that the Chinese don't have disease of the heart and blood vessels is what we like to call a vampire myth—it simply refuses to die. The myth that low-fat, high-carbohydrate diets are healthy lives on and on.

For example, in an otherwise excellent book (by a faculty member of a prestigious Ivy League medical school), the author, after bemoaning the sorry state of the American diet, sees a ray of hope in the future. He writes:

> America's table is, slowly but surely, becoming leaner. In the 1970s and 1980s, we witnessed some encouraging changes in the American diet. Beef consumption declined for the first time in the history of the country. The consumption of leaner chicken and fish rose. The word *fiber* entered everyday parlance, as did *cholesterol* and *oat bran*. Despite a confused chorus of experts recommending different strategies, a lot of Americans still got the message: eat less fat and more fruits, vegetables, whole grains, and fiber. [Italics in original.]

The author is correct. Beginning with the back-to-the-earth movement of the late 1960s and early 1970s, various authorities have pounded the low-fat drum until the message finally thudded into our national collective consciousness. And the message has

---

1. In both rural and urban China the majority of deaths from cardiovascular disease are from stroke, whereas the majority of cardiovascular deaths in the United States are from heart attack. Urban-dwelling Chinese males have about half the rate of heart attack of American males but almost six times the rate of stroke; urban Chinese females have about three-quarters the rate of heart attack of their American counterparts and almost five times the rate of death from stroke.

been heeded by most Americans. The entire populace has been counting fat grams and fat percentages for the past twenty years or so. The food-processing industry, discovering a new way to increase sales, has ridden the low-fat wave shamelessly, employing cadres of food technologists who have figured out ways to engineer almost every food available into a low-fat or nonfat variety, wrapping them all in packaging proclaiming their low-fat/no-fat, no-cholesterol status. And America has bought it. Sales of low-fat products have blasted into the stratosphere. People are reading labels in the aisles of supermarkets everywhere in order to purchase only those products containing minimal fat, or better yet, no fat (and, typically, minimal taste, but that doesn't really matter in the great American quest to cut the fat). After loading the car with grocery bags of low-fat foods, it's off to jog or to the health club to work out. As we approach the turn of this century, we've become Mark Twain's fitness buff of the turn of the last century who "eats what he doesn't want, drinks what he doesn't like, and does what he'd druther not, all the while smugly announcing himself to be energetic, joyful, and certain of long life, and exhorting his errant neighbor to reform."

And where has this passion for dietary austerity gotten us? We have become the people characterized by the humorist P. J. O'Rourke, who in a recent magazine article described "the American people" as "masses waddling into airports, business offices and churches dressed in drooping sweats or fuchsia warm-up suits or mainsail-sized Bermuda shorts, each with a mobile phone in one ear and a Walkman in the other and sucking Diet Pepsi through a straw."

According to the latest statistics, gym and spa memberships have almost doubled over the past ten years, while government surveys show that more and more Americans are "eating more healthily" by buying less meat and making every effort to cut the fat from their diets.[2] For the past two decades there has been a

---

2. As measured by the Healthy Eating Index (HEI), developed by the United States Department of Agriculture in 1989. This index measures the consumption of grains (by their standards healthy), vegetables, fruits, and meat (by their standards unhealthy) in the average American diet and assigns an overall score, with 100 being the gold standard. The American Dietetic Association dubbed the HEI "the most accurate measure-

concerted effort by the government, the medical profession, the drug companies, food manufacturers, and the nutritional establishment to wean us from dietary fat. "Authorities" on all fronts have cautioned us that fat in the diet is the cause of obesity, heart disease, type II diabetes, too much cholesterol in the blood, numerous types of cancer, and a host of other problems. If we zealously exterminate the fat from our diet, we've been told, we can protect ourselves against all of these diseases. And oh, have we listened.

According to government statistics we have reduced the fat consumption in the United States by almost 25 percent over the past fifteen years[3] (see below). By all rights this decline in the consumption of fat should have increased the health of Americans by quantum leaps. But has it? Have obesity, diabetes, cancer, and all the rest of the diseases laid at the door of dietary fat been reduced by a commensurate amount? Hardly. During this same time period we have seen in this country an almost epidemic increase in these disorders. The incidence of adult obesity has increased by almost 30 percent in the past decade alone. Childhood obesity has *doubled*. Type II diabetes has increased by a factor of more than *ten*. Heart disease deaths, after more than ten years of decline, took a turn for the worse in 1992 and have slowly been increasing since. An accurate measure of the increase in cardio-vascular diseases can be seen in the rates of discharge from the hospital of patients with that diagnosis, which, according to the American Heart Association, have increased by 25 percent since 1976. The incidence of stroke is on the rise, and cancer continues its relentless and increasing toll with the very cancers most often blamed on fat consumption—cancer of the breast and prostate—leading the charge.

---

ment to date on how Americans eat." In 1996 the HEI was 63.8, which was an improvement over the 61.5 calculated in 1989. Of course this index measures an improvement in healthy eating only if you consider a lot of grains and starchy vegetables and not much meat as healthy, which we don't. You can find all you would ever want to know about the HEI on the Internet at www.usda.gov/cnpp/hei.htm.

3. The third National Health and Nutrition Examination Survey (NHANES III) researchers found that a cross section of Americans ate 33 percent of their calories as fat in 1997, down from the 43 percent found during the NHANES II study in 1987.

Fat Intake and Prevalence of Overweight Among U.S. Adults

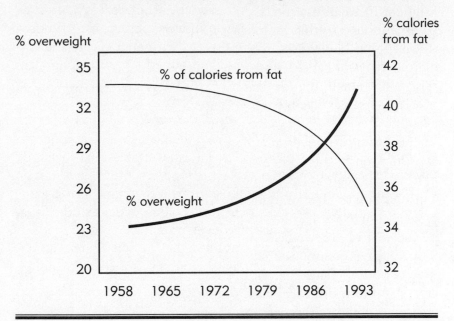

Clearly the low-fat diet hasn't been the panacea that many had hoped for; in fact, it has turned out to be a dismal failure, a fact admitted publicly in 1996 by most of the world's experts in nutritional research. And we were on hand to hear it. We attended the Second International Symposium on Dietary Fats and Oil Consumption in Health and Disease hosted by Southwestern University Medical School in Dallas, Texas, in April 1996, at which nutritional researchers from around the world presented their findings on the effects of fat in the human diet. After the presentations showing that study subjects following the low-fat diet hadn't gotten rid of their obesity, hadn't lowered their cholesterol levels,[4] had lowered their HDL levels (the good cholesterol),

---

4. The only positive finding was that the low-fat diet *sometimes* lowered LDL cholesterol (the so-called bad cholesterol), but even that finding was negated by the fact that this lowered LDL cholesterol was converted—under the influence of the low-fat diet—into a subtype that is actually more dangerous.

and had increased their blood levels of triglycerides (a major risk factor for heart disease; see chapter 4), the moderators of the symposium pronounced the low-fat diet a failure.[5] When asked by audience members (most of whom were physicians, scientists, or nutritionists) how they should treat their patients now that the low-fat diet is not the cure-all we had hoped for, the moderators responded that they didn't know for sure what did work, but they definitely knew what didn't.[6]

The *American Journal of Clinical Nutrition* published as a supplement to their March 1998 issue all the papers presented at this symposium along with some of the formal discussions that took place. The following quotes from this supplement will give you an idea of the thinking of the symposium participants: "At this stage there is no conclusive evidence from epidemiologic studies that dietary fat intake promotes the development of obesity more so than other macronutrients"; "Within the United States, a substantial decline in the percentage of energy from fat consumed during the past two decades has corresponded with a massive increase in obesity"; "Diets high in fat are not the primary cause of the high prevalence of excess body fat in our society, nor are reductions in dietary fat a solution"; "Numerous publications dating back to the preinsulin era showed that low-fat, high-carbohy-

---

5. As attendees at this conference we can tell you how resolute were the moderators and most of the speakers in their emphatic denunciations of the low-fat diet. We were surprised—but then again not really—when the published version of this conference had the following lukewarm conclusion in the editorial overview of the meeting: "In summary, this supplement brings the role of macronutrient composition as a determinate of nutritional health into focus. It calls into question but does not necessarily negate the recommendations for a change in eating habits to reduce the percentage of fat in the diet."

6. Interestingly, despite the attendance and participation of a great number of the world's experts on diet and nutrition at this symposium, it garnered zero press coverage. The week after this meeting, however, a researcher from Iowa published a paper in the *Journal of the American Medical Association* that indicated that people who ate hamburger more than thirty-two times per month developed non–Hodgkin's lymphoma (a type of blood cancer) at a slightly greater rate than those who ate hamburger less frequently. The *New York Times* and *USA Today* reported these findings, and we heard the researcher interviewed on National Public Radio. You tell us which is the most important and the most newsworthy: the world's nutritional experts renouncing the low-fat diet or the study about hamburger? Conspiracy buffs, take note.

drate diets increase serum lipids"; "Replacement of saturated fat by carbohydrates adversely affects plasma HDL [good cholesterol]"; "It is clear that compared with high-carbohydrate diets, high-monounsaturated-fat diets improve lipoprotein profiles as well as the glycemic profile."

The astounding thing about the whole low-fat-diet disaster is that the entire country (actually, the entire world, at least that part of it that was boneheaded enough to take it seriously) took part in a long-term scientific study based on theories—not fact, but theories—that turned out to be wrong. It's mind-boggling that the medical and nutritional scientific hierarchy encouraged all 250 million or so of us to participate in this experiment by constantly exhorting us for the sake of our health to cut, cut, cut the fat from our diets without a shred of hard evidence that it would work. Walter Willett, M.D., Ph.D., professor of medicine and chairman of the Department of Nutrition at the Harvard School of Public Health, said in a recent interview, "Low-fat has been like a religion. But it was just a hypothesis to begin with."[7] So, the low-fat diet was foisted on Americans as if it were a proven road to health when it was nothing but a hypothesis. A theory. An idea. In reality, an educated guess.

But isn't it pretty clear that fat in the diet and cholesterol at least cause heart disease? Not really. The whole idea that fat and cholesterol cause heart disease is just that: an idea. The idea has a name: it's called the lipid hypothesis. Not the lipid fact, but the lipid hypothesis. It's a hypothesis instead of a fact because no one is exactly sure what does cause heart disease. A hypothesis becomes a fact when enough experimental evidence accumulates to confirm the hypothesis, which hasn't happened by a long shot yet with heart disease. In fact, there are a number of hypotheses about what causes heart disease, some of the more prominent of which are listed below in no particular order of importance: the homocysteine hypothesis, the trans-fatty-acid hypothesis, the infectious hypothesis, the hemodynamic (blood flow) hypothesis, the magnesium-deficiency hypothesis, the heated-milk-protein hy-

---

7. Interview in *U.S. News and World Report,* 12 January 1998, 57.

pothesis, the sugar hypothesis, the vegetable-oil hypothesis, and the vitamin C–deficiency hypothesis.

These are but a few of the many theories of why we develop heart disease at such great rates, and we'll touch on some in greater detail in later chapters. When scientists finally find the answer it will probably be a combination of circumstances, not a single cause. An interesting common feature about these theories is that they all, except maybe the infectious hypothesis, argue that heart disease is a function of our Western diet in some respect. Another interesting particular about these hypotheses is that those that get media attention are the ones that drug companies can develop medications to fix: the lipid hypothesis (cholesterol-lowering drugs); the infectious hypothesis (new antibiotics); the homocysteine hypothesis (proprietary vitamin combinations); and the hemodynamic hypothesis (anticoagulants).

Surely, though, saturated fat, the bane of all nutritionists and dietitians, has been implicated as a risk factor for heart disease and a host of other maladies, hasn't it? Absolutely. But just being *implicated* is not the same as being a *cause*. However, with all the finger pointing going on, you would think saturated fat had been caught red-handed and had had its guilt proven beyond the shadow of a doubt. But, alas, even with poor old much maligned saturated fat, such is not the case. A recent paper that reviewed all the other papers published on the role of saturated fat in heart disease concluded that "there is little evidence that SFA (saturated fatty acids) as a group are harmful."[8] So, the low-fat diet has been a disaster, and even saturated fat isn't as bad as we thought it was. Recent nutritional research further attests to this truth. Let's take a look at a study published a couple of years ago that not only demonstrates the innocence of fat as a cause of cardiovascular disease but also illustrates a number of things you should look for in interpreting the medical literature.

---

8. U. Ravnskov, "The Questionable Role of Saturated and Polyunsaturated Fatty Acids in Cardiovascular Disease," *Journal of Clinical Epidemiology* 51, no. 6 (1998): 443–460.

The Spanish Paradox

When a group of scientists evaluated the changing dietary patterns in Spain over the past twenty-five years, they found that the consumption of bread decreased, the consumption of fruits and vegetables decreased, and the consumption of even olive oil decreased.[9] Over the same time, Spaniards increased their consumption of dairy products and meat of all kinds. In other words, the diet of the average Spaniard—at least by our misguided modern nutritional standards—degenerated; he ate more high-fat foods of animal origin, while at the same time low-fat, high-carbohydrate foods went lacking. According to the prevailing pyramid paradigm of what good nutrition is (again, misguided in our opinion), people throughout Spain should be dropping like flies from cardiovascular disease. What the researchers found, however, was that the rates of death from heart disease declined dramatically over this period. Since this didn't fit with what the researchers expected to find, they, as all good researchers do, tried to find some way to reconcile their data with what they "knew" to be true. They reckoned that perhaps some isolated areas in Spain contained unenlightened people who ate a lot of meat, fat, and dairy products, fouling up the statistics for the rest of the country. And when they did evaluate consumption on a region-by-region basis they found exactly that, but, unfortunately for their hypothesis, the high-meat-eating regions had the *greatest* declines in the rates of death from heart disease. In their words, "it is also paradoxical that regions demonstrating the highest increases in fat intake displayed the lowest rates of CHD [coronary heart disease] mortality." So uncooperative were their data that these researchers wrote the whole thing off as a quirk and called it the Spanish Paradox. They added a caveat that we're sure would never have been added had their data not blown up in their faces but that is most important and needs to be heeded whenever evaluating a

---

9. L. Serra-Mejam et al., "How Could Changes in Diet Explain Changes in Coronary Heart Disease Mortality in Spain? The Spanish Paradox," *American Journal of Clinical Nutrition* 61, suppl. 6 (June 1995): 1351s–1359s.

study of this type: "Observational studies on populations are only useful for formulating hypotheses and they cannot provide convincing evidence of cause-and-effect relations."

This caveat is the first of two that we recommend you heed whenever you evaluate medical studies. This type of study is called an epidemiological study, which is a study of the disease patterns of large groups of people as a function of a particular activity, such as diet, exercise, or smoking. You see epidemiological studies all the time reported in the media. For instance, when you read the report of a study that shows that Greeks who consume large amounts of olive oil live longer than those who don't, the inference that you draw from such a study is that olive oil promotes longevity. Actually such a study tells you nothing other than that olive oil consumption may promote longevity and that the theory should be evaluated in a controlled study designed to eliminate as many of the other variables as possible. The reason you can't use the epidemiological study to prove this hypothesis is that there are way too many variables in a free living group of people to be able to dissect only olive oil consumption out of the mix and keep everything else equal.

Looking at epidemiological studies always reminds us of a story we read somewhere about a kid taking a test in college. One of the questions went something like this: You are in a tall building and you have an altimeter. How can you use it to determine the height of the building? The obvious answer is to subtract the altitude reading on the ground from the reading at the top of the building. The kid, however, listed a number of unorthodox methods using the altimeter. He pointed out that he could tie the altimeter to a string and hang it off the building until it touched the ground, then measure the string. He could drop the altimeter from the top and time its fall, then calculate the height. He went on to list a host of other novel ways to use the altimeter to find the answer and ended his answer by writing that he could simply take the altimeter to the architect who designed the building and say, "I'll give you this really cool altimeter if you'll tell me how tall the building is." Researchers doing an epidemiological study have, just like this kid, a thousand different ways of looking at the problem. And they often pick a solution that confirms their bias.

The second caveat is never, never, never rely on only one study. Whenever you see a single study hailed in the media as the proof of anything, remember this caveat. All scientists have biases, and more times than not they design the study (and, after all, it is their study) to show exactly what they want to show. Whenever we see a study that purports to prove a benefit of meat, we have to fight down the impulse to wave it in the face of anyone who disagrees with us. But that's not good science. Rather, what we do is evaluate the study carefully, looking at all the "fine print," which is the manner in which the study was designed and carried out, looking at the raw data, and only then looking at the researcher's conclusions to see if they indeed do follow from the procedures and data. If after our analysis the study looks sound, and if it is corroborated by other studies,[10] only then do we wave the study in the face of everyone.

So, where do we go from here? Now that it has become clear that the low-fat diet is not the answer to our nutritional prayers, what is? What kind of diet should we follow to maximize our health and longevity? A vegetarian diet? A high-protein diet? A low-protein diet? A macrobiotic diet? A low-calorie diet? What *is* the best way to eat to maintain our health and to prevent or reverse the diseases that we've come to associate with aging? And since the low-fat diet was such a bust despite the many assurances we had from almost all the health authorities, how do we know that another diet will be any better in the long run? What should we eat?

---

10. A sometimes exception to the one-study caveat is what are called meta-analysis and review studies. These are studies in which a researcher knowledgeable in the field evaluates the data from a large number of studies performed over several years in a variety of laboratories looking for trends and statistical significance. One such study in the *Journal of the National Cancer Institute* evaluated seventy-two different studies on the link between tomato consumption and the risk of various cancers. It appears from this analysis that there is a statistically significant link between high levels of tomato consumption and lower risk for prostate, lung, and stomach cancer. This type of study obviously is more reliable than just one study showing this same link, but you've still got to be careful because a biased researcher can include only those studies "proving" his point of view. See E. Giovannuci, "Tomatoes, Tomato-based Products, Lycopenes, and Cancer: Review of the Epidemiological Literature," *Journal of the National Cancer Institute* 91, no. 4 (17 February 1999): 317–331.

Part of the answer can be found in the writing of anthropologist Mark Nathan Cohen: "The field of medicine often appears naïve about the full range of human biological experience, basing conclusions about human health—even what is 'normal'—on the comparatively narrow experience of contemporary Western society." The scientists and nutritionists who promoted the low-fat diet got waylaid because they based their recommendations on a few preliminary studies (and a whole lot of bias) involving a few thousand subjects while remaining oblivious to, or ignoring, the vast amount of anthropological data accumulated on the health and dietary habits of humans living over many millennia.

In the coming chapters, we'll examine the diet that our ancient ancestors ate and the lifestyle that they lived and reconcile that with our modern existence, trying to take into account the best of both worlds.

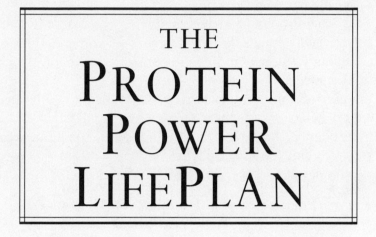

THE
PROTEIN
POWER
LIFEPLAN

All truth passes through three stages. First, it is ridiculed. Second, it is violently opposed. Third, it is accepted as being self-evident.
—ARTHUR SCHOPENHAUER

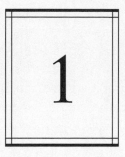

MAN THE HUNTER

The deviation of man from the state in which he was
originally placed by nature seems to have proved to him
a prolific source of diseases.
—EDWARD JENNER (1749–1823)

I n our living room on the coffee table sits one of our most
prized possessions, a fifteen-to-twenty-thousand-year-old cave-
bear skull that we got from Russia. From back of the head to
snout the skull measures almost two feet in length and sports ca-
nine teeth that are three inches long. The entire animal would
have been about seven to eight feet tall and weighed close to a
thousand pounds. Examination of this skull shows a huge ridge
running along the top, where the muscles that worked the jaws
were connected. From here they ran along the face and attached
to bony protrusions (called the mandibular rami) on the lower
jaw. The larger the mandibular ramus, the greater the mass of the
muscle attached to it and the greater the closing force of the jaws.
The mandibular rami of our cave bear are about the size of a
child's hand, and when you compare them to the size of the rami
of a human jaw, or even a dog's jaw, which are both about the
size of a dime, you can imagine the crushing strength in the jaws
of this creature.

Cave bears used to roam the fields and forests of prehistoric Europe, until they were hunted to extinction by early man. As we gaze at our skull and envision the eight-foot, thousand-pound beast with the three-inch teeth, the four-inch claws, and the jaw strength to snap a man in two, we can begin to appreciate how great our primeval ancestors' need for meat must have been. To think of this creature, snarling and gnashing its teeth, slashing with giant claws, charging and roaring, it almost defies imagination that people just like us went after them with not much more than sharpened sticks. But they did, and did it so well that cave bears are no more. And we are still here and carry in our genes this same need for meat that drove our forebears to brave tooth and claw to get it.

Despite these facts, we still regularly receive letters that question exactly what kind of diet our ancient ancestors actually ate. Although in anthropological scientific circles, there's absolutely no debate about it—every respected authority will confirm that we were hunters—many people still believe in the "dangers" of meat eating in light of our supposed vegetarian past. We've had at least twenty people send us copies of the same table published in an anti-meat book from the 1970s showing how sundry parts of our anatomy or physiology are more like those of herbivores than of carnivores, thus "proving" our vegetarian inclinations. We are, of course, neither. We're *omnivores,* able to subsist on meat *and* plants—hence the intermediate size of our intestinal tracts. Recently we received a newsletter clipping quoting a well-known doctor on the subject of our vegetarian past, as well as an e-mail from a *Protein Power* devotee in Italy whose physician had forbidden him to eat meat because it was "a silent poison." We even had one indignant reader tell us in no uncertain terms that she was abandoning our program unless we could answer to her satisfaction the questions that were raised by the quote, boldly circled in red, in her church bulletin, which she enclosed. The little blurb pronounced with great authority that the human body was designed to eat only food of plant origin and that meat "putrefies" in the human colon, becoming a poison. The physician from the (as always) prestigious medical school who had made this statement was someone totally unknown to us, and after a diligent search, we discovered he had been dead for over a hundred years. Such are the myths and misconceptions about what we humans were designed to eat.

Our meat-eating heritage—a topic we thought we'd covered sufficiently in our previous book—is an inescapable fact. But to be certain that this time we leave no room for doubt, we will delve back into the issue more deeply and lay out the facts of the matter so that you'll be armed with the truth and prepared to defend your nutritional choice with authority.

You'll hear it said, usually by those espousing vegetarianism for ideological reasons, that primitive tribes that eat a mainly plant-based diet enjoy better health. For instance, such authorities frequently cite the lower-than-the-average-American cholesterol levels of a typical male of the !Kung tribe (a commonly studied, contemporary chiefly vegetarian hunter-gatherer society) as proof of the health benefits of meatless living. While it's true that some predominantly vegetarian hunter-gatherer groups (a minority of such groups, as we shall see later) have low rates of the "chronic diseases of affluence," it doesn't necessarily follow that this good fortune is a result of their diet. Consider the Masai, for example. The Masai, another intensively studied group of African pastoralists who subsist mainly on meat, milk, and the blood of the cattle they herd, are famous and famously studied because of their incredibly low cholesterol and blood pressure levels even into advanced age despite their enormous intake of fat.[1] Here we've got two totally diverse diets—the !Kung and the Masai—and the followers of both have a low incidence of chronic diseases. Obviously there are other factors at play in the development of these diseases besides just diet, so let's take a closer look at the issue.

Anthropologists have known for decades that the health of humanity took a turn for the worse when our ancestors abandoned their hunter-gatherer means of subsistence in favor of the farm somewhere between eight thousand and ten thousand years ago. The fossil record leaves little doubt that compared to their

---

1. The latest government statistics show that adult Americans consume on average about 100 grams of fat per day; the average Masai consumes around 300 grams of fat per day, most of it of the saturated variety.

farming successors, the hunters were more robust, had greater bone density, decreased infant mortality, a longer life span, a lower incidence of infectious diseases and iron-deficiency anemia, fewer enamel defects, and little or no tooth decay.

Humans have followed a Paleolithic diet for a few million years and a "modern" agricultural diet for only a few thousand years. The not too gentle forces of natural selection have spent millennia shaping and molding our evolving line, weeding out those offshoots and mutations that didn't thrive on the available fare, reinforcing those traits that improved our survival, until we emerged as modern humans some one hundred thousand years or so ago. Since our modern form and physiology today is the same as that of these one-hundred-thousand-year-old ancestors,[2] it stands to reason that we should function best on the diet they— and we, their descendants—were designed to eat, not necessarily the "prudent" diet recommended by modern nutritionists, which is often composed primarily of foods that weren't even in existence for the vast majority of our time on earth. It is by turning to the vast amount of anthropological data that we can determine what our ancestors ate for the three to four million years that we have been recognizable as humans.

In a Word: Meat

In anthropological research if you follow the trail of meat consumption, you'll find the history of our earliest ancestors, because there is no real debate among anthropologists about early man's history as a meat eater and his evolution into a skilled hunter; the only debate is about when this hunting ability became fully developed.

Upon the discovery of the first fossils of our earliest upright ancestors anthropologists postulated that these creatures, the australopithecines, and those that followed until the advent of agriculture were "bloodthirsty, savage" hunters. As archeologists developed more technologically sophisticated means of analyzing

---

2. Using known rates of DNA change, geneticists estimate that modern man's genes are 99.998 percent the same as those of man before the agricultural revolution.

their collections of bones and tools, thinking drifted from the idea of early man as hunter to that of early man as scavenger. Gone was the notion of groups of skilled hunters stalking, bringing down, and butchering large herbivores; in its place was the vision of groups of hominids[3] coming upon the kills of large carnivores and stripping the remaining bits of flesh from the carcasses and using primitive tools to pummel and break into the cavities of the long bones and skulls to get at the marrow and brains within. The mainstream archeological and anthropological view posits that this scavenging lifestyle predominated until the last one hundred thousand years or so, coinciding with the arrival on the scene of anatomically modern humans. But, thanks to recent findings, this view is changing—and changing in almost flashback fashion to the ideas of the earlier anthropologists. Our ancestors from a long, long way back indeed appear to have been skilled hunters.

New excavations in Boxgrove, England, and Atapuerca, Spain, reveal that hominids as far back as five hundred thousand or more years ago were exquisitely skilled hunters. Archeologists at Boxgrove found evidence of numerous kill and/or butcher sites of extinct horses, rhinoceroses, bear, giant deer, and red deer—all large mammals requiring a great deal of skill and fortitude to bring down with primitive implements. Researchers know these animals were hunted and not just found and scavenged, not only because of the arrangement of bones at the butcher site, but through microscopic evidence as well. When analyzed under a microscope, the bones of scavenged carcasses typically show the cut marks from the tools of the scavengers lying over the tooth marks of the carnivores that actually made the kill, indicating that the scavenging came later. At Boxwood, archeologists found just the opposite. The cut marks from the flint tools on the bones show evidence that tendons and ligaments were severed to remove muscles from the bones. The cut marks compare to those produced by today's butchers using modern tools. In the words of

---

3. Hominids are members of the family Hominidae, which includes all species in our human lineage from us, *Homo sapiens sapiens,* to our ancestors after the split with the apes. Although modern humans are hominids, archeological and anthropological writers typically use the term to describe not modern man but all forms of early man all
Australopithecus

Michael Pitts and Mark Roberts, two of the primary excavators at Boxgrove, "every animal for which there is any evidence of interference by the hominids has been carefully, almost delicately, butchered for the express purpose of consuming the meat."

Further evidence of hunting comes from several actual wooden spears found throughout Europe that have proven to be the oldest wooden objects of known use found anywhere in the world. Archeologists have dated an almost sixteen-inch-long spear tip carved of yew wood found in 1911 in Clacton, England, to be somewhere between 360,000 and 420,000 years old. Another spear, also made of yew, that is almost eight feet long and dated to 120,000 years old was found amid the ribs of an extinct elephant in Lehringen, Germany, in 1948. A few years ago excavators in a coal mine near Schöninger, Germany, found three spruce wood spears shaped like modern javelins, the longest of which measured over seven feet, that proved to be 300,000 to 400,000 years old. And at one of the butcher sites at Boxgrove, excavators actually found a fossilized horse scapula that shows what appears to be a spear wound.

The excavation at Boxgrove provided archeologists with another surprise. It had long been thought that such stone tools as arrowheads and hand axes, once fashioned, were carried around by their makers and used as needed, much as we do today with modern hunting knives and other camp tools. Researchers who have practiced making prehistoric tools and arrowheads from flint—flint knapping, as it's called—found the task tedious, difficult, and fraught with the constant risk that one wrong strike could destroy the tool in the making. As a result, the thinking was that the effort put into making quality stone tools was so great that the makers would surely value them and keep them as long as they could. Amazingly, it appears from the meticulous examination of these ancient sites that these hominid hunters were so adept at making flint tools for butchery that they knocked them off on the spot, used them to skillfully dismember their prey, and left them at the site rather than carry them around. And these weren't just crude flint chips; these were some of the finest flint hand axes ever found. Modern attempts to reproduce the quality of these tools have usually fallen far short of the mark. Obviously

these ancient hominids were skilled enough to whip out a flawlessly made butchering tool at a moment's notice, a fact that implies a lifetime of hunting, butchering, and meat consumption.

We know from these European sites that hominids were
actively hunting and eating meat as far back as five hundred
thousand years ago, but what about before that? The earliest
stone tools date to around 2.6 million years ago and have been
found in association with extinct animals' bones from the same
period. Some of these have cut marks with overlying carnivore
teeth marks, indicating hunting, while others have carnivore teeth
marks with overlying cut marks, implying scavenging. The most
probable conclusion is that protohumans back at least 2.6 million
years ago—a time corresponding to the appearance of the genus
Homo—were engaged in the consumption of meat by either scavenging or hunting activities and probably a combination of the
two.

Prior to 2.6 million years ago the human line was represented
by australopithecines, which have been believed to be primarily
fleshy fruit eaters. So, it was thought, the human line developed
the taste for meat sometime between the plant-eating australopithecines and the appearance of *Homo,* but even that time
frame has now been pushed back. Anthropologists Matt Sponheimer and Julia Lee-Thorp from Rutgers University and the
University of Cape Town, respectively, performed an ingenious
analysis on the remains of four three-million-year-old *Australopithecus africanus* specimens found in a cave in South Africa.
Bones of this age are always fossilized, thus preventing researchers from extracting living material from them for analysis, but not
so for the tooth enamel; tooth enamel persists relatively unchanged through the millennia and lends itself to testing for organic content. Whatever is incorporated into the developing
enamel stays there—in this case for three million years. By testing
for variations in the carbon atoms making up the tooth enamel
researchers can determine what the owner of the tooth ate because different food sources contain specific carbon isotopes.
When Sponheimer and Lee-Thorp analyzed the australopithecine
enamel for the content of Carbon-13, a heavy isotope typically
found in grasses and in the flesh of grass-eating animals, they

found plentiful amounts, indicating that these hominids ate either a fair amount of grass or grass-eating animals or both. Analysis of the surfaces of the teeth, however, didn't show the specific scratches that are the telltale signs of grass eaters, leading the researchers to conclude that australopithecines at least as far back as three million years ate meat.

We have evidence tracking back three million years for meat eating by our ancestors and at least a five-hundred-thousand-year history of skillful hunting. In terms of generations this means that we modern humans are the result of one hundred fifty thousand generations of meat eating, twenty-five thousand generations of skilled hunting, but only a mere four hundred to five hundred generations of agriculture.[4] Since geneticists calculate that it takes at least two thousand generations for even minimal changes to be manifest, it should be apparent that eons of meat eating forged our physiology and metabolism to respond optimally on a diet containing significant amounts of meat. A low-fat, high-carbohydrate diet, the real fad diet in evolutionary terms, limits the consumption of the meat we were designed by nature to eat and replaces it with starchy foods that our bodies haven't had the time to adapt to. It's no wonder the low-fat diet wasn't what it was cracked up to be. It's far too new for our bodies to know what to do with.

Brain Food

Not only was meat a principal source of nutrition for developing man, it actually was the driving force allowing us to develop our large brains. For years anthropologists argued that we humans got our large brains because we had to develop them to learn hunting strategies to capture and kill game much larger, faster, and meaner than ourselves. Anthropologists Leslie Aiello and Peter Wheeler turned that idea on its head in a brilliant paper postulating that we were able to develop our large brains not to

---

4. And only about ten generations since the Industrial Revolution, and one, or maybe two at most, generations since the introduction into our diets of highly processed foods.

learn to hunt but because the fruits of our hunting—nutrient-dense meat—allowed us to decrease the size of our digestive tracts.[5] The more nutrient dense the food, the less digestion it needs to extract the nutrients, and consequently the smaller the digestive tract required. (The human digestive tract, while longer than true carnivores, is the shortest of any of the primates.[6])

Is meat really that nutritionally dense? Let's take a look at a few examples of meat compared to plant foods and see. First, let's look at protein. Protein is the only truly essential macronutrient. Fat is also essential, but you can go a lot longer without fat than you can without protein. (Carbohydrates, the third macronutrient, are totally unessential to human health.) So, if you are trying to get protein you could eat 8 ounces of elk meat, a small amount by Paleolithic standards, and get about 65 grams of it. Or you could eat almost 13 heads of lettuce to get the same amount. Or 56 bananas or 261 apples or even 33 slices of bread. If you're trying to get methionine, an essential amino acid that the body uses to make glutathione, its major antioxidant, you could eat the same 8 ounces of elk, or you could eat any of the following: 22 heads of lettuce, 127 bananas, 550 apples, or 46 slices of bread. In almost any nutrient category you want to look at, meat is going to come out a winner because of its incredible nutritional richness that doesn't require much digestive activity to get to.

Table 1.1 shows the difference between the digestive tract of a sheep, which is a true herbivore, and a dog, which is primarily a carnivore, and a human. Let's take a look and see where our species falls in the spectrum from carnivorous to vegetarian traits.

---

5. L. Aiello and P. Wheeler, "The Expensive Tissue Hypothesis: The Brain and the Digestive System in Human and Primate Evolution," *Current Anthropology,* 36, no. 2 (April 1995): 199–221. Meat eating simply gave us the metabolic room to have a larger brain, and, quite obviously, humans have brains much larger than other carnivores. What other researchers have postulated is that the ability to use the hands allowed early human and prehuman ancestors to obtain essential fats found in large concentrations in the brains of other animals, an area pretty much off-limits to other carnivores because of the thickness of the bony skull. (See chapter 3, "The Fat of the Land," and chapter 11, "Calisthenics for the Brain.")

6. Interestingly enough, the primate with the largest digestive tract and the smallest brain for its body size is the gorilla, which is a total vegetarian.

TABLE 1.1

Functional and Structural Comparison of Man's Digestive Tract with That of a Dog and Sheep

	MAN	DOG	SHEEP
Teeth			
Incisors	Both Jaws	Both Jaws	Lower Jaw Only
Molars	Ridged	Ridged	Flat
Canines	Small	Large	Absent
Jaw			
Movements	Vertical	Vertical	Rotary
Function	Tearing-Crushing	Tearing-Crushing	Grinding
Mastication	Unimportant	Unimportant	Vital Function
Rumination	Never	Never	Vital Function
Stomach			
Capacity	2 Quarts	2 Quarts	8½ Gallons
Emptying Time	3 Hours	3 Hours	Never Empties
Interdigestive Rest	Yes	Yes	No
Bacteria Present	No	No	Yes—Vital
Protozoa Present	No	No	Yes—Vital
Gastric Acidity	Strong	Strong	Weak
Cellulose Digestion	None	None	70%—Vital
Digestive Activity	Weak	Weak	Vital Function
Food Absorbed From	No	No	Vital Function
Colon & Cecum			
Size of Colon	Short-Small	Short-Small	Long-Capacious
Size of Cecum	Tiny	Tiny	Long-Capacious
Function of Cecum	None	None	Vital Function
Appendix	Vestigial	Absent	Cecum
Rectum	Small	Small	Capacious
Digestive Activity	None	None	Vital Function
Cellulose Digestion	None	None	30%—Vital

	MAN	DOG	SHEEP
Bacterial Flora	Putrefactive	Putrefactive	Fermentative
Food Absorbed From	None	None	Vital Function
Volume of Feces	Small-Firm	Small-Firm	Voluminous
Gross Food in Feces	Rare	Rare	Large Amount
Gall Bladder			
Size	Well Developed	Well Developed	Often Absent
Function	Strong	Strong	Weak or Absent
Digestive Activity			
From Pancreas	Solely	Solely	Partial
From Bacteria	None	None	Partial
From Protozoa	None	None	Partial
Digestive Efficiency	100%	100%	50% or Less
Feeding Habits			
Frequency	Intermittent	Intermittent	Continuous
Survival Without			
Stomach	Possible	Possible	Impossible
Colon and Cecum	Possible	Possible	Impossible
Microorganisms	Possible	Possible	Impossible
Plant Foods	Possible	Possible	Impossible
Animal Protein	Impossible	Impossible	Possible
Ratio of Body Length to:			
Entire Digestive Tract	1:5	1:7	1:27
Small Intestine	1:4	1:6	1:25

From Walter L. Voegtlin, M.D., F.A.C.P., *The Stone Age Diet* (New York: Vantage Press, 1975), 44–45.

But What If I'm a Vegetarian?

A larger percentage of our patients than you might imagine are vegetarian to some degree. With some modifications, the *Protein Power LifePlan* works fine for vegetarians, but before we start patients on the vegetarian version we always inquire as to their rationale for following such a diet. If they are vegetarians because they believe it a more healthy way to eat, we disabuse them of that notion quickly.[7] If, on the other hand, they are vegetarians for ideological reasons, we have no quarrel with that and we help them modify our program to solve their health problems within the limits of their ideology. We do, however, encourage them to read a fascinating little book entitled *The Covenant of the Wild* that goes a long way toward removing many of the inhibitions that some people have about using animals for food.[8]

Were We Hunter-Gatherers or Gatherer-Hunters?

What about the gathering that went along with the hunting? Don't we have a history of a fair amount of plant consumption along with our meat eating? How about the ancient potatoes that went along with our mastodon steak? Until the advent of fire about five hundred thousand years ago, it was fairly difficult for our predecessors to get enough calories from plant foods because the plants themselves fought back by evolving anti-nutrients. Anti-nutrients are chemicals within the plants that bind with the nutrients, making them unavailable for absorption by potential herbivorous predators. (See chapter 6, "The Leaky Gut: Diet and the Autoimmune Response," for more details.) Often we lose sight of the fact that, like humans and other species, plants evolve, too. The inner goal of plants is to live long, prosper, and disseminate as many seeds as possible in order to propagate the species. If a particular plant is tasty and easy to harvest (we're talking about plants in the wild, not hybrid plants that we put in gardens

---

7. See the following references from the medical literature to learn the hazards of vegetarian diets: J. T. Dwyer, "Nutritional Consequences of Vegetarianism," *Annual Review of Nutrition* 11 (1991): 61–91; E. C. Burke et al., "Multiple Nutritional Deficiencies in Children on Vegetarian Diets," *Mayo Clinic Proceedings* 54, no. 8 (August 1979): 549–550; T. Remer et al., "Increased Risk of Iodine Deficiency with Vegetarian Nutrition," *British Journal of Nutrition* 81, no. 1 (January 1999): 45–49. Also see the web site www.beyondveg.com for both the science and the pseudoscience pertaining to vegetarianism.

8. Stephen Budiansky, *The Covenant of the Wild* (New Haven: Yale University Press, 1999). This little book is a real gem. It is written by a small-time farmer who has witnessed the red-in-tooth-and-claw characteristics of nature firsthand and who makes a scientifically valid case for the use of animals for food.

today), it doesn't last long and certainly doesn't get much of a chance to spread its seeds. Plants, however, that develop (via natural selection) a means to keep from being eaten, whether by growing protective thorns or stickers, acquiring a particularly nasty taste, or producing anti-nutrients, survive to reproduce and multiply. The variety of plant foods available to the vast majority of evolving humans simply wasn't enough to nourish them without a generous amount of meat in the diet. In fact, Cambridge anthropologist Robert Foley says that hunter-*gatherers* "along with modern agriculturalists . . . are an evolutionarily derived form that appeared towards the end of the Pleistocene [ten thousand or so years ago] as a response to changing resource conditions." In other words, according to Dr. Foley, gathering, like agriculture, is a recent phenomenon, not a lifestyle that has its roots in several million years of evolution. That said, it's interesting to find, however, that hunter-gatherers (low-fat proponents always want to call them gatherer-hunters) are primarily meat eaters.

Most of the commonly accepted information about hunter-gatherers comes from a paper by R. B. Lee that was presented at a 1968 symposium in Chicago called, strangely enough considering the data presented, "Man the Hunter." Using the 1967 edition of Murdock's *Ethnographic Atlas,* a compilation of data about 862 of the world's societies, Lee concluded that the average hunter-gatherer got about 65 percent of his calories from plants and the remaining 35 percent from animals. This paper with its 65:35 plant-to-animal-food ratio has been quoted extensively in both the medical and the anthropological literature and used as the basis for the calculations of the prehistoric diet by innumerable authors who have promoted the idea that the diet of evolving man was mainly plant based. Unfortunately it is incorrect.

A colleague and good friend of ours, Loren Cordain, Ph.D., professor at Colorado State University, one of the world's experts on the Paleolithic diet, and one of the most industrious human beings we've ever known, sensed that there was something not quite right about Lee's paper and decided to investigate the data himself. Dr. Cordain's first clue that something was amiss was unbelievably basic and had been overlooked by all the researchers who had used Lee's paper as the basis of their own work. He simply ran a computerized nutritional analysis of a typical hunter-gatherer diet using the 65:35 plant-to-animal-food ratio. He discovered that for a human to get the calories needed to live on a diet of this nature using plants commonly available to a hunter-gatherer, he would have had to gather approximately twelve pounds of vegetation daily, an unlikely scenario, to say the least.

After making this discovery, Dr. Cordain reviewed Lee's original paper and calculations and unearthed some startling facts. Lee only used 58 of the 181 hunter-gatherer societies listed, and he didn't include animal foods obtained from fishing in his calculations. Moreover, he classified the collection and consumption of shellfish as a gathering activity. The *Ethnographic Atlas* itself considers the collection and consumption of small land fauna (insects, invertebrates, small mammals, amphibians, and reptiles) gathering and categorizes them as such, in so doing ascribing many of the actual animal-derived calories to the plant category.[9]

Dr. Cordain turned to the 1997 update of the *Ethnographic Atlas,* which represents 1,267 of the world's societies, 229 of which are hunter-gatherers, and did his own calculations. Using all the hunter-gatherer societies listed and putting fishing and shellfish gathering into the appropriate hunter category, he found that the 65:35 values of Lee were flipped. Dr. Cordain calculated the actual plant-to-animal-food ratio to be 35 percent plant, 65 percent animal. He found that the majority of hunter-gatherers throughout the world get over half their subsistence from animal foods; only 13.5 percent derive more than half their food from gathering plants. And these figures would lean even more in the direction of animal food were it not for the bias built into even the updated *Ethnographic Atlas* by the inclusion of small animals, reptiles, worms, grubs, etc., in the plant category.

Our primitive ancestors, whether hunters or hunter-gatherers, by all accounts lived fairly prosperous lives, at least by their standards. They lived in small, closely knit groups, and compared to the early farmers that followed them, they had much better

---

9. Dr. Cordain's scientific "hunter-gatherer" paper describing his findings is currently in press at the *American Journal of Clinical Nutrition* (reference unavailable at this book's press time). Those interested in his work should read his "magnum opus" on the dangers of cereal grain: L. Cordain, "Cereal Grains: Humanity's Double-Edged Sword," *World Review of Nutrition and Diet* 84 (1999): 19–73.

health, greater stature, more children reaching maturity, and a longer life span.[10] Turning to an agricultural existence forced the reliance on fewer numbers of foods, and since no single plant food provides a full complement of all the nutrients humans need, many people suffered nutritional deficiencies. And if the crop failed, famine set in—an experience foreign to most of the hunter-gatherer populations because they were always on the move, traveling to where there were plenty of game and fertile fields for gathering. A system in which large groups of people lived in close proximity, at least where early man was concerned, wasn't really all that advantageous. Most of the infectious diseases that have caused so much misery throughout history—smallpox, cholera, tuberculosis, and a host of other bacterial and viral infections—became problems only after the advent of the agriculture and the development of cities. All this begs the question, why did humans ever settle down and become civilized? Why did they leave their Garden of Eden, give up their hunting jobs requiring only a few hours of work per day, and submit to the backbreaking toil of an agricultural life? It just doesn't make sense.

This question has been pondered ever since anthropologists figured out that humans made this transition, and, as you might

---

10. Another misconception is that prehistoric man usually died when he was twenty years old, so it didn't matter how much meat or fat he ate because he didn't live long enough to develop heart disease or any of the other disorders that meat and/or fat supposedly cause. The twenty-year figure that is often used as the average age of death for prehistoric man is precisely that: the average age of death. That figure tells us nothing about the rate of aging or the maximum life span of prehistoric man. A much more reliable figure that has been developed and used by those scientists studying aging is the mortality rate doubling time (MRDT), the time it takes for the mortality rate, i.e., the probability of dying each year, to double. For example, if your probability of dying this year is set arbitrarily at one, and it takes eight years before your probability of dying is double what it is now, your MRDT is eight, which is about what it is in humans. Someone thirty years old, therefore, is twice as likely to die at age thirty-eight, four times as likely to die at age forty-six, and eight times as likely to die at age fifty-two, and so on. The MRDT of mice is about three months; a fruit fly's about ten days. Dr. Steven Austad from the Univerity of Idaho has been able to determine that the MRDT of prehistoric man was about the same as ours. Prehistoric man had the capability to live as long as we do, he just didn't have as gentle an environment, so what we're comparing when we compare our average age at death to his is the relative hostility of our two environments.

expect, almost as many hypotheses have been forwarded as there are anthropologists. Greg Wadley and Angus Martin, researchers at the University of Melbourne in Australia, have put forth an engaging theory that makes a lot of sense to us.[11] They point out that there exists a considerable amount of research establishing the fact that cereal grains, especially wheat, maize, and barley, and, to a slight extent, dairy products contain opioid substances called exorphins. Opioid substances are those that have an opium-like effect, stimulate the opioid receptors in the brain, and are to varying degrees addictive. When bands of primitive people stumbled onto patches of wild grains and consumed them they discovered the reward from consuming "addictive" substances, i.e., comfort foods. People quickly developed ways of making these foods even more edible by grinding and cooking them. As the grains become more palatable through processing, the more they were consumed and the more important the exorphin reward became.

In the words of Wadley and Martin, "At first, patches of wild cereals were protected and harvested. Later, land was cleared and seeds were planted and tended, to increase quantity and reliability of supply. Exorphins attracted people to settle around cereal patches, abandoning their nomadic lifestyle, and allowed them to display tolerance instead of aggression as population densities rose in these new conditions." According to these researchers, then, grains were the first opiate of the masses!

Whether this theory is the correct one or not, there is no question in our minds that carbohydrate foods cause cravings and are, to a certain degree, addictive, particularly those of cereal grain origin. If you look at any list of the top ten foods consumed by Americans you will find bread, crackers, chips, breakfast cereals, and other high-carbohydrate, grain-based products. We have all experienced the addictive nature of carbohydrates and their ability to override the feeling of fullness. Think back to the last time you were at a restaurant or at someone's house for dinner and

---

11. G. Wadley and A. Martin, "The Origins of Agriculture—A Biological Perspective and a New Hypothesis," *Austrialian Biologist* (June 1993): 96–105. This article can be found on the Internet at www. vegan-straight-edge.org.uk/GW_paper.htm.

you ate until you were stuffed. If one of your dinner mates asked you to try just a bite of the delicious swordfish (or any other meat dish), you no doubt begged off, saying, "I'm just too full; I couldn't possibly eat another bite." But then, if your host or your waiter arrived bearing dessert, you probably said, "Oh, well, dessert, sure. I'll have some cake"—or ice cream, or tiramisu, or cobber, or whatever. You are able to eat the dessert, which is always rich in carbohydrates, because just the thought of the carbohydrates overrides your brain signals telling you that you're full. Carbohydrates fail to trigger our off switch. That's why people who binge always do so on carbohydrates. No one binges on steak or eggs or pork chops; they always binge on cookies and candies and other carbohydrate junk foods. Having taken care of as many carbohydrate junkies as we have over the past fifteen years, we recognize that cereal grains and products made from them have an allure that transcends the mere taste bud stimulation they provoke. As Wadley and Martin point out, "The ingestion of cereals and milk, in normal modern dietary amounts by normal humans, activates reward centres in the brain. Foods that were common in the diet before agriculture . . . do not have this pharmacological property. The effects of exorphins are qualitatively the same as those produced by other opioid . . . drugs, that is, reward, motivation, reduction of anxiety, a sense of well-being [i.e., comfort foods], and perhaps even addiction. Though the effects of a typical meal are quantitatively less than those of doses of those drugs, most modern humans experience them several times a day, every day of their adult lives."

It should be clear by now that whichever way you look at it, the majority of our time as humans or our sort-of-human predecessors on this earth has been spent eating meat. The adoption of agriculture with its dependence on a grain-based diet is a recent phenomenon, in fact just a second in evolutionary time. The forces of natural selection haven't yet had anywhere near the time necessary to mold us to function optimally on a grain-based diet. We are still operating with forty-thousand-to-one-hundred-thousand-year-old biochemistry and physiology. Geneticists have evaluated the DNA sequences of humans and our closest relatives, the chimpanzee, and found the difference to be a mere 1.6 percent of genes, meaning we have 98.4 percent of genes in common with chimpanzees. By determining the rate of genetic change since we split away from chimpanzees, scientists have been able to calculate the rate of genetic mutation in humans, which turns out to be on the order of about a half a percent per million years. That means that over the past ten thousand years—the time since the advent of agriculture—we have changed genetically to the tune of about 0.005 percent. That's not much at all. In fact, that means that we have 99.995 percent of our genes identical with those of our big game–hunting ancestors. We are they. We have Fred Flintstone bodies living in a George Jetson world. And therein lies the root of our problems.

In our medical/nutritional practice we view modern diseases in our patients through the lens of their Paleolithic ancestry and use the Paleolithic diet and lifestyle with some twentieth-century modifications as a template to restore their health. (Throughout this book, we'll hold up that lens to the Paleolithic world to give you a look at where and how your modern lifestyle and diet may conflict with it.) We care for patients who have heart disease, elevated cholesterol and triglyceride levels, diabetes, obesity, high blood pressure, gastroesophageal reflux, various autoimmune disorders, and a number of other problems by using a protein-based diet containing a fair amount of meat.[12] Patients are constantly amazed at how quickly they improve and often believe that it is nothing short of miraculous. The reality is that we are just getting them to follow a diet they were intended to eat. We were designed to function optimally on a particular diet, we stray from this diet, we develop disease, we return to the correct diet, and the disease disappears. It's basically as simple as that.

One of the primary ways in which a Paleolithic nutritional regimen works to resolve these problems is by lowering insulin levels. Virtually every food our prehistoric ancestors had available (with the exception of honey) is one that doesn't stimulate the body to

---

12. Another of the most common vampire myths is that our program is a high-protein diet. Our program is actually an adequate-protein, moderate-fat (good-quality fat), carbohydrate-restricted diet that contains an enormous variety of berries and melons, green and colorful vegetables, nuts, and other plant foods that would have been found on the Paleolithic table.

produce much insulin, whereas the vast majority of foods we eat in today's world do just the opposite and send insulin levels through the roof. In the next chapter we'll take a look at this most powerful of our metabolic hormones and learn the havoc it can wreak when we stray from our ancestral bill of fare.

BOTTOM LINE

The overwhelming mass of scientific evidence supports the notion that for most of our time on earth, humans and their prehuman ancestors have eaten meat. By all reputable scientific accounts, we've been hunting and gathering (with heavy reliance on the hunting) for the better part of three million years. Eons of natural selection and human development molded our metabolic machinery to succeed on this ancient dietary scheme that appears to have included about 65 percent foods of animal origin and about 35 percent foods of plant origin. Only about ten thousand years ago (at most) did we settle down to cultivate grains and begin to include them as food in our diets. The metabolic changes necessary for humans to adapt to this dietary change—in short, to be able to use these "new" foods well—would reasonably take a few thousand generations (or about forty thousand or fifty thousand years). We're simply not there yet—and won't be anytime soon.

Turning to the use of grains allowed humans to settle in large cooperative groups necessary to build great civilizations, but at a price to the individual members of the group. While we can subsist on grain-based diets, we don't as a species thrive on them; the fossil record shows that after the adoption of agriculture human health, stature, and longevity went into sharp decline. In the last century in the Western world, thanks to a general increase in dietary protein, we've begun to recover our stature, but because of our continued heavy reliance on cereal grains, metabolic health still lags. We're riddled as a society with epidemics of diabetes, high blood pressure, heart disease, and obesity, all of which we inherited when our ancient ancestors abandoned their successful hunting-and-gathering lifestyle in favor of the addictive lure of grains (components of which indeed do stimulate the narcotic centers of the human brain).

In our medical/nutritional practice, we care for people with all components of this epidemic of modern diseases. To restore their health, we advocate a return to the basic nutritional principles of our ancestral hunting-gathering lifestyle by prescribing a diet of nutrient-dense foods—meat, fish, and poultry, rich in protein and good-quality essential fats; fruits, berries, and vegetables, rich in antioxidants and cancer-fighting substances—and limiting what early humans never knew existed—grains, refined sugars, and other concentrated starches.

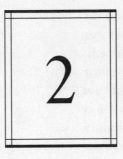

THE INSULIN CONNECTION

Certains foods make for fat. . . . To a scientist, there is
nothing so tragic on earth as the sight of a fat man
eating a potato.
—VANCE THOMPSON, *Eat and Grow Thin,* 1914

The human body has rendered up its secrets at a much slower rate than has the rest of the universe. Over two thousand years ago the ancient Greeks laid the foundation for modern physics, mathematics, and philosophy; at the same time, Greek physicians thought the arteries carried air instead of blood. Just a couple of centuries later the Greek physician Galen performed his dissections and wrote his great treatise on anatomy—mainly incorrect—that influenced physicians until the fifteenth century. He did figure out that blood instead of air flowed through the arteries, but he believed the liver pumped it instead of the heart. In the seventeenth century Isaac Newton was grappling with how the planets moved and deriving his laws of motion, while Gottfried Wilhelm Leibniz and René Descartes worked out differential equations and analytical geometry. At about the same time, the English physician William Harvey finally determined that it was the heart that pumped the blood. By the late 1800s scientists knew the speed of light, the motion of the planets, and, to an incredibly close approximation, the forces that moved them. Immanuel Kant had written his *Critique of Pure Reason,* one of the supreme intellectual achievements of all time, and Arthur Schopenhauer had fine-tuned it. And medical scientists still didn't know that insulin, the primary hormone of all metabolism, even existed.

Although the ancient Egyptians had written about diabetes as early as 1500 B.C., it wasn't until the dawn of the twentieth century that medical scientists had a clue to its cause. In 1889 in his laboratory in Strasbourg, Austria, researcher Oskar Minkowski accidentally discovered that the pancreas produces a substance that controls blood sugar. He found that when he removed the pancreas from a dog, it developed diabetes. Prior to Minkowski's discovery, other renowned researchers had decreed that diabetes resulted from injuries to or diseases of the kidneys, stomach, blood, nervous system, or liver.

In 1905 Albert Einstein published his three papers on Brownian motion, the photoelectric effect, and the special theory of relativity that changed the world of physics. At the same time, medical researchers were feeding extracts of raw pancreas to patients with diabetes in a futile effort to help them. For the next fifteen years the only even marginally effective treatment afforded diabetic patients was the "proven" two-step therapy of starvation coupled with intensive exercise, both of which we now know increased the effectiveness of what little insulin these unfortunate patients could themselves produce.

The team of Frederick Banting and Charles Best in 1921 isolated and purified insulin, the substance in the pancreas that lowers blood sugar, and used an injection of this "new" substance to successfully treat a diabetic dog. In January of 1922 they treated their first human patient, an eleven-year-old severely diabetic boy, who improved dramatically. In the years since, insulin has saved the lives of millions. People with diabetes who would otherwise have perished after enduring short, miserable lives now, thanks to insulin, enjoy almost the same life expectancy as those without the disease. But still, insulin has many secrets left to reveal.

Now, at the turn of the twenty-first century, while physicists are busy breaking the atom into not only protons, neutrons, and electrons but also quarks (six types in all, with the names up, down, strange, charm, bottom, and top), neutrinos (particles so small that they could pass through millions of miles of lead without the least effect on their motion), muons, taus, muon-nutrinos, and tau-nutrinos and, as if this were not enough, discovering that all these particles have anti-particles acting in opposite fashion, medical researchers are arguing over what constitutes a healthy diet. And a huge debate rages over whether too much insulin is a cause or an effect of disease. There is no doubt in the minds of medical researchers the world over that too much insulin in the blood causes problems, but the molecular mechanisms of exactly how it does still elude precise description. Would that the secrets of the body lent themselves to discovery as readily as those of the greater universe. But while there's still no consensus in much of nutritional medicine and there are many medical frontiers left to explore, medical science does understand a thing or two. Let's take a look now at what research scientists have discovered (and what we've learned through years of clinical practice treating patients) about the role of excess insulin in disease.

The Metabolic Insulin-Resistance Syndrome

If you were to run a computer search looking for insulin and disease, you'd find over twenty thousand research papers in the medical literature. There is no question that insulin plays a large role in the development of disease—there's medical consensus at least on that point—but the debate still rages on *how* it plays this role. The medical world can't even come to a consensus on what to call the ever-growing cluster of disorders related to insulin, variously dubbing them collectively as Syndrome X, the Hyperinsulinemia/Insulin-Resistance Syndrome, the Diseases of Civilization, the Metabolic Syndrome, and our new favorite, the Metabolic Xyndrome (a tongue-in-cheek term coined by University of Southern California researcher Dr. Richard Bergman and introduced at a recent scientific meeting we attended on this issue). What was once called the Deadly Quartet, referring to the newly identified syndrome of four diseases (hypertension, diabetes, elevated triglycerides, and obesity), could now be rightly thought of as a Deadly Big Band, with the ever-growing number of disorders now included in it (more about which in a bit).

Entire textbooks have been written just on insulin, insulin resistance, and hyperinsulinemia, so there's no lack of talk about the subject in the literature. However, while most of these books and papers discuss how insulin exerts its influence on a particular disease process, precious few (in fact only about one hundred of the twenty thousand) address the treatment of the underlying insulin problem.

But that is precisely what our years of clinical practice dealing day to day with these problems has taught us to do: treat the problem. By reducing the excess insulin in the blood of our patients, which is the driving force behind their medical problems, we are successful in the vast majority of cases. It would be an impossible task to cover in a single chapter all the aspects of insulin and the diseases its excess causes. Consequently, we've chosen to give you just a basic brief description of how elevated insulin influences an ever-growing cluster of metabolic disorders and then describe effective ways of treating these problems.

Introducing the Players in the Deadly Big Band

Medical researchers have implicated excess insulin as the cause of or, at the very least, a major driving force behind the development of a majority of the diseases that afflict many of us as we grow older. And although space limitations won't permit us to fully discuss all of them, here's the current list of insulin-related disorders; it reads like a *Who's Who* of the diseases of modern man: heart disease, elevated cholesterol, elevated triglycerides, high blood pressure, blood clotting problems, colon cancer (and a number of other cancers), type II diabetes, gout, sleep apnea, obesity, iron-overload disease, gastroesophageal reflux (severe heartburn), peptic ulcer disease, polycystic ovary disease.

It may not seem possible that one hormone could cause or be a major factor in all these disparate diseases, but it makes more sense when you realize that insulin is the primary hormone driving all of metabolism and influencing the actions of virtually every cell in the body. Before we see how insulin exerts its powerful effects, let's define some terms that we'll be using throughout this chapter and the rest of the book as well.

Insulin: A hormone made in the pancreas and released into the blood under a number of circumstances. Insulin is the major nutrient-storage hormone. Along with its other many duties it drives excess blood sugar, proteins, and fats into the cells for storage. Insulin's primary minute-to-minute job is to keep the blood sugar from going too high. Whenever the blood sugar rises, the pancreas pumps insulin into the blood to drive the sugar into the cells and reduce the amount in the blood, thus lowering the blood sugar level. Insulin performs this feat by binding to and activating the insulin receptors located throughout the body, but mainly on the muscle cells.

Insulin receptors: Proteins that reside on the surface of various cells and bind to insulin circulating in the blood. When insulin binds to these receptors it activates them, causing them to perform their specific tasks. For example, by binding to the insulin receptors on muscle cells, insulin stimulates them to move glucose (sugar) from the blood into the muscle cells for storage. You can think of insulin receptors as tiny sugar pumps that are turned on by insulin. Without insulin to activate them, these receptors won't work and sugar will accumulate in the blood, leading to all kinds of disastrous consequences if not treated, a problem faced by juvenile-onset, or type I, diabetic patients who make almost no insulin. These patients can't activate their insulin receptors (which work fine, they just need insulin), and as a result they build up high levels of sugar in their blood, which can be deadly if allowed to get out of hand. These diabetic patients treat themselves with injections of insulin to supply the insulin they themselves can't make.

Hyperinsulinemia: A condition in which there is too much insulin in the blood.

Insulin resistance: A condition in which the insulin receptors require more than the normal amount of insulin to make them work. Insulin resistance leads to hyperinsulinemia. And, as we shall see, hyperinsulinemia leads to insulin resistance.

Insulin sensitivity: A situation to be desired. The opposite of insulin resistance. When the insulin receptors are sensitive, they require very little insulin to make them work, and hence, people who are insulin sensitive have low levels of insulin in the blood. The lower the insulin level in the blood, the lower the risk for insulin-related disorders.

How Does Insulin Resistance Occur?

Let's look briefly at how insulin works. When you eat, the food travels from your mouth, through your stomach, and into your small intestine. The job of your digestive system is to break the food down into its various molecular components—the protein into amino acids, the fats into smaller fatty acids, and the carbohydrates into glucose (sugar)—so that they can be absorbed into the body. Your body can't absorb complex carbohydrates as they are; it can only absorb them once they're reduced to their basic subunits—sugar molecules. Each carbohydrate food, then, has a sugar equivalent. A medium potato, for example, contains a little over 50 grams of starch and other carbohydrates. When you eat a potato, your digestive tract breaks the complex carbohydrate starch into its sugar molecules, which you can then absorb. The 50 + grams of carbohydrate becomes 50 + grams of sugar, or a little more than a quarter of a cup.

When you consume over a quarter of a cup of sugar—whether it started out as a potato or a soft drink matters little—it goes through the walls of your small intestine into your bloodstream. If you add a quarter of a cup of sugar to the amount already in your blood, your blood sugar level will rise. Your body doesn't really like it when your blood sugar level goes up; in fact, your body likes to keep your blood sugar in a fairly narrow comfort zone—neither too high nor too low—and operates complex metabolic machinery to keep it there. When your blood sugar jumps up out of this comfort zone, as it surely does when you eat the potato or drink the soft drink, this elevated sugar level puts in the call to the pancreas asking for insulin. When your pancreas gets the message that the blood sugar is too high, it begins to release its stored insulin and starts making more.

The insulin travels through the blood, washing over the insulin receptors on the surfaces of the cells, and binds to them. When the insulin binds to these receptors it activates them, and they begin to pump the sugar out of the blood, where it can cause trouble, and into the interior of the cells, where it can be used or stored. Your pancreas continues to make and release insulin for as long as your blood sugar is above the comfort zone. As soon as the insulin-activated receptors have pumped enough sugar into the cells to reduce your blood sugar level back into the comfort zone, the high blood sugar signal to your pancreas ceases, your pancreas stops releasing the large amounts of insulin, and the system goes back into idle awaiting the next load of sugar it will have to deal with. When you eat another potato, sweet roll, bagel, ear of corn, or any other carbohydrate food, the cycle starts over again.

As long as this system works as it's supposed to, you do fine. You could even eat sugar straight from the sugar bowl, and it would go from the spoon to your mouth to your bloodstream then rapidly into your cells, all under the direction of a tiny spurt of insulin working smoothly and efficiently. (Not, of course, that spooning sugar into your mouth would do you much good in the long run; it just wouldn't hurt in the short run if all's working efficiently.) But, if there is a hitch in the system—and there are hitches of some magnitude in the systems of about 75 percent of us—you've got problems. What kinds of problems? Let's see.

You eat your potato, your digestive tract breaks the potato into its quarter cup of sugar and moves it through into the blood. Your blood sugar level rises and sends a signal to your pancreas. Your pancreas releases insulin. So far, so good; everything is working as it should. The insulin washes over the insulin receptors but isn't able to activate them. If the insulin receptors aren't activated, they can't pump the sugar out of the blood. If the sugar doesn't get pumped out of the blood, your blood sugar level stays high. Your high blood sugar level continues to badger your pancreas for more insulin. Your pancreas obliges and makes and releases more. More insulin now surrounds your receptors, but they still refuse to work. Your blood sugar remains elevated, and as long as it does, your pancreas continues to discharge insulin until it finally puts out enough to goad your stubborn insulin receptors to action, and they begin to work—grudgingly. At this point, the level of sugar in your blood begins to fall slowly as the receptors pump it into the cells. Finally, your blood sugar is back to normal, but not without the effort of a whole lot of insulin to get it there.

Your pancreas compensated for your sluggish, stubborn insulin receptors by producing more insulin to flog them into working. Over eons of time nature has endowed your body with countless such systems, all designed to compensate for the failure of other systems; the one whereby excess insulin overpowers resistant receptors is just one. But it's an important one because if our blood sugar stays too high for long we develop a host of problems in short order. What kinds of problems? Blurred vision, excessive urination, thirst, dehydration, dizziness, coma, and even death.

Insulin's main minute-by-minute function is to keep the blood sugar from going too high, but that's not its only job. As we've said before, insulin is the major metabolic hormone in the body, so it has many, many other functions. But since the regulation of blood sugar is its most important job for our immediate survival, all its other functions take a backseat to it. If blood sugar gets way out of whack, you could be dead in twenty-four hours, so insulin is going to focus its attention there first and worry about its other duties later. Excess insulin circulating throughout the body, bullying resistant insulin receptors into line, causes other problems of a less immediate, but ultimately no less deadly, nature. Among them are the problems that make up the list mentioned above: heart disease, diabetes, elevated cholesterol and triglycerides, high blood pressure, and all the others that cause most of the disease misery we modern humans suffer as we age.

Why do our receptors become stubborn and when? That's the $64,000 question that medical researchers are wrestling with today—one of those areas in which lots of research effort has failed to bring about a consensus. Many theories abound, but none has so far been unequivocally proven. The actual question should perhaps be, what comes first? Hyperinsulinemia or insulin resistance? In other words, do resistant receptors cause the high insulin levels required to make the receptors work in their resistant state, or does the pancreas release high insulin levels that somehow cause the receptors to be resistant? For a long time we put our money on the first explanation, but now—though the actual reason is far from proven—the preponderance of the evidence to the contrary has changed our minds. It appears—at least based on presently available information—that the elevation of insulin levels occurs first.

You may be wondering at this point, how could insulin injure the very receptors it requires to do its job? And the answer—in medical parlance—is that it causes them to *down-regulate.* Let's explore that notion in a bit more depth.

Insulin receptors aren't fixed things on the surfaces of the cells. They're made inside the cells in response to a need for insulin action. When there's not much insulin around, sensors within the cells take note and *up-regulate* the production of docking stations for insulin, transporting them to the cell surface to lure and capture any insulin passing by. On the other hand, when there's lots of insulin in the blood, the cells don't need to make as many docking stations—a process called, logically enough, down-regulation. The more insulin receptors available, the better insulin works; the fewer receptors, the less efficiently insulin works.

You've probably experienced a phenomenon similar to up- and down-regulation yourself. Think about what happens when you walk into a room where something smells really awful. At first the odor just about knocks you down, but then after you have stayed in the room for a while, you don't really notice the smell any longer. If you leave the room and stay outside for a few minutes, then walk back into the smelly room, BAM, there is the horrible odor in full force again. The odor in the room doesn't change—only your perception of it does. Why? Because just as insulin receptors do when bombarded by excess insulin, smell receptors become blunted, or down-regulated, when they are bombarded by an overwhelming odor. When the pancreas overproduces insulin, this excess insulin drives the cells to down-regulate the number of insulin receptors, resulting in insulin resistance. In order for the insulin to work effectively and lower blood sugar, the pancreas must produce more and more, which then results in more receptor down-regulation. The whole process becomes a vicious cycle leading to more and more insulin in the blood and more and more down-regulation of the insulin receptors. By the same token, creating a situation nutritionally in which insulin levels stay down allows the receptors to begin to resensitize and up-regulate.

But how does it all start in the first place? No one really knows, but it appears to be a hereditary disorder activated by excess carbohydrate intake. Why do we think this? One clue comes from the research that has been done on relative newcomers to the high-carbohydrate diet, which provides some interesting insights. For example, a number of extensively studied groups of people—the Austrialian aborigines and the Pima Indians, to name a couple—have developed severe insulin resistance since being subjected to a more modernized carbohydrate-rich diet. When these people follow their traditional low-carbohydrate diets, they don't develop insulin resistance or hyperinsulinemia. In fact, the aborigines can actually reverse their insulin-related disorders when they revert to their traditional diet even for just a few weeks.

Another clue that the disorder is hereditary comes from looking at the very young, who should, by all rights, be metabolically healthy. When researchers study the children of people who have diabetes, high blood pressure, obesity, and a number of other symptoms of too much insulin, they find that these children already have significantly more insulin in their blood than do their friends of the same age whose parents are healthy. These same hyperinsulinemic children, however, may outwardly appear to be just as healthy as their friends who have low insulin levels. They don't have the high blood pressure, elevated cholesterol levels, or elevated blood sugar levels of their parents yet, but the writing is on the wall. Their excess insulin is already starting to down-regulate their insulin receptors, setting them up for insulin resistance, more severe hyperinsulinemia, and a lifetime of fighting all the problems they will surely develop as a consequence if they stuff themselves with sugar, starch, and bad fats. If, however, these kids eat a more carbohydrate-restricted diet, they can reduce their insulin levels, up-regulate their receptors, and not go on to develop the full-blown insulin-resistance syndrome.

Unfortunately what we usually hear from the parents of these children goes something like this: "Oh, I have to really watch my diet to keep my weight off and my cholesterol down, but my kids are lucky. They can eat anything they want and never gain weight.

Of course, I was like that when I was their age, too." We always remind these parent-patients that if they, themselves, had not eaten everything they had wanted when they were kids, they wouldn't be in our office being treated. The best time to start eating properly is in childhood, before the problem really gets a foothold. But sadly, the syndrome has already begun to get that foothold; it's showing up in ever younger age groups. Adolescent obesity continues to skyrocket—doubling in the last decade. And now, what we once called adult- or maturity-onset diabetes occurs in schoolchildren as young as eight and ten years old. How big is this problem of insulin-resistance? Let's look.

You've Got Your Facts Right . . . It's Your Conclusions We Question

If you read many magazine articles on diet and health you will sooner or later come across a health writer who says, "Oh, sure, insulin resistance is a problem all right, but only for a small percentage of people. Studies have shown that only 25 percent of individuals have an insulin problem." This commonly quoted 25 percent figure comes from a 1987 paper written by Claire Hollenbeck and Gerald Reavan, Stanford University researchers and pioneers in the field of insulin resistance and hyperinsulinemia. In this study Hollenbeck and Reavan did a glucose-tolerance test on a group of young healthy adults, but with a twist. Instead of simply slugging them with sugar syrup and then measuring blood sugar levels over a couple of hours, these researchers also looked at insulin levels over the same period of time. They found that, as expected, these healthy subjects all had normal glucose-tolerance curves. But the surprise came when they plotted the insulin levels: their insulin curves were all over the place. Some of the subjects required very little insulin to keep their blood sugar levels in check; others needed much more insulin to do the same job. The researchers divided the subjects into quartiles (groups of 25 percent of the subjects) based upon their insulin levels and produced the graphs shown in figure 2.1. As you can see from the graph on the left, all the subjects had the same amount of glucose in their

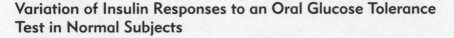

FIGURE 2.1

Variation of Insulin Responses to an Oral Glucose Tolerance Test in Normal Subjects

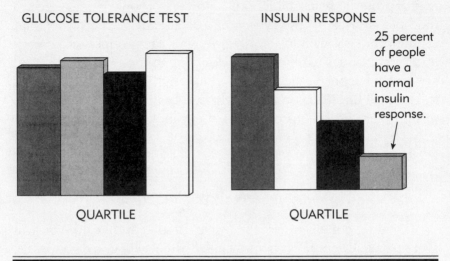

GLUCOSE TOLERANCE TEST

INSULIN RESPONSE

25 percent of people have a normal insulin response.

QUARTILE   QUARTILE

Modified from: C. Hollenbeck and G. M. Reavan, *Journal of Clinical Endocrinology and Metabolism* 64 (1987): 1169–1173.

blood, but from the graph on the right you can see that the amounts of insulin required to maintain these similar glucose levels varied greatly. The tall column on the far left is the group that required the most insulin to keep their blood sugars normal; the short column on the right denotes those requiring the least insulin. Since the tall column represents the 25 percent requiring the most insulin, many people have stated that only this quarter of people overproduce insulin, and hence the oft quoted "only 25 percent of people have insulin problems."

We look at this study a little differently. We look at the column on the right and say that that group of 25 percent has a normal insulin response, while the other three columns reflect the fact that 75 percent of people overproduce insulin *to some degree.* In our experience, we have found that being overweight is a fairly sensitive indicator of hyperinsulinemia, and this 75 percent figure is in complete accordance with a recent Harris Poll (February 1996) showing that 74 percent of adult Americans are overweight *to some degree.* Look around you at the people you work with, at your friends, at your adult family members, and we think you'll agree. At least 75 percent of these people are overweight to some extent—some hugely so, others with a little excess beer belly. And others still have one or more of the other problems of excess insulin. So, although we agree with Hollenbeck and Reavan's facts, our conclusion is that the real number of people suffering some degree of hyperinsulinemia is at least 75 percent, not the 25 percent that you hear all the time.

Another interesting thing about this study is that the subjects were *young,* "healthy" adults, yet 75 percent of them had an exaggerated insulin rise when they were given sugar. Since it is an established fact that people become more insulin resistant as they age,[1] we expect this 75 percent figure would have been even greater if the study subjects had been in their fifties. Again, you can confirm this by the eyeball method. Just go to a mall, a county fair, or any other gathering of people and look at them. We're sure you'll agree that the number of adults who could stand to lose a few pounds is greater than 75 percent—and many of them could stand to lose *quite* a few.

Insulin and Illness

We've now seen how insulin affects blood sugar, how it makes the receptors down-regulate and become resistant, and how the state of hyperinsulinemia develops. But none of this explains how excess insulin causes all the other problems that it does, so let's take a brief look at some of the many insulin-related disorders and see what the research has so far shown in how insulin figures in.

HEART DISEASE

What causes a diseased heart? In fact, the most common affliction of the heart is not a disease of the heart muscle per se but of the arteries that feed the muscle. Therefore, a more accurate

---

1. At least they do in Western societies. Studies of groups still living their traditional low-carbohydrate lifestyles remain insulin sensitive throughout their lives.

reflection would be to call it coronary artery disease. It occurs, as you may well already understand, when hard material builds up inside the normally slick and elastic arteries that carry blood to feed the heart muscle—the disorder we know as arteriosclerosis. Theories for the cause or causes of this buildup would fill a book—indeed, have filled quite a number of them. Currently in vogue are theories that run the gamut from infection caused by the chlamydia bacterium (the infectious theory of heart disease) to elevated levels of the amino acid homocysteine (the homocysteine theory of heart disease), the iron-storage theory, the elevated cholesterol theory, the oxidized cholesterol theory, and the hemodynamic (blood flow) theory, which explains heart disease (actually quite convincingly) as occurring in areas where the rate of blood flow slows, such as at bends or forks in the arterial tree. All these theories have merit and all of them have their strong proponents and none of them have yet been proven unequivocally correct. Our own theory—and that of a number of other research scientists—is that the chief instigator in the heart disease saga is elevated insulin levels. Let's examine the ways that insulin has been shown to contribute to the narrowing of coronary arteries.

1. Insulin stimulates the growth of smooth muscle cells in the walls of arteries, thickening them and narrowing the interior blood passageway.
2. Insulin stimulates the growth of the fibrous connective tissues that gives structure to the earliest forming plaques inside the arteries.
3. Insulin promotes an increased oxidation of the LDL particles and in the insulin-resistant state, a higher average blood sugar, which together result in a greater degree of LDL damage by the caramelization process (the irreversible attachment of blood sugar to the LDL lipoprotein). Both these events increase the likelihood that the altered LDL will become misdirected into the arterial walls. In its migration through the walls of the blood vessels, damaged LDL will attract the attention of immune fighters (macrophages) in the vicinity, which will attack it, feed on it, and ultimately incorporate the damaged cholesterol into the forming arterial plaque.

4. Insulin increases the production of fibrinogen, the blood substance that begins the process of clot formation by forming weblike strands to snare the red and white blood cells that pass by, thickening the blood and making it more prone to clot.
5. Insulin drives the kidneys to waste magnesium and potassium, which can in time lead to ionic imbalances within the heart's cells that predispose to abnormal heart rhythms, potentially fatal fibrillation of heart muscle, and death.

TYPE II DIABETES

In the course of developing insulin resistance, in order to keep the blood sugar within a normal range, the body will call on its insulin-production factory, the pancreas, to step up its output to meet the increased demand. If it takes more insulin to make the sluggish receptors work, then the body will simply crank out more insulin. However, if the syndrome continues, a point will ultimately be reached at which the amount of insulin necessary to overcome the building resistance will be more than the pancreas can possibly make, even working triple shifts. At that point, diabetes ensues. It is the ultimate expression of insulin resistance, signaling that the need for insulin's action has finally outstripped the capacity of the pancreas to respond.

Excess insulin—largely the consequence of eating a diet that contains much more sugar and starch than a stone-aged metabolism, unfit to the task, can contend with—sets the stage for down-regulation of the insulin receptors and the development of insulin resistance and finally, if left unchecked, potentially diabetes. Given our modern predilection for subsisting largely on carbo junk—cookies, candies, cakes, ice cream, pies, muffins, doughnuts, bagels, breads, pasta, rolls, sugar-sweetened cereals, french fries—and the insulin rise such foods occasion, it should come as no surprise that the incidence of diabetes has risen tenfold in the last thirty years. Amazingly, the standard treatment for diabetes in the last several decades has been the high-carbohydrate, low-fat diet. Fat was seen as the enemy of diabetics, and a high-carbohydrate diet (which as you now know really means a diet high in sugar) as the remedy. We've always questioned that approach—which by the way is dismally unsuccessful—reasoning that if diabetes is a disease of too much sugar in the blood, how can you treat it by putting more in? Clearly, you can't. And thankfully, for the sake of diabetic sufferers everywhere, the tide has begun to take a sensible turn toward a diet of higher protein, higher fat, and less carbohydrate. The most recent recommendations of the American Diabetes Association—which once recommended a 60 percent carbohydrate diet for treatment—now basically say, "Whatever works between patient and doctor on an individual basis." In effect, they're finally catching up with what we (and a few others) have been doing successfully for our own diabetic patients for years . . . using a diet (such as *The Protein Power LifePlan*) that feeds their bodies what they need and limits what they don't. It's simply a matter of applied biochemistry—if excess insulin is causing the problem, reduce the insulin levels, and lo and behold, people get better.

HIGH BLOOD PRESSURE

Elevated blood pressure is a complex disorder and although insulin resistance plays a role in a fair amount of it, we'd be the first to say that other causes unrelated to insulin can also be blamed. But we do understand several of insulin's roles at present. For example, research has shown that insulin stimulates the kidneys to hold on to salt and water. In a closed system—such as the human vascular tree—increasing the volume of liquid within the system drives the pressure up. Furthermore, if you then squeeze the pipes of that system, making them tighter and smaller inside—which elevated insulin does by causing an increased constriction of blood vessels—it's like crimping the end of a water hose: the pressure of what's flowing goes up. As a wise old engineer (MDE's dad, to be precise) would have said, "It's all a matter of physics, sugar."

From a hormonal standpoint, insulin excess causes the body to release more of the stress hormones, including cortisol and aldosterone, both of which exert what's called in medical terms a pressor effect, meaning that they raise blood pressure. And recent research has shown that squeezing the kidneys from outside— such as would happen, potentially, with an excess of internal fat stored around them—can elevate blood pressure. So in effect, because insulin is a fat-storage hormone—a role that we'll discuss in more detail in a bit—and because it especially promotes the storage of fat within the abdominal cavity, the elevated blood pressure associated with the metabolic insulin-resistance syndrome may, at least in part, occur in response to the external pressure on the kidneys, caused by the buildup of thick layers of fat around them. This is another intriguing slant on insulin's role in disease, and one that jibes nicely with the fact that in obese hypertensive people it often doesn't take much weight loss to effect a drop in blood pressure. Since abdominal fat responds rapidly— being among the first fat depots harvested during weight loss—it stands to reason that shedding the excess around the kidneys would occur pretty early in the game.

But possibly the most important of insulin's actions related to hypertension involves its promotion of the loss of magnesium, about which we've written an entire chapter (see chapter 9, "The Magnesium Miracle"). Suffice it to say here that the magnesium wasting brought about by excess insulin strongly promotes the constriction of blood vessels and persistently elevates blood pressure. In fact, replacing magnesium directly into the vein will quickly return an elevated pressure to normal levels.

OBESITY

One of insulin's jobs as the primary nutrient-storage hormone is to transport fat into the fat cells. When we eat a meal, the various nutrients are absorbed into the blood, and the levels of sugar, fat, and amino acids in the blood rise. As we've already discussed, insulin drives the sugar into the cells to be burned as a fuel, but it will also drive any excess to be stored away either as muscle starch (called glycogen) or as fat; it also drives amino acids into the muscle cells and fat into the fat cells. If we are insulin resistant it takes more insulin to overcome the stubborn receptors and move the sugar into the cells—the first and most important of insulin's jobs. The surge of insulin required to accomplish that task leaves an excess available to move fat into the fat cells. Each time an insulin-resistant person eats a high-sugar, high-starch insulin-raising meal, they're buying a one-way ticket for excess calories of any kind to be moved into their fat cells. As the process continues over the years, the fat-storage depots (called adipose tissue) become more and more engorged with fat, and ultimately obesity results. And so it's not surprising that most people who are insulin resistant and hyperinsulinemic are also obese to some degree; obesity—like elevated blood pressure, high cholesterol or triglycerides, or diabetes—is simply another consequence of their metabolic disorder, not a cause of it.

If an individual develops insulin resistance and hyperinsulinemia and has excess insulin in the blood stuffing fat into the fat cells all the time, why doesn't that individual get more and more obese until he weighs in at 800 pounds? Some few actually do, but most people with insulin resistance and hyperinsulinemia gain anywhere from just a few pounds to 70 or 80 pounds of excess fat, then stabilize at that point and gain very little and very slowly from that point on. Why? Because they ultimately develop resistance to insulin's ability to store fat just as they developed resistance to insulin's ability to store sugar. At first, while the insulin resistance is developing and the pancreas is making excess insulin to overcome the resistance to the storage of sugar, the excess insulin easily transports fat into the fat cells. At this stage of the game people notice that they are putting on weight. As the insulin resistance and hyperinsulinemia worsen, the excess weight piles on faster and faster. But then it slows down and begins to stabilize because the fat cells are becoming resistant to insulin's ability to transport fat into them. Some people develop fat-cell resistance sooner, and so don't gain a tremendous amount of weight as a consequence of their insulin disorder; other people have fat cells that hold on to their sensitivity to insulin's action longer, leaving them prey to a much more significant degree of obesity.

We see a number of patients in our clinic who have hyperinsulinemia and many of the symptoms that go along with it, such as high blood pressure, elevated triglycerides, low HDL (good) cholesterol, and any number of others, but who are normal weight or even thin. These patients are extremely insulin resistant at the level of the fat cells and can't really store much fat. We also see patients who weigh 500 to 700 pounds and are morbidly obese. When we measure these patients' insulin levels, often they aren't much higher than our thinner patients', but the obese patients obviously haven't developed the same degree of insulin resistance in their fat cells. As you can see from this example, it's not just the amount of insulin involved that causes the effect; it's the amount of insulin in the blood in combination with the degree of insulin resistance in the various tissues.

<h2 style="text-align:center">INSULIN AND SEX</h2>

Okay, maybe that title misleads slightly, but not entirely so. Insulin resistance, indeed, does have an impact on the production of various reproductive hormones. For example, the body takes the cholesterol molecule and from it builds various hormones, such as DHEA, androstenedione, estrogen, progesterone, testosterone, cortisol, and aldosterone.

FIGURE 2.2

Synthesis of the Sex Hormones

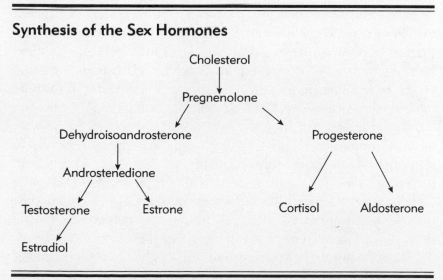

As you can see from figure 2.2, the body processes cholesterol in a stepwise fashion that leads ultimately to the male sex hormone testosterone, and from there to the female sex hormone estradiol (an estrogen). When the system works smoothly, people of both sexes produce appropriate amounts of these hormones; however, insulin resistance upsets this balance. Men, who don't normally transform much of their testosterone to estrogen in the final step of this production scheme, will do so when they become insulin resistant. This increased transformation to estrogen compounds results in what's termed feminization; in other words, under the influence of higher levels of estrogen than is normal for them, insulin-resistant men will begin to take on some body characteristics usually associated with women: muscle wasting in the shoulders and chest, loss of some facial and body hair, a slight broadening at the hips. Conversely, under the influence of insulin resistance, women do just the opposite. Whereas they would normally carry the final production step on to transform most of their testosterone into estradiol, this step falters, leaving them with higher than normal levels of testosterone. This relative excess of male hormone causes masculinization—the growth of some facial hair, coarser body hair, a broadening of the shoulders, chest, and back, a deepening of the voice. (This same process occurs in women with polycystic ovary disease, many of whom struggle with insulin-driven storage of excess body fat as well.) The altered production of the sex hormones can be made more pronounced when people take hormonal supplements, such as androstenedione, the sports performance enhancer, and DHEA, the "youth" hormone, which have recently received so much attention in the media. These "mother hormones" are the forerunners of testosterone, estrone, and estradiol in the production scheme; when people take them as supplements, what happens depends on their level of metabolic balance. Insulin-resistant men can gobble DHEA or androstenedione pills till they're blue in the face and what they may get for their trouble is more estradiol or estrone, which have been linked to cancer development in men. Insulin-resistant women will reap more testosterone. Although taking such supplements has become fashionable—in the wake of sports enhancement by pro athletes who've endorsed such products—we'd counsel against it until you've first rehabilitated your metabolism through proper diet. Otherwise, you might get an effect you didn't count on. Fortunately, reversing the insulin resistance reverses these hormonal shifts, too.

And that brings us to the meat of the matter: how to effectively reverse insulin resistance and restore metabolic balance.

In our practice we treat all the diseases associated with the metabolic syndrome by focusing on what we feel is the underlying problem: insulin resistance and hyperinsulinemia. We understand that the connection between insulin resistance and hyperinsulinemia and all these disorders has not been proven to the satisfaction of every scientist in the world, but we know from many years of practice and many, many thousands of patients that if we treat our patients as if excess insulin causes their problems, they get better. There are a number of effective ways to treat insulin resistance and hyperinsulinemia, which we will address shortly, but first let's look at how we determine if a patient actually has insulin resistance or hyperinsulinemia.

How Do You Know? Testing for Insulin Resistance

The gold standard for determining insulin resistance and hyperinsulinemia is the euglycemic-clamp test. In this test, which is done only in specially equipped research labs under careful, careful supervision, researchers give insulin and blood sugar intravenously at the same time to determine glucose disposal, which is a measure of how efficiently insulin works. You will never get this test in your doctor's office because it is too time consuming and expensive and even a little dangerous. Because the euglycemic-clamp test is too expensive and cumbersome even for most research labs, scientists developed a way to approximate the values they would get from the euglycemic-clamp test using a mathematical model. This test, called the Bergman Minimal Model, involves giving glucose intravenously, then measuring the blood sugar and insulin frequently over the next couple of hours. As with the euglycemic-clamp test, the Bergman Minimal Model is used mainly for research purposes, and as such doesn't offer much in the way of useful information to a doctor and patient in an office setting.

But there are other ways of determining insulin resistance and hyperinsulinemia that can easily be done in a physician's office.

The three methods we use in our clinic are the fasting insulin level, the two-hour post-glucose insulin, and what we call the insulin-challenge test.

The simplest one, the *fasting insulin level,* involves merely drawing a sample to measure the amount of insulin in a patient's blood after an overnight fast. It's quick, inexpensive, and provides a fair amount of information if carefully handled and performed by a reliable lab. We consider normal fasting insulin levels to be anything under 10 milligrams/deciliter. Anything above 10 mg/dl we consider to be abnormal and an indication of insulin resistance and hyperinsulinemia.

In the second kind of test, a *two-hour post-glucose insulin evaluation* or *two-hour insulin,* we give patients who have fasted overnight a measured amount of glucose to drink, then draw blood two hours later to measure both insulin and glucose levels. This test will uncover those people who oversecrete insulin in response to food, an important bit of information, since many people who have normal fasting insulin levels will have a much higher than normal two-hour insulin level. A major study has shown that, in general, men with insulin resistance will usually have an elevated fasting insulin level, while women with insulin resistance tend to have much higher two-hour insulin responses. So people, especially women, with a normal fasting insulin level but whose symptoms or history suggest insulin resistance should have a two-hour insulin test done.

The test that we do that has the most utility and that we think gives the most information as to an individual's insulin-resistance status is the *insulin challenge test.* While it's a pretty easy test to do, it does require experienced personnel and instructions before attempting it, which we're happy to provide to professional colleagues.[2] To perform this test we first measure the blood sugar of patients who have fasted overnight. Then, based on their weight, we administer a small dose of regular insulin intravenously. We then measure their blood sugar response regularly over the next

---

2. Check our web site at www.eatprotein.com for the specific instructions on how we perform the insulin challenge test, or have your physician write our clinic at the address listed in the appendix.

fifteen minutes. Since insulin drives sugar into the cells, in people with normal sensitivity to insulin, we would expect to see the blood sugar level fall to half of what it was before the insulin. For example, a patient with good insulin sensitivity might have a beginning blood sugar level of 90 mg/dl, which would then fall to around 50 mg/dl after the administration of insulin. Insulin-resistant patients, however, may scarcely get any drop in blood sugar at all. A patient with insulin resistance with the same 90 mg/dl blood sugar level might well see a drop to only 80 mg/dl after the same dose of insulin.

We find the insulin challenge test valuable because we can repeat it periodically to see if patients are becoming more insulin sensitive with our treatment. After six to eight weeks of nutritional therapy, a patient whose blood sugar initially dropped from 90 mg/dl to only 80 mg/dl after insulin administration might see a fall in blood sugar to 50 mg/dl on a repeat of this test. Such a response verifies both to us and the patient that the treatment is working and that the insulin receptors are up-regulating and becoming more sensitive. Along with this improved insulin sensitivity we usually see an improvement in other lab values that go along with an increasing insulin sensitivity and reduced hyperinsulinemia.

Reversing Insulin Resistance

We now know how to test for insulin status, but how do we treat the problem? How do we increase insulin sensitivity? What do we do to get the receptors to upregulate and become more sensitive? There are basically seven methods we use in our practice to improve insulin sensitivity, and all but the last are a part of the *Protein Power LifePlan*.

1. decrease carbohydrate intake
2. decrease caloric intake
3. exercise
4. alter the dietary fat profile
5. supplements
6. deplete the body of excess stored iron
7. medications

The most important and most effective method is the first—decreasing carbohydrate intake—and we'll explain why in the pages that follow. In the chapters ahead, we'll explain why these various methods work and show you how to incorporate these strategies into your lifestyle. In chapter 13, "*LifePlan* Nutrition," you'll learn just how to change what you eat for maximum health and well-being. You'll discover how exercise lowers insulin levels and improves insulin sensitivity in chapter 12, "Born to Be Fit." You'll learn how to alter your dietary-fat profile in chapter 3, "The Fat of the Land." You'll find out how excess iron storage—now tied to the insulin-resistance syndrome—may lead to sluggish functioning of the thyroid gland, the pancreas, and the liver, creating metabolic mayhem, how to determine if it's a problem for you, as well as how to easily rid yourself of it if it is in chapter 8, "The Modern Iron Age." Although we'll discuss a few of the supplements here, you'll want to focus on chapter 9, "The Magnesium Miracle" and chapter 11, "Calisthenics for the Brain," where you'll learn yet more about the supplements we have found most useful in treating our patients. But first, let's explore why reducing carbohydrate is the backbone of the *Protein Power LifePlan*.

KNOCKING THE STARCH OUT OF YOU

If we examine all the possible strategies to reduce insulin and improve insulin sensitivity to see where we can get the most bang for our buck in terms of insulin lowering, we need to look no further than this: restrict carbohydrates. This strategy is without a doubt the single most effective way you can increase your insulin sensitivity and lower your insulin level. We have tried every way imaginable in our clinic to improve insulin sensitivities in our patients (and in ourselves), and we haven't found anything that compares to just plain old carbohydrate restriction. It makes sense if you think about it, because insulin is released in response to dietary carbohydrate, excess insulin blunts the receptors, blunted receptors require more insulin to make them work, and so on. If you simply quit putting excess carbohydrates into the system, the process moves in the other direction. Less sugar (simple and complex carbohydrates) in the mouth means less sugar in the blood, less sugar in the blood requires less insulin to deal with it, and less insulin bombardment of the receptors means that the receptors will up-regulate and become more sensitive. More-sensitive receptors means that it takes less insulin to make them work, and less insulin makes even more-sensitive receptors. It leads to whatever the polar opposite of a vicious cycle would be. A beneficial cycle?

We have heard amazing stories from our patients and readers of how they went about changing their diets to accomplish carbohydrate restriction—without much else in the way of guiding nutritional principles—and the astounding improvements they achieved in their overall health. To our horror, patients have reported increasing their intakes of all manner of horrible processed fats, consuming diet drinks by the dozens, eating all kinds of deep-fried foods, practically wallowing in oxidized cholesterol–filled, fat-drenched scrambled eggs—but all the while keeping their carbohydrate intake low—and they have had spectacular results. Despite their prodigious intake of trans fats and lipid peroxides (see chapter 3, "The Fat of the Land"); despite their not eating a diet rich in antioxidants, other than the precursors for glutathione (see chapter 5, "Antioxidant Use and Abuse"); despite their consumption of God only knows how much aspartame and other artificial sweeteners (see chapter 7, "How Sweet It Is . . . Not!"), they got better simply because they reduced their carbohydrate intake and became more insulin sensitive. Is this the kind of nutritional strategy we recommend? Absolutely not, although you might think so to read the propaganda regarding *Protein Power* that's appeared in some venues over the years— these critics clearly haven't read the book and write only from misguided bias.

But because the power of carbohydrate restriction brings about such rapid beneficial changes and is so potent and easy to implement, it is the basis of the Hedonist approach to the *Protein Power LifePlan* (see chapter 13, "*LifePlan* Nutrition"). Although we don't allow Hedonists to run totally amok and eat everything that isn't red hot or tied down as long as it doesn't have many carbohydrates in it, we do allow them to enjoy a fairly wide range of foods, many of which probably aren't the absolute best choice for perfect health, but hey, they're hedonists. The point is that by simply restricting carbohydrates you can go a long, long way toward improving your health.

UNFORTUNATELY, CALORIES DO COUNT, TOO . . . BUT NOT AS MUCH

Another way to increase insulin sensitivity and to reduce insulin levels is to cut calories. Cutting calories is not nearly as effective as cutting carbohydrates if you're trying to reduce insulin, but it does work. Let's take a look at a reliable study that was done a few years ago that shows the difference between cutting carbohydrates and simply restricting calories à la the old low-fat diet. We say reliable because the subjects in this study were hospitalized throughout the course of the study and were under close and continuous observation. The hospital's metabolic kitchen weighed and measured the food so that the study subjects got exactly what they were supposed to get, no more and no less. Studies done on an outpatient basis requiring subjects to record their food intake in food diaries are almost worthless. A number of studies have shown that even conscientious and highly motivated subjects uniformly underestimate the amount of food they eat and overreport the amount of exercise they perform. Inpatient studies of this sort are worth their weight in gold because the data is reliable.

Researchers at the Geneva University Hospital in Geneva, Switzerland, in collaboration with researchers at Stanford University studied a group of forty-three obese adults who had been unable to lose weight as outpatients. The researchers randomized these patients into two groups and put both groups on 1,000 calories per day, a low-calorie diet by anyone's estimation. The higher-carbohydrate group got their 1,000 calories as 115 grams of carbohydrate, 30 grams of fat (about 26 percent of total calories, so a low-fat diet), and 73 grams of protein. The low-carbohydrate group got about the same amount of protein, about double the amount of fat, and about a third less carbohydrate than the other group. (See table 2.1 for the exact figures.) After six weeks on 1,000 calories per day the higher-carbohydrate group had dropped their insulin levels by about 8 percent, which is indeed

TABLE 2.1

	LOW-CARBOHYDRATE GROUP		HIGHER-CARBOHYDRATE GROUP	
	% OF CALORIES	GRAMS	% OF CALORIES	GRAMS
protein	32%	79 grams	29%	73 grams
carbohydrate	15%	38 grams	45%	115 grams
fat	53%	59 grams	26%	30 grams

an improvement and looks promising until you compare it to the results of the low-carbohydrate group, who dropped their insulin levels by a whopping *46 percent* over the same period and on the same number of calories. And as you might expect, all the other lab values that go along with an increase in insulin sensitivity were greatly improved on the lower-carbohydrate diet, prompting the authors of the study to note that "fasting plasma glucose, insulin, cholesterol, and triacylglycerol [triglyceride] concentrations decreased significantly in patients eating low-energy diets that contained 15 percent carbohydrate, but neither plasma insulin nor triacylglycerol concentrations fell significantly in response to the higher-carbohydrate diet." Although the group on the low-carbohydrate diet lost a little more weight than did the higher-carbohydrate group, the difference wasn't statistically significant. We find it both interesting and telling that the authors chose to entitle the report of their study "Similar Weight Loss with a High- and Low-Carbohydrate Diet." The only result in these two groups that *was* similar was weight loss. In every other way, the low-carb group fared better. They could have more honestly entitled their work "Reduction of Insulin, Triglycerides, Cholesterol, and Blood Sugar Markedly Better on Low-Carbohydrate Than High-Carbohydrate Diet." Even so, the authors of the study did go so far as to say that given that the low-carbohydrate diet was vastly superior to the low-fat diet in improving all other parameters evaluated, they felt it "reasonable to question the advocacy of this [low-fat] dietary approach."

Reasonable indeed!

So, What Causes Weight Loss?

Is it carbohydrate restriction or calorie restriction? It's clear from studies such as the one we just discussed as well as many others that carbohydrate restriction leads to much greater improvement in blood lipid and insulin values, but what about just plain old weight loss? Based on our years of clinical experience we believe that if you compare two diets of equal calories but different carbohydrate contents, the one containing the fewest carbohydrates will result in a slightly greater weight loss, but it's a tough hypothesis to unequivocally prove. The indisputable fact that the lower-carbohydrate diet reduces insulin, cholesterol, triglycerides, and all the rest to a much greater degree than the higher-carbohydrate diets do clearly means that something is going on metabolically with the lower-carbohydrate diet that isn't with the other. But these types of things are terribly difficult to study with any precision, because of all the variables involved.

Let's say we want to study a diet to see what changing the different macronutrients does to a specific set of parameters, much as the researchers did in the Swiss study mentioned above. If you reduce carbohydrates and keep the calories the same, you've got to replace the carbohydrates with something, so you replace them with fat or protein and see what happens. Whatever happens, you can't say with any surety that it happened because the carbohydrates were restricted any more than you can say it happened because the fat or protein was increased. If you want to eliminate the effect of the increased fat or protein, then you've got to keep them the same and only reduce the carbohydrate content of the diet . . . but then you decrease the calories. And who can say whether or not the resulting changes come from the carbohydrate restriction or from the decreased calories? As you can see, it's truly a difficult business to design a study to evaluate the difference made by changing only one macronutrient. What we end up having to do is rely on our knowledge of biochemistry and physiology and our clinical experience to make a judgment that we feel is valid. That judgment is that carbohydrate restriction works better than caloric restriction alone. But there is yet another twist in the carbohydrate-calorie story.

Carbohydrate restriction actually aids in the calorie-restriction process. A number of studies both in humans and in animals have demonstrated that when presented with unlimited quantities of foods containing high, moderate, or low amounts of carbohydrate, the group given the high-carbohydrate foods will eat more calories than the group given the low-carbohydrate foods, with the group given the moderate-carbohydrate foods falling somewhere in the middle. Since these studies didn't limit the amount of food that the subjects could eat, then it follows that the lower-carbohydrate foods were more filling on a per-calorie basis than the higher-carbohydrate foods. In other words, restricting carbohydrates is a clever way of restricting calories. Much has been made of this phenomenon by health writers who portray our program as merely a low-calorie diet in disguise. The only reason its followers lose weight, they write, is because they're on fewer calories than before, so there is no magic. Well, we never claimed that there was any magic to it, only good, solid nutrition that, depending on the individual, might or might not be low-calorie. But if our ancient physiology responds to a low-carbohydrate diet by turning off the hunger center in our brains sooner than it does with a higher-carbohydrate diet, why not take advantage of this difference and exploit it for our benefit?

But caloric restriction alone doesn't explain it all. Remember that our old friend (or enemy) insulin is a nutrient-storage hormone. After we eat, blood levels of insulin rise in an age-old call to begin packing away any excess (of sugar *or* fat) in our storage depots in case we might need it later. But that's not insulin's only action here. Not only does insulin store fat in the fat cell, it also prevents the fat that is already in the fat cell from coming out (a process that makes sense because if insulin only put fat in and didn't prevent its exit, it would be like trying to fill up a bucket with a hole in the bottom). This is an important point because it explains the difference in weight loss between a high-carbohydrate and low-carbohydrate diet of equal caloric content. A high-carbohydrate diet is going to stimulate the release of more insulin than a low-carbohydrate diet of equal calories, so the excess insulin is going to make it a little more difficult for the fat cells to release their fat content, even with the caloric deficit. This resistance brought about by the higher insulin levels is why we believe that low-carbohydrate diets encourage a more rapid weight loss.

OPENING THE DOOR OF THE FAT CELL

If insulin levels are low enough, then fat storage pretty much shuts down. It almost doesn't matter how much you eat—it's not going to get into the fat cells without the assistance of insulin. And furthermore, with insulin kept low, fat (both from dietary sources and from the body's fat stores) gets into the muscle cells much more easily, where it can be burned for energy. We see this phenomenon in action all the time. Patients come into the clinic or send us their diet diaries indicating that they have been keeping their carbohydrate intake within the prescribed limits, or even lower, and they haven't been losing weight, and they want to know why. We question them or look at their diaries and often find that they have indeed been keeping their carbohydrate intake low but at the same time have been eating enormous quantities of food. To give you an example, a woman from the northeastern part of the country sent a diary showing her daily low-carbohydrate fare and demanding to know why she had only lost 4 pounds over the first few weeks on the program. Her diet was as follows:

BREAKFAST: a four-egg omelet with cream cheese, five or six pieces of bacon or sausage, and coffee.

MID-MORNING SNACK: 4 ounces of nuts and 2 to 4 ounces of cheese.

LUNCH: a large bowl of tuna or ham or chicken salad made with real mayonnaise, a bag of pork rinds, and a diet drink.

MID-AFTERNOON SNACK: nuts and cheese again.

DINNER: a 16-ounce piece of prime rib, a green vegetable, and a small salad.

DESSERT: sugar-free gelatin with whipped cream and coffee.

If you calculate this, you'll find that she indeed was well below her 30-to-40-gram daily carbohydrate restriction, but she was eating somewhere in the neighborhood of 5,000 calories each day. The remarkable, even stunning, realization is not that while she was eating all this food she lost only 4 pounds but that she didn't gain 30 pounds! The point is that she kept her insulin low by keeping her carbohydrates restricted and wasn't able to store the fat that she ate. Had she added 100 grams of insulin-stimulating carbohydrate—a mere 400 more calories—to this regimen, her weight would no doubt have skyrocketed. We can take home a couple of lessons from this example. The first is that although cutting carbohydrates doesn't necessarily mean you will lose a lot more weight than you would on a high-carbohydrate diet of equal calories, it does mean that if you eat a huge number of calories in low-carbohydrate form, you will be prevented from gaining the weight you would on a high-carbohydrate diet of the same number of calories. The second lesson is that if you want to *lose* weight, you have to watch the calories—even on a low-carbohydrate diet—particularly if you're a small person. Remember, low-carbohydrate intake means a lower insulin level; and, a lower insulin level means that you can easily unload fat from your fat cells. But, if your body has no need to use any of the fat from your fat cells because it has more than enough fat to meet all its needs coming in from your diet, it's not going to go after your stored fat, and you won't lose weight. To lose weight, you've got to create an energy deficit. For the vast majority of people, simply following a low-carbohydrate diet will easily create enough of a caloric deficit to bring about a reasonable weight loss. But small people have to be careful because they can easily eat enough calories despite keeping their carbohydrate intake low to meet their small caloric needs without ever creating a deficit.[3] The good news is that if you are trying to lose weight, the minute you do reach your goal, you can increase your calories substantially without the fear of gaining weight—as long as you keep your carbohydrates restricted enough to keep your insulin level low. This will be an easier task

---

3. The foods that give these people the most trouble are foods that, although low in carbohydrates, contain a large number of calories. The worst offenders are nuts, cheese, and nut butters. Almonds, for example, contain 330 calories in ¼ cup along with less than a gram of available carbohydrates. Cheddar cheese has close to 500 calories in 4 ounces and a little less than 2 grams of carbohydrates.

than when you started because after your period of carbohydrate restriction you will have increased the sensitivity of your insulin receptors, allowing you to eat more carbohydrates than before while still keeping your insulin controlled.

GILDING THE LILY: THE ADDED BENEFIT OF SUPPLEMENTS

Although the vast bulk of the health improvement our patients achieve on the plan derives from simply changing the foods they eat, we often also recommend the use of a few supplements that research has established will help to improve insulin sensitivity. We make this recommendation especially for people who have heart disease, diabetes, or hypertension—or who have been taking cholesterol-lowering drugs of the "statin" group (see chapter 4, "Cholesterol: The Good, the Bad, and the Ugly"). Here are the ones we've found most useful in our clinical practice and the average amounts we recommend: magnesium (400 to 600 mg per day), chromium picolinate (200 to 1000 *micro*grams per day), vitamin E (400 to 800 IU per day), alpha-lipoic acid (200 to 600 mg per day), and coenzyme Q10 (100 to 300 mg per day). This is not meant to be a comprehensive list of every supplement ever reported to increase insulin sensitivity, nor a comprehensive list even of every supplement we use in our practice. It is an overview of some of the supplements that we have had extensive firsthand experience with and that we use every day in our treatment of insulin-resistant patients. You'll also find a chart in the appendix called Micronutrient Round-up, compiling all our basic recommendations for supplementation for various conditions. For additional details about the supplements we use and why, see chapter 4, "Cholesterol: The Good, the Bad, and the Ugly," chapter 5, "Antioxidant Use and Abuse," chapter 9, "The Magnesium Miracle," and chapter 13, "*LifePlan* Nutrition."

PHARMACEUTICALS

With our insulin-controlling nutritional strategy and the occasional use of supplemental nutrients, we rarely find need for the use of prescription medications to control the metabolic disorders in our patients. We view our role as one of getting people *off* medications, not prescribing more of them. But a couple of them are worthy of mention.

There are a couple of drugs on the market that have been shown to increase the sensitivity of the insulin receptors and lower insulin levels. One is a relatively new drug called troglitazone, marketed under the trade name Rezulin, which initially showed some promise as a drug to reduce insulin but unfortunately resulted in reports of liver damage in some of the people who took it. These reports clouded its safety profile sufficiently to result in its temporary withdrawal from the market. Although it's now back on the market, we still have some reservations about its safety and so prefer to rely on a different anti-diabetic medication whenever possible. (There are several new "glitazone" cousins now coming onto the market. Their manufacturers claim they do not cause liver damage, but only time will tell if that's indeed the case. And it wouldn't surprise us for time to also tell what untoward effects they *do* cause.) Metformin, marketed under the trade name Glucophage, already has an extensive track record in Europe and Canada, where it's been in wide use for over twenty years. We've used this drug extensively and much prefer it to troglitazone for effectiveness, even without the specter of liver damage in the picture. It's the drug we turn to on the rare occasions when lowering blood sugar levels in type II diabetics requires a drug. Unlike other oral diabetic medications (particularly those in the sulfonylurea class) that whip the already fatigued and struggling pancreas to make more insulin—an action, by the way, that will almost invariably lead to what's called beta-cell burnout, the point at which the pancreas simply gives up trying to produce insulin at all—metformin increases the insulin sensitivity of the liver cells. The reason that this action is important is that the sugar in your blood comes not just from the breakdown of the carbohydrates in the food you eat but also from the glucose your liver produces every day from amino acids. Normally, rising insulin acts to block the liver's sugar production, but when the insulin receptors in the liver become resistant, that action fails and the liver cranks out sugar unabated. This liver output accounts for the phenomenon seen in some diabetics whose blood sugar upon retiring to bed may be a well-controlled 95 mg/dl and then will mysteriously rise to 140 mg/dl by morning, when they've eaten nothing during the night. Metformin can pick up the slack by heightening the sensitivity of the liver's insulin receptors, thereby reducing the liver's output of sugar—and thus helping to achieve better sugar balance. When it's needed, we'll recommend doses of 850 to 1,500 mg, usually taken at bedtime, based on the degree of blood sugar control needed. Usually as the beneficial effects of our nutritional program begin to show and blood sugar stabilizes, we can taper the dosage of metformin and in most instances discontinue it altogether. Again, we want to caution people with diabetes to *never, never* undertake changes of diet, diabetic medications, or dosages except under the express guidance of their personal physician.

And that, in a nutshell, is the way we combat the insulin-related disorders that we inherited with our adoption of the civilized agricultural lifestyle. Before humankind settled down to sow, reap, and mill—at least with the certainty that paleoscientists can now ascertain—our early ancestors had about as much familiarity with diabetes, high blood pressure, and heart disease as they did with quarks and neutrinos. None. Their natural lifestyle provided them a regimen that included most of the precepts we now use to prevent and treat these disorders: they ate a diet that kept their insulin controlled and their blood sugar stable, one generally low in carbohydrates, devoid of grain starch and sugar; they lived actively, exercising in bursts of high intensity, interspersed with rest and revelry, which improved insulin sensitivity as well; they could obtain plenty of natural antioxidants in the berries, nuts, and seeds their surroundings provided; their water supply, rich in magnesium, kept their insulin receptors working smoothly; and the wild game and fish they ate provided a far superior fatty-acid profile than most modern humans eat today, keeping their cell membranes fluid and functional.

But the natural lifestyle that was available to them is also available to you—and by applying its principles today, you can break the insulin connection, heal your insulin receptors, improve your insulin sensitivity, and enjoy the wellness you were born to have.

BOTTOM LINE

▼

Abnormal metabolism of a single hormone, *insulin*, lies at the root of heart disease, diabetes, hypertension, cholesterol and triglyceride elevations, and a host of other disorders that occur more and more commonly in Western cultures. Although they do not appear to have occurred prior to our adoption of an agricultural civilization, these are not new diseases—descriptions of diabetes and heart disease occur in ancient Egyptian texts written twenty-five hundred years ago; however, our rudimentary understanding of what causes them is fairly recent. The discovery of insulin occurred fewer than eighty years ago, in 1921.

Nutritional science is still in its infancy in many ways. For example, even at the close of the twentieth century, scientists can agree that too much insulin causes problems but still debate exactly how. At a time when physicists describe the character and function of subatomic particles, nutritional scientists still cannot agree on what constitutes a healthy diet. There isn't even agreement on what to call the cluster of disorders caused by insulin excess, which goes under a baker's dozen titles: the Metabolic Syndrome, the Hyperinsulinemia/Insulin-Resistance Syndrome, Syndrome X, the Deadly Quartet, the Diseases of Civilization, and on and on. A library search for information about insulin and its roles in disease will yield well over twenty thousand research articles; a similar search for how best to treat the underlying condition will yield fewer than one hundred.

Insulin's main job in the body is to keep blood sugar in the normal range. When we eat, blood sugar rises, signaling the need for insulin to bring it back down. Insulin does this job by activating special insulin receptors on the surfaces of the cells, which then pump the sugar out of the blood and drive it into the cells, where it can be either burned for energy or stored for later use. On a diet high in sugar and starches (which the digestive tract turns into sugar immediately in order to absorb it) the body must produce a large amount of insulin to handle the load. We know that elevated levels of insulin in the blood precede the development of the Metabolic Syndrome—a phenomenon that has been shown to occur early on in the children of adults with the syndrome—and that continued high levels can damage the system, making the cells resistant to insulin's action. As this resistance develops, the job of keeping blood sugar within the normal range requires even more insulin and a vicious cycle begins. Although research has yet to clearly establish exactly how the insulin receptors become resistant, research does show that it occurs quite commonly; about 75 percent of adults will overproduce insulin to some degree in response to eating carbohydrates. Since in the last few decades, Americans have turned to diets higher in carbohydrate and lower in fat, it should come as no surprise that these Diseases of Civilization—unheard of before the adoption of agricultural lifestyle—have skyrocketed.

We spent many pages in our last book, *Protein Power*, detailing insulin's roles in the development of these diseases, and here we focus mainly on our treatment of them. What follows is a brief review of how insulin excess promotes the development of this cluster of diseases.

Insulin promotes heart disease by thickening the artery walls (especially dangerous in the small arteries that feed the heart); by increasing the tendency of the blood to clot; by promoting cholesterol damage through both increased oxygen and sugar in the blood, making it easier for it to attach to the artery walls; and by promoting the excess storage of iron in the tissues (a relatively newly identified important risk for heart attack).

In the case of high blood pressure, insulin excess stimulates the kidneys to retain sodium (salt) and water, expanding the blood volume. Insulin also increases the tension in the walls of the arteries, making them stiffer and less able to expand to accommodate the increased blood volume, driving the pressure within the system higher. Some recent research even suggests that insulin may play a role in elevating blood pressure by increasing the storage of fat around the kidneys that may put pressure on them from outside, driving the blood pressure up.

Diabetes (type II, or adult-onset) is but insulin resistance carried to its extreme; when the cells become so resistant to insulin's effect that it takes more insulin than the pancreas can possibly produce to lower blood sugar, diabetes results.

Under the influence of insulin, the liver increases its production of cholesterol, resulting in more of the "bad" LDL cholesterol, less of the "good" HDL type, and higher levels of triglycerides in the blood—a blood profile that spells increased risk for heart disease.

In relation to obesity, insulin is a storage hormone—it puts fuels, both sugar and fat, away for later use. High levels of insulin tell the fat cells to store fat and keep it there. In order to get the stored fat out of the fat cells and burn it for energy—that is, to lose fat—insulin levels must fall. In order for insulin levels to fall, the system must become more responsive to insulin's effects; in short, to solve any of the disorders related to insulin resistance—whether to lose weight, to lower cholesterol or triglycerides, reduce high blood pressure, or stabilize blood sugar and control diabetes—you must improve the workings of the insulin receptor. The only effective ways to achieve this goal are to reduce carbohydrates, reduce calories, or increase exercise. Of the three, the most effective method by far is to reduce carbohydrates.

We've spent the last decade and more treating these disorders effectively with our *Protein Power* nutritional regimen, which keeps insulin levels down by restricting dietary sugars and starches, by encouraging the types of exercise that lower insulin levels and improve insulin sensitivity, and by the judicious use of a few critical nutrient supplements (chiefly magnesium, chromium picolinate, alpha lipoic acid, and coenzyme Q10) that improve insulin receptor function. In the pages ahead, we devote specific chapters to exercise, the benefits of magnesium and sunlight, the dangers of excess iron storage, the damaging effects of grains, the best types of fat to eat for your health, the truth about cholesterol and heart disease, and to the outlining of your nutritional plan. You'll want to read at least the Bottom Line condensations of each of these chapters to fully understand how all these disorders intertwine, but you'll also want to examine the entire nutritional plan to see how to put it to use.

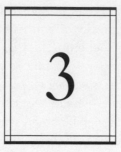

THE FAT OF THE LAND

And ye shall eat the fat of the land.
—GEN. 45:18

As humans and prehumans, we've been consuming the "fat of the land" for about three million years, but what we consume now, as modern humans, varies greatly from what our ancestors ate. To get an idea of the kinds of fats we humans consumed for most of the eons we've been on this planet, let's look at a report from the records of a scientific expedition to Arnheim Land in 1948. Arnheim Land is a remote area of over thirty thousand square miles in the Northern Territory of Australia that was set aside as a reserve for the "use and benefit of the aboriginal inhabitants of northern Australia," to allow them "to pursue their natural mode of life in their own land without dependence on the European economy." The multinational research team that undertook the expedition lived with and carefully described every facet of aboriginal life, which they described in multiple volumes of research papers.[1] What follows is

---

1. *Anthropology and Nutrition,* vol. 2 of *Records of the American-Australian Scientific Expedition to Arnheim Land,* ed. Charles P. Mountford (Melbourne: Melbourne Univer-

58

their description of how the aborigines prepared and ate a wallaby. It's fairly graphic, so those of you with weak stomachs may wish to skip ahead.

> A large fire was made in a depression in the sand, and stones and shells were heated. Small green branches were placed on top of the stones and the wallaby was flung on these. After 5–10 minutes it was taken off the fire, placed on a layer of green leaves, and the singed fur was removed with a tomahawk. [Just the fur, not the skin.] Although the women sometimes did this preliminary treatment, a man always did the subsequent cutting up, which was done with a metal spear blade.
>
> The first cut was made horizontally on the ventral [belly] surface at the level of the anus, and the next on the dorsal [back] surface along both sides to sever the leg muscles. Another cut was then made from the anus to the neck. The viscera were pulled out; and the kidneys, liver, heart and lungs, and the omental and mesenteric fat [the fat surrounding the intestines] were separated from the rest, and cooked on the hot stones and coals for 5 minutes. The cooked lungs were used to soak up the blood inside the carcass and then eaten. The offal was regarded as a delicacy by everybody and a certain amount of squabbling always followed its distribution.
>
> The tail was cut off, and during the cooking was put on or alongside the body. The carcass was laid flat, dorsal side downwards, on the hot stones and ashes and the body cavity was filled with hot stones. Sheets of paperbark formed a cover over the animal, and sand was scooped out to make an oven. Wallabies weighing 15–20 pounds were cooked for 25–35 minutes. Everything edible was eaten except the stomach and intestines. The skull was cracked open to get the brain, and the bones were broken to extract the marrow.

If you were to look through our research files you would find many more such examples of what true hunter-gatherers routinely

---

sity Press, 1960). This report is a couple of hundred pages long and makes fascinating reading for anyone interested in how true hunter-gatherers live.

ate. American Indians butchered and ate the entire buffalo, sans, of course, hooves, horns, hide, and bones. Eskimos left no parts of the carcasses of seals, walruses, and caribou uneaten, except, again, the truly inedible portions. The same goes for hunters in Africa, New Guinea, South America, and everywhere else native populations have been studied. All these groups ate the whole animal, whereas we more modern, more finicky types tend to eat only the muscle meats. As a result, when we try to make assessments of the nutritional content of primitive diets, we could be— and have been—way off the mark. If, for example, we were trying to determine the fat content of the Arnheim Land aboriginal diet, and we assumed that the aborigines ate only the muscle meat from the wallabies (as most of us would, we imagine, if we were presented with a wallaby to cook and eat), our calculation of the fat content would be abysmally low. The fact that the muscle meat of most wild animals contains a much smaller percentage of fat than does that of domestic animals has led many a researcher to seriously underestimate the fat content of the primitive diet. To really appreciate how much and what kind of fat primitive man ate, we have to have whole-carcass analyses of wild animals, not just analyses of their steaks. And guess what? Those studies haven't been done.[2] But based on some preliminary work, we know the percentage of fat calories in the diets of early humans is a whole lot higher than researchers have previously calculated.

The point of all this is that we spent a lot of years evolving on a diet that was loaded with fat. And, not only loaded with fat but loaded with fat of a different kind than we eat today. If you try to follow a Paleolithic diet by eating a steak, you'll get most of your fat as saturated fat, with a little monounsaturated and polyunsaturated fat thrown in. If, on the other hand, you follow a Paleolithic diet by eating an entire elk, you'll get an entirely different range of fats.

Since we do not now eat the whole carcass of anything, except

---

2. We are currently involved in such a study with our colleagues at Colorado State University. We are performing whole-carcass analyses for nutrient composition on at least twenty elk from the front range of the Rocky Mountains. The results of this study should be published in mid to late 2000.

maybe sardines, we miss out on a large amount of certain types of fat that evolution has designed us to function optimally on. In fact, next to the adoption of a grain based-diet, the change in the amount and types of fat we eat is the most dramatic alteration we've made in our subsistence since Paleolithic times. And, even compared to the relatively recent changeover to a grain-based diet, the change in the amounts and types of fat has happened just yesterday in an evolutionary time frame. We've been eating grains for about eight to ten thousand years but began eating the fats we do only about a hundred, or at most, a couple of hundred years ago.

In 1910 we consumed 83 percent of our fat as animal fat and only 17 percent as vegetable fat, and practically all of that came from eating the actual vegetables. Now, we get three times the amount of vegetable fat we did then and a little more than half the animal fat. And we have added a new kind of fat, an unnatural, processed fat called *trans* fat, to the mix. *Trans* fat, widely used for baking, turn up in all kinds of processed foods; unfortunately, according to the second National Health and Nutrition Examination Survey (NHANES II) done nearly twenty years ago, the largest contributors of calories to the U.S. diet are white bread, rolls, crackers, doughnuts, cookies, and cakes, so we consume—at least those of us who follow the typical American diet—a hefty dose of these unnatural fats. Think about this. *The largest contributors of calories to the U.S. diet are white bread, rolls, crackers, doughnuts, cookies, and cakes*—i.e., junk. That's pitiful. It's no wonder there is so much obesity, heart disease, diabetes, and all the rest. We evolved eating like the Arnheim Land aborigines, and now the largest category of calories we eat comes from cellophane-wrapped packages of cereal grains and processed fats, neither of which we ever saw during 99.8 percent of our time on earth as hominids or humans. As you might imagine, this horrendous dietary change has come at an enormous health cost.

PUFA, the Magic Dragon, and Friends

Fat is a catchall word with a lot of different meanings. For the purposes of this book we will refer to fatty acids in their large groupings: saturated fatty acids (SFAs), monounsaturated fatty acids (MUFAs), and polyunsaturated fatty acids (PUFAs). Within these larger groupings we will discuss a few specific fats, and in the PUFA grouping in particular we will discuss the truly essential fats, members of the omega-3 and omega-6 families.

What about a fat distinguishes it as belonging to one or another of these groups? For the most part, it's the way it's put together. For example, all fats are composed of chains of carbon atoms strung together in various lengths. Short-chain fats have a few carbons, medium-chain fats have more carbons, and long-chain ones have the most carbons. The carbons attach to one another with chemcial-electrical attractive forces called *bonds*. Each carbon has four potential spots on its surface to which it can bond to its neighboring carbons or to some other sort of atom or group of atoms. The most common atom to bond to the bonding sites on the carbons in fat molecules is hydrogen. (That's why, in chemical parlance, they're called *hydrocarbons*.) The basic skeleton of a fat molecule might look like this:

$$-\overset{|}{\underset{|}{C}}-\overset{|}{\underset{|}{C}}-\overset{|}{\underset{|}{C}}-\overset{|}{\underset{|}{C}}-\overset{|}{\underset{|}{C}}-\overset{|}{\underset{|}{C}}-\overset{|}{\underset{|}{C}}-\overset{|}{\underset{|}{C}}-\overset{|}{\underset{|}{C}}-\overset{|}{\underset{|}{C}}-\overset{|}{\underset{|}{C}}-$$

On all sides of the carbons—where they're not attached to other carbons—the atom can accept a hydrogen atom, so that the two on the ends could take three hydrogens (one above, one below, and one to the side) and the interior carbons could accept two (one above and one below), as shown below:

$$H-\overset{\displaystyle H\,H\,H\,H\,H\,H\,H\,H\,H\,H\,H}{\underset{\displaystyle H\,H\,H\,H\,H\,H\,H\,H\,H\,H\,H}{C-C-C-C-C-C-C-C-C-C-C}}-H$$

When every possible site for bonding is occupied by a hydrogen, the fat is said to be saturated, meaning that it has all the hydrogen it can take. In such a configuration, the fat is very stable electrically and chemically and is rigid, or solid, at room temperature. Butter, lard, coconut oil, and palm kernel oil contain saturated fats.

Sometimes, however, one or more hydrogen molecules are missing from the structure. When this occurs, the empty spot will develop a weak attraction to a neighboring carbon, forming a double bond, a much less stable chemical-electrical attraction. This means that the carbon atom at that spot is not fully saturated—rather it's unsaturated with hydrogen atoms. When the molecule contains a single double bond, it's termed monounsaturated; when it has two or more, it's termed polyunsaturated.

Monounsaturated fats, found richly in such foods as olives and olive oil, avocados, nuts, lard, and poultry fat are relatively stable fats. Polyunsaturated fats—those with several double bonds—remain as liquids at room temperature, but because of the unstable nature of their structure, they tend to oxidize easily and become rancid quickly. They must be fiercely protected from damage in the body by antioxidants (see chapter 5, "Antioxidant Use and Abuse," for more details) or they, themselves, will become harmful lipid peroxides.

Some members of the polyunsaturated-fat family are crucially important to your health—most notably members of the omega-3 family of fatty acids, the fatty acids called DHA (docosahexanoic acid) and EPA (eicosapentanoic acid). The omega designation refers to the spot in the carbon chain where the first double bond occurs. (The first carbon on the left is designated number 1, so an omega-3 fat has its first double bond between the third and fourth carbons in the chain. An omega-6 has its first one between number 6 and number 7.) The location of this bond imparts special characteristics to the fat. Omega-3 fats are made by plants (primarily by cold-water algae) but in the food supply occur primarily in the fat of cold-water fish, such as sardines, wild salmon, herring, mackerel, and tuna that feed on these plants. The omega-6 fats also occur primarily in the plant kingdom and turn up in large concentrations in the vegetable oils that currently make up such a huge share of the fat intake of modern man, as well as in arachadonic acid (AA), an omega-6 fat found in meat and eggs. Let's see what the intake of these various kinds of fats means for the body.

You Are the Fat You Eat

Fatty acids function in many ways throughout the body but nowhere more importantly than in the cell membrane. Cells can be thought of as minute factories designed and constructed to perform specific tasks in the body. Raw materials have to be fed into the cells, waste has to be taken away. The cell membrane, the "skin" around the cells, acts not only as a barrier to the flow of contents into and out of the cell but as the vital housing for the multitude of protein structures—receptors, transporters, pumps, etc.—that serve the cell. Protein structures in the cell membrane are responsible for moving the raw materials in and the waste out while the cell membrane maintains the integrity of the cellular structure. Cell membranes are composed primarily of two rows of fatty-acid molecules, called a lipid bilayer, arranged so that their outer surfaces attract water and their interior repels it. The fatty-acid core of the bilayer prevents molecules that dissolve in water, such as blood sugar (glucose), from passing through the cell membrane.

Glucose's chemical structure allows it to dissolve in water, not fat, and effectively prevents it from passing, without assistance, through the fatty-acid core of the bilayer. Although the blood sugar of individuals with type I diabetes can go sky high, it can't penetrate the lipid bilayer and make it into the interior of the cells. In order to get into the cells, glucose must be transported in via the action of the insulin receptor, a protein on the surface of the cell membrane. Along with insulin receptors many other proteins on and in the cell membrane perform thousands of vital functions involving moving materials into and out of cells. (See figure 3.1.) In order for these crucial protein structures to perform optimally they must be able to move and shift and rotate and reconfigure—each twist and turn dependent upon the fluidity and suppleness of the lipid bilayer in which they work. The fluidity and suppleness of the bilayer is a function of the types of fatty acids that make up its core. And, in turn, the types of fatty acids in the bilayer core are, in great measure, a consequence of the types of fatty acids in the diet. Good dietary fatty acids make for supple, fluid membranes, allowing the resident protein structures

FIGURE 3.1

The Lipid Bilayer

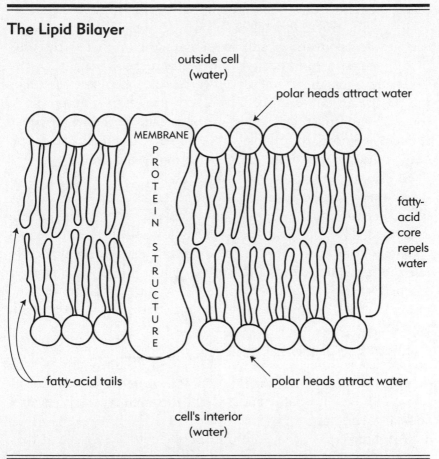

to do their jobs efficiently; bad fatty acids do just the opposite, making stiff, rigid membranes that restrict the necessary movement of the protein structures, hindering their proper function. So, good fats make good membranes. But what are good fats? And bad fats? Actually, with one exception—trans fatty acids, more about which we'll discuss below—there are no good or bad fats: it's a question of amount rather than kind.

Quod Nutrit Nutrimentum Est

The expression "You are what you eat" is truer with fats than with any other nutrient. When you eat protein your digestive tract breaks that protein down into its amino acid components and sends them to the various protein-needy tissues for reassembly into protein structures that have no resemblance to the protein you ate. Carbohydrates are the same. When you eat carbohydrates, your body breaks them down into their basic sugar components and burns them for energy, reassembles them as long chains for storage, or converts them to fat. Dietary fat, however, is absorbed pretty much as it goes in and is then burned for energy, stored as adipose tissue, or incorporated into cell membranes and other tissues in just about the same form in which you ate it.

If you go out to the ball game and eat a hot dog, the next day the now unrecognizable protein in the hot dog is completely reformulated into enzymes, bone, muscle, and other protein structures. The carbohydrate in the bun—and in the hot dog if you ate a cheap hot dog—is already burned, stored, or turned to fat. But if you look in the mirror, the fat in the hot dog will be staring back at you, unchanged, in the lipid bilayers of your skin, in the whites of your eyes, and even in your brain. That's why it pays to be careful about the types of fat that you eat.

Actually, it's not quite true that fats aren't changed in the body, because some types, but not all, are transformed to varying degrees. Before we discuss the importance of these transformations, let's look at what happens to the different types of fats after you eat them.

All three types of fats are transported into the cells and then into the mitochondria within the cells to be burned for energy. The fats not earmarked for burning are incorporated into various structures in the tissues, including the lipid bilayer, in their same configuration. Polyunsaturated fats keep the membranes supple; saturated fats (along with cholesterol) provide the structural stability of the bilayer membrane. If we have the right mix, then we have optimal fluidity with just the right amount of stability. How do we get this optimal mix? By the consumption of the right ratio of saturated to unsaturated fats? Not entirely. Fortunately the body has the ability to transform the fats we eat—and the fats we make from carbohydrate—into the fats we need.

Specific enzymes in the mitochondria can lengthen and even add a double bond to a saturated fat and make it a monounsaturated fat. These enzymes, called elongases and desaturases, are incredibly important in the modification of fatty acids, especially the polyunsaturated fatty acids. Monounsaturated fats can undergo the same elongations and desaturations to convert them to longer-chain polyunsaturated fats. Both the omega-3 and omega-6 families of polyunsaturated fats are elongated and desaturated to make the absolutely vital fatty acids that we require for life. But no matter how much desaturation and elongation the saturated and monounsaturated fats sustain, they can never become members of the omega-3 or omega-6 families of fats. Humans don't have the specific desaturase enzymes to convert other fatty acids to omega-3 or omega-6 fatty acids—only plants have those enzymes. We must get our omega-3 and omega-6 fatty acids either directly from plants or indirectly, by eating animals that have eaten plants.

As long as we get plenty of the omega-6 and omega-3 families of fats and as long as our desaturase enzymes are working, then we can transform the saturated fats we eat into the unsaturated fats we need. The problem is, how do we keep our desaturase enzymes humming along in top form?

Scientists have developed a measurement of the amounts of unsaturated fats in tissues and even in foods called the unsaturation index (UI). The lower the UI, the greater the amount of saturated fat in whatever is being measured. The UI of pure saturated fat is 0, while the UI of pure DHA (a highly unsaturated fat) is 600. A number of studies have been done using the UI to determine what effect various types of dietary fats have on the degree of unsaturation of the lipid bilayer. Most of the study subjects consuming a diet with a UI of around 80 (typical of the standard Western diet) were found to have muscle cell lipid bilayer UIs in the neighborhood of 160 to 170. This large increase in the degree of unsaturation means that the desaturase enzymes are hard at work. It also means that we don't have to eat only unsaturated fats to keep our membranes supple as long as our desaturase enzymes are working efficiently. We'll see a little later in this chapter the steps we can take to ensure that our desaturase enzymes desaturate away at maximal efficiency; doing so helps to improve our insulin sensitivity.

The more supple and flexible your cell membranes are, the greater will be your insulin sensitivity, and the lower will be your blood insulin level. This all makes sense because the insulin receptor is a protein that resides in and on the cell membrane, and as the cell membrane becomes more fluid, the insulin receptor can function better. When the insulin receptor functions better, it becomes more sensitive and less insulin is required to make it work. So to increase the sensitivity of your insulin receptors you can eat more unsaturated fat and/or increase the activity of your desaturase enzymes.

If we look at our Paleolithic past to try to determine the best kind of fat for us to eat, we find that although early man ate all kinds of fats, the one he probably ate the most of was monounsaturated fat. We say this because it is clear from the anthropological data that earliest man was a scavenger and usually got to the carcass after the large predators had their fill of it. He was left with the skull and the long bones of the legs, neither of which the largest predators could crack. With the help of a large rock—the first technological advance—he could, and did, split the long bones and the skull and eat the contents. Based on the limited analyses that have been done, it appears that monounsaturated fats make up the majority of the marrow fat in most wild animals and about a third of the fat in the brain. Since brain and marrow were the first foods of animal origin our earliest ancestors ate large quantities of, it can be said that we cut our evolutionary teeth on monounsaturated fat. Knowing this it makes sense that the so-called Mediterranean diet, with its emphasis on the monounsaturated fat olive oil (and pork; lard contains significant amounts of monounsaturated fat), would promote better blood lipid values in those who follow it than the typical American diet, with its emphasis on processed, saturated, and omega-6 PUFA vegetable fats.

Along with the large amount of monounsaturated fat, our ancient relatives consumed a radically different ratio of the omega-6 to omega-3 fats than we modern offspring do. Remember, humans can't make omega-6 and omega-3 fats from other fats because we don't have the necessary desaturase enzymes. Plants do have the enzymes necessary to produce the omega-3 and omega-6 families of fats but not exactly the ones we need. The omega-3 and omega-6 fats that we actually need are arachadonic acid (AA), an omega-6 fat, and eicosapentanoic acid (EPA) and docosahexanoic acid (DHA), both omega-3 fats. We can get these fats from eating plants containing their omega-3 and omega-6 precursors and let our own desaturase and elongase enzymes convert them to AA, EPA, and DHA, or we can get them preformed from animals that have already converted them for us. The latter way is by far the easiest.

The parent to the whole family of omega-6 fats is linoleic acid (LA), a fatty acid found in the seeds of most plants. The parent to the line of omega-3 fats is alpha-linolinic acid (ALA), which sounds confusingly similar to LA. ALA is found primarily in the chloroplast of green, leafy vegetables instead of in the seeds—with the exception of flax, fig, and raspberry seeds, which contain a large amount. The various desaturase and elongase enzymes work on these parent fats adding carbon-carbon double bonds and lengthening them until LA is ultimately converted to AA, and ALA is converted to EPA and DHA. (See figure 3.2.)

Flax seed oil is a rich source of ALA. If all the desaturation and elongation enzymes are working in top order, the body converts the ALA in flax seed oil to EPA and DHA just fine. If, on the other hand, these enzymes aren't working up to snuff, then there can be problems. Most of our patients have disorders that interfere with the proper function of these enzymes and, therefore, don't respond particularly well to flax seed oil because it's not the flax seed oil itself that they need. It is the EPA and DHA end products of flax seed–oil conversion. We have much better results with our patients when we give them the actual EPA and DHA directly. For these reasons, we wrote in *Protein Power* that we didn't like flax seed oil and didn't recommend it. And we got more criticism from more people for that one little section than we got for the rest of the book in its entirety.

We have reevaluated our position on the flax seed–oil controversy that we unwittingly started. If people are reasonably healthy, we don't have a problem giving them flax seed oil. We actually take it ourselves sometimes. But, we still think it is preferable to take the end products EPA and DHA, which we actually need, than to take the parent fat, ALA, in the form of flax seed oil and

FIGURE 3.2

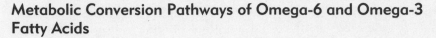

Metabolic Conversion Pathways of Omega-6 and Omega-3 Fatty Acids

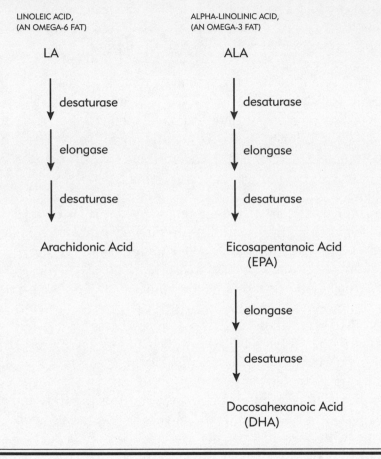

let our bodies do the conversion. Some people refuse to take the EPA and/or the DHA because they can't stand the taste or they are vegans and refuse to eat food of animal origin. For these folks, flax seed oil is great. It gives them a good source of omega-3 fats that they otherwise wouldn't get. But taking flax seed oil is kind of like buying crude oil and running it through your home distillery to make gasoline for your car. If that's the only way you can get gasoline, then that's what you have to do. If you can buy the gasoline already distilled, however, it's much more efficient to do that and avoid all the hassle of the home-distillation process. Before we get into how you can take the EPA and DHA directly, let's take a look at why it's important for you to get them in the first place.

Supplying the Eicosanoid Factory

The saturated fats, monounsaturated fats, and even some polyunsaturated fats that we eat are burned for energy, stored, or incorporated into the lipid bilayer or other structures. The omega-3 and omega-6 fats have much different functions. Fatty acids from either of these families can be burned, stored, or dragooned into work in the lipid bilayer just like all the other types of fat, but unlike the other fats only these omega-3 and omega-6 fats can be transformed into eicosanoids. Eicosanoids are twenty carbon (thus their name, from the Greek *eikosi,* "twenty") biologically active substances—some even say the most biologically active of all the substances made in our own bodies—that act at the level of the cell and within the cell to initiate all sorts of reactions. Eicosanoids can cause the blood to clot or cause it to be more thin; they can cause an inflammatory response or an anti-inflammatory response; they can cause smooth muscles to contract or to relax. All these functions and many, many more are mediated by eicosanoids, all of which are made from either omega-3 or omega-6 acids. In short, eicosanoids control just about any physiological function that you want to talk about.

Eicosanoids usually act like the accelerator and the brakes on a car. Eicosanoids derived from one family of fatty acids act in one way; eicosanoids coming from the other family of fatty acids in the opposite direction. The two types of eicosanoids working in concert can achieve extremely fine control of various psychological processes. For example, eicosanoids derived from the omega-3 family of fatty acids act as blood thinners. Those derived from the omega-6 family do just the opposite—they cause the blood to be more prone to clot. If everything works as it's supposed to, the first group of eicosanoids keeps the blood flowing smoothly through the tiniest arterioles and capillaries while the second group makes sure that the blood doesn't thin so much that it flows out through the walls of the blood vessels. If there is a cut, then the omega-6 family springs into action and helps the clotting process to proceed so that there is minimal blood loss.

In general, the eicosanoids from the omega-6 family of fats cause blood to clot, promote the rapid growth of cells, induce smooth muscle cells to contract,[3] bring about an inflammatory response, cause pain, and have a whole host of other effects. In general, the eicosanoids from the omega-3 family have pretty much the opposite effects of their omega-6 counterparts. As long as these two groups of eicosanoids are in balance, the system hums along beautifully. If they get out of balance, however, and one side starts to exert more influence, then there will be trouble.

Since the fat from wild animals contains about equal amounts of omega-6 and omega-3 fats, people eating that meat get these two fats in about equal amounts. If they eat a few seeds and certain kinds of nuts along with the meat, they will get a tiny bit more omega-6 fats but not much. If they eat some shoots or berries or other kinds of nuts, they will get a little more omega-3 but not much. In virtually all of the analyses of the Paleolithic diet it has turned out that our predecessors ate about twice the amount of omega-6 as omega-3. That gives us our model of what we ought to do to achieve a balance of these fatty acids and their corresponding eicosanoids and reap the health benefits. But do we? Well, of course not. When you analyze the typical American diet you find an omega 6–to–omega 3 ratio of not double, not triple, not even ten times that of Paleolithic ancestors, but a whopping *twenty to fifty times* greater. We routinely eat twenty to fifty times more omega-6 fatty acids than we do omega-3 . . . and we pay the price. Remember, the omega-6 eicosanoids are the ones that cause the pain, inflammation, smooth muscle contraction, blood clotting, etc. And when you've got twenty to fifty times more of the omega 6s than you do of the omega 3s working their way

---

3. Asthma is an example of too much smooth muscle contraction. In the presence of too many omega-6 eicosanoids the tiny smooth muscles around the small airways in the lungs can overcontract, causing a narrowing of the airways and the wheezing and difficulty of breathing that is all too familiar to asthma sufferers.

through your system, it should come as no surprise that you'll get pain, inflammation, and all the rest. But why is there this enormous discrepancy in intake?

If you routinely dined on the whole carcass of roasted wallaby, like our Arnheim Land aboriginal friends that we discussed earlier, you would get a more balanced ratio of omega-6 to omega-3 fatty acids, but you don't. You eat steak and salad and bread and cereal and, God forbid, french fries, and a whole lot of other stuff that your Paleolithic ancestors never encountered. Remember, omega-6 fatty acids are found primarily in seeds, so if you eat grains and grain products, you get a lot of omega-6 fatty acids. When cattle are fed out on a feedlot to fatten them up, they eat grain that contains omega-6 fatty acids, which are incorporated into their fat. Grain-fed beef has an omega 6–to–omega 3 ratio of 15:1 or so, instead of the 2:1 found in the meat of game. So even eating beef—if it's grain-fed—gives you an increased omega 6–to–omega 3 ratio. Almost all salad dressings are made with oils high in omega-6 fats, and french fries and other similar foods are deep-fried in vegetable oils containing a high percentage of omega-6 fats.

Countless studies have correlated an increased level of omega 6s in the diet with increased rates of heart disease, insulin resistance, cancer, diabetes, and the rest of the diseases that go along with getting older. As we as a society consume more and more omega-6 fats without a corresponding increase in omega-3 fats to balance them out, we will see increases in the incidence of these disorders along with a tendency for them to begin occurring earlier.[4] In most cases it takes twenty or thirty years for the system to break down because during youth the enzymes work efficiently. The desaturase and elongase enzymes that convert the EPA and DHA from the parent omega-3 fat work overtime to produce enough of these end products to maintain a semblance of balance in the corresponding eicosanoid production. As age creeps on, however, these enzymes begin to lose their vitality and the production of the omega-3 family of eicosanoids declines, leaving the

---

4. We are beginning to see cases of adult-onset diabetes in children who haven't even reached their teens.

enormous numbers of the omega-6 eicosanoids unopposed. When this happens, the problems start.

How can we deal with this situation? Easy. Eat more omega-3 fat and less omega-6 fat. One way that you can get more omega-3 fat is to take flax seed oil, but an even better way is to get the actual DHA and EPA. One of the best ways to do so is to eat sardines. All cold-water fish contain EPA and DHA, and you can get these fats from eating salmon, mackerel, and other large cold-water fish, but you have to eat a fair amount. You've also got to be sure that the fish aren't farm raised, because farm-raised fish don't have the same levels of these fats as do wild fish of the same kind. If you get the actual wild fish, then you have to worry a little about the contamination to which free-living ocean fish are exposed. The toxins—mercury, PCBs, etc.—tend to concentrate in the larger fish, because each time one fish eats another, the predator retains all the toxins of the prey. If a large fish eats five smaller fish, then the fish doing the eating ends up with five times the amount of toxins in its flesh compared to each of the smaller fish. A large salmon gets large by eating many, many smaller fish and consequently has the potential of containing large amounts of mercury and other fairly nasty compounds. For this reason, we're reluctant to have people eat huge amounts of large ocean fish to get their EPA and DHA—the toxins will accumulate in them just as they do in the large fish.

Sardines are a much better choice because they are small and low on the food chain, so they haven't had time to accumulate many toxins. They are caught and rapidly put in cans, so air and light—both of which will destroy EPA and DHA—can't get to them. And they contain a large amount of these good omega-3 fats. The best sardines to get are also the most difficult to find—the ones packed in sardine oil. We don't know why these are so difficult to find, but they are. We find them in the grocery store once in a blue moon and buy them all. The next best choices are those packed in olive oil or in spring water. You want to avoid the ones packed in soybean oil or cottonseed oil because these oils have a fair amount of omega-6 fats in them, the very fats we're trying to avoid.

If you don't like sardines—and many people don't—then you can give cod-liver oil a whirl. People often refuse to take sardines as medicine because of the taste but will gladly slurp down a dose of cod-liver oil—maybe not gladly, but at least more willingly than they will eat sardines. Fortunately, there is a cod-liver oil on the market that has almost no taste. It is Carlson's Cod Liver Oil, and it is available at most health food stores. It comes in a green bottle that is shaped like a hip flask, and the oil has a slight lemony flavor. Its delicate omega-3 oils are protected by a layer of inert gas that prevents oxygen from contaminating the oil. Once it's opened, however, you should store it in the refrigerator and use it quickly, discarding any that's left after two or three weeks. If you can't choke down the sardines, make a run for the Carlson's. There are other cod-liver oil products available that will do just fine if you can't find the Carlson's, but it's been our experience that compliance is much, much better with the Carlson's than with any other product we've found.

How about fish-oil capsules? Well, it's time to air some more *Protein Power* dirty laundry. In the chapter on fats in *Protein Power* we recommend that readers take fish-oil capsules to get their essential fats; we put patients on them and we took them ourselves, so it was a valid recommendation. But then, shortly after the book was published, we came across a couple of medical articles that changed our view. Researchers had pulled bottles of fish-oil capsules off the shelves of health food stores and checked them for rancidity. They found that in almost 50 percent of the cases some of the capsules in a given bottle were rancid. When fish oil becomes rancid it doesn't go from being a good fat to being a neutral fat, it becomes a harmful fat. The same properties that make EPA and DHA good for us—their extreme degree of unsaturation—also makes them prone to rancidity. Rancid fats become substances called lipid peroxides that cause all kinds of problems once they get inside us. As we will see in chapter 5, "Antioxidant Use and Abuse," a huge portion of our immune system is devoted to dealing with the lipid peroxides we make ourselves. We don't need to make the job even harder by adding them to our diets!

However, if you just can't stand sardines and you can't get

down the cod-liver oil, then you *can* take fish-oil capsules if you obey the following rules. First, buy only fish-oil capsules that come in glass bottles. Plastic is permeable to air, and air is death to fish oil. When you bring the capsules home, put them in the refrigerator so that you will slow down any untoward chemical reactions that may be causing rancidity. And the most important rule of all: every two or three days chew a capsule to make sure the supply hasn't started to go bad. If the capsules are fresh, they will taste slightly fishy; if they are not fresh, you will know it. If the latter is the case, pitch the whole bottle and start over. But, you may be asking yourself, if I have to chew the fish-oil capsules periodically, how is that different from just taking the cod-liver oil straight? That's what we ask, too, but it's been our experience that many people would rather chew a capsule a few times a week than take the oil every day. If you can't (or won't) eat the sardines, take the cod-liver oil, or take fresh capsules, then at least take flax seed oil. For our money, however, Carlson's Cod Liver Oil is a lot less objectionable than flax seed oil. Everyone has different tastes, so see what you like—but whatever you do, get your omega 3s.

Another way to increase the amount of omega-3 end products is to increase the activity of the desaturase and elongase enzymes that convert them from ALA, the parent omega-3 fat. Before we get into how we can do this, however, let's look at a different kind of fat, one that actually inhibits the actions of these important enzymes.

Trans Fatty Acids

Trans fatty acids are like Woody Allen's mythical beast that has the head of a lion and the body of a lion but is somehow not a lion. Trans fatty acids have the head of a fat and the body of a fat, and they taste like a fat, but, unfortunately, they are definitely not a natural fat. Trans fatty acids are processed fats, a product of technology, not of nature. To make trans fatty acids, food technologists start with good-quality unsaturated fats that they heat to a high temperature. They then add a nickel catalyst to the heated fat and pump hydrogen gas into the mixture. What comes out the other end of this process called partial hydrogenation is a trans fatty acid, a fat that looks like a natural fat but doesn't act like one.

Food technologists developed the partial-hydrogenation process to convert vegetable fats, which are normally liquid at room temperature, into fats that act more like saturated fats and have a much longer shelf life than the polyunsaturated fats from which they were converted. An unsullied polyunsaturated fatty acid looks something like A in figure 3.3. A trans fatty acid looks like B.

FIGURE 3.3

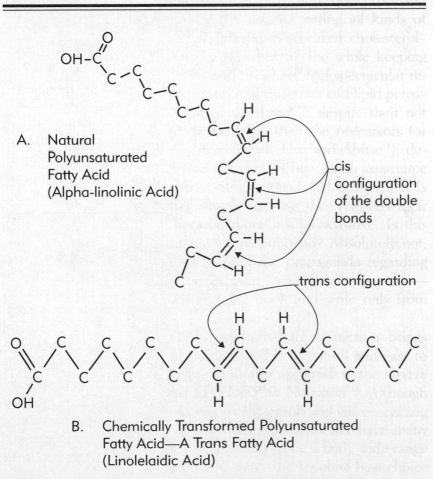

A. Natural Polyunsaturated Fatty Acid (Alpha-linolinic Acid)

cis configuration of the double bonds

trans configuration

B. Chemically Transformed Polyunsaturated Fatty Acid—A Trans Fatty Acid (Linolelaidic Acid)

As you can see, the long linear configuration of the trans fatty acid lends itself to being packed more closely together with other trans fatty acids then does the polyunsaturated fatty acid. The crooked, wiggly shape of the polyunsaturated fatty acid makes these fats difficult to pack tightly together and is the reason these fats are liquids at room temperature. Because of their ability to pack tightly and because of their longer shelf life, trans fatty acids were the choice for food manufacturers even before the recent craze to avoid saturated animal fat. Now that everyone seems to be avoiding saturated fats in general and animal fats in particular, food manufacturers have stumbled into a bird's nest on the ground. They can use a fat that they can call an unsaturated fat but that has a shelf life of forever and all the properties of a saturated fat save one: it isn't good for you.

Since trans fatty acids are unnatural fats, the body hasn't developed a specific way to deal with them, so it treats them like real fats and just does the best it can. Unfortunately, thanks to a sinister quirk of biochemistry, the body tends to incorporate trans fats into the lipid bilayer in preference to good-quality unsaturated fats, especially during times of essential-fatty-acid deficiency. Since most of us have a deficiency in omega-3 essential fats—especially if we're eating a diet containing a lot of trans fats—and a surplus of omega-6 fats, what we end up with is a lipid bilayer made of trans fats and omega-6 fats, a real recipe for disaster. What kind of disaster? Read on.

Mary G. Enig, Ph.D., a research scientist at the University of Maryland, has devoted a great deal of her career to the study of trans fatty acids. She has developed a state-of-the-art laboratory and has analyzed countless products for trans-fatty-acid content. Her scientific papers provide a frightening glimpse into the world of dangers wrought by the food-processing industry. She has published a list of some of the "physiological alterations" resulting from the consumption of trans fatty acids that she and other researchers have found to be "important because of their potential impact on health."[5]

---

5. Published in *Trans Fatty Acids in the Food Supply: A Comprehensive Report Covering 60 Years of Research,* Mary G. Enig, 2nd ed. (Silver Spring, Md.: Enig Associates, Inc., 1995). This publication is available from Dr. Enig through her website www.enig.com.

Trans fatty acids lower HDL (the good cholesterol) in a dose-response fashion; that is, the more trans fats you eat, the lower your HDL will be; they raise LDL (the bad cholesterol); they raise lipoprotein(a)—in fact, trans fatty acids are one of the only substances known for sure to raise the levels of this mysterious, but dangerous, lipoprotein; and they raise total cholesterol in the serum by 20 to 30 milligrams/deciliter.

And that's not where the damage stops. Trans fats interfere with the reproductive system, too, by decreasing the levels of testosterone in male animals, increasing the numbers of abnormal sperm.[6] In the female, elevated levels of trans fats decrease the amount of cream in human breast milk, reducing the overall quality available to nourish the growing infant, which correlates with low birth weights. They also inhibit the function of a number of enzymes, in particular the delta-6 desaturase enzyme, one of the enzymes responsible for conversion of both omega-3 and omega-6 fats into their more unsaturated products, as well as altering the activities of the enzyme system that metabolizes toxic chemicals, carcinogens, and medications; and to add insult to injury, they even weaken the immune response while they increase the production of free radicals. (See chapter 5, "Antioxidant Use and Abuse.")

But for our purposes in restoring balance to the beleaguered insulin system, trans fats wreak even more havoc by decreasing the response of the cells to insulin. In other words, trans fats contribute to the development of insulin resistance directly as well as causing hyperinsulinemia. They hamper proper function of the insulin receptor by changing the fluidity of the lipid bilayer and other cellular membranes and even cause alterations in the size of adipose tissue cells, their number, and their fatty-acid composition, further worsening the effects of essential-fatty-acid deficiency.

As you can see from this list, trans fatty acids cause a plethora

---

6. There have been a number of articles in both the scientific press and the lay press on the documented decrease in both the amount and quality of human sperm over the last forty years. Could this be in large part because of increased intake of trans fatty acids over this same period of time? That's where we would put our money.

of damaging effects throughout the body. We—or, more precisely, food manufacturers—have made a real Faustian bargain: we've traded a longer shelf life for a shorter human life.[7]

We know what trans fatty acids are and what they do, but where do we find them? What kinds of food are they in? And how much trans fats do we really consume? Let's answer the last question first. By most calculations trans fatty acids represent 7 percent of the fats of the average American diet. And by our calculations, this figure may *underestimate* the intake; we believe the consumption is much higher than that. If you assume the average American diet to be about 3,000 calories in which 35 percent are from fat, and each gram of fat is 9 calories, you come up with the 7 percent supposedly from trans fat equals a little over 8 grams of trans fatty acids per day. This sounds plausible until you realize that one medium order of french fries in a fast-food restaurant contains about 7 grams of trans fatty acids. Kids and especially adolescents, who eat enormous amounts of processed foods, consume huge amounts of trans fatty acids. We have seen teenagers bolt down half a dozen doughnuts at a sitting or eat an entire package of cookies or a bag or two of potato chips—and these are all just snacks, just a small portion of what a typical teenager eats in a day. If you do the trans-fatty-acid calculations on teenage diets, you will find that the trans-fatty-acid intake is more like 40 to 50 grams per day; in a 3,000-calorie, 35 percent–fat diet, that would be closer to 40 percent of fat calories. We wouldn't be surprised if it were even higher than this.

Trans fatty acids are found in all sorts of processed foods. They are in margarines, salad oils, bakery goods, potato chips, corn chips, crackers, and in all sorts of candies. And this is just the short list. When Dr. Enig's group analyzed various foods for trans-fatty-acid content, they discovered that the "highest levels

---

7. We say this in a speculative sense because statistically people are living longer now than ever before. But the ones who are long lived now, the ones that are setting the curve, grew up during an era of few trans fats. Their mothers cooked with lard, not processed vegetable shortenings, which contain large amounts of trans fatty acids. With the widespread development of diabetes and other insulin-related disorders at younger and younger ages, it may prove difficult for the advances in medical technology to keep up with the end results of the deterioration of the quality of our food.

of trans fatty acids in bakery goods were found in sandwich cookies, vanilla wafers, animal crackers, and honey graham crackers." How many times have we given our children these items as snacks? How many times have we had them for snacks ourselves?

Trans fatty acids are everywhere, and, unfortunately, there are no labeling laws on the books at this time forcing food manufacturers to divulge the amount of these fats in their products. You can be sure, however, that if you buy any kind of vegetable oil or vegetable-oil product that doesn't have a dark colored bottle and that doesn't require refrigeration after it's been opened, you've got a trans fat. Commercially made salad dressings, for example, contain a significant amount of trans fatty acids. If you look at the label, you will often see that it's made of soybean oil, not a particularly bad oil in its fresh state, but one that food manufacturers love to partially hydrogenate and convert to a "plastic" food. According to Mary Enig, approximately 70 percent of the soybean oil consumed in this country has been partially hydrogenated. That means that if you see soybean oil as an ingredient in a product you're eating, the odds are that it's been hydrogenated. The hydrogenation process converts soybean oil from having no unnatural fats to a substance containing over 53 percent chemically altered fats. We always keep a sharp eye out for any products containing soybean oil and avoid them; we recommend that you do the same.

Once you realize what horrible products trans fatty acids are and how widespread is their use in processed foods, it becomes easy to understand why most people see such an improvement in their health no matter what kind of diet they go on. There is no physician, nutritionist, or dietitian I know who recommends a diet high in trans fatty acids. Virtually everyone recommends avoiding candy, cakes, doughnuts, french fries, cookies, etc. Despite the fact that many diet gurus preach the low-fat, high-carbohydrate diet, which we believe goes contrary to our own metabolism, their recommendations do their followers good because they decrease the amount of trans fatty acids. Vegetarians, however, in their zeal to avoid animal fat will often substitute partially hydrogenated vegetable fats. Some studies have shown an increase in the intake of trans fatty acids in diets of people trying assiduously to avoid animal fats.

How Do I Avoid Trans Fats?

The best way to avoid trans fatty acids is to become a devoted label reader. Look for the words *partially hydrogenated* and avoid any products that contain them. Avoid processed foods. If you never eat a processed food, you won't get enough trans fat to spit at. Avoid foods that have been deep-fried, unless you deep-fry them yourself—and if you do deep-fry yourself, make sure that both the oil you use and the food you fry are fresh. There have been a few papers published asserting that keeping oil at a high temperature as is done in restaurants with deep fryers can convert unsaturated fats into trans fat. According to Mary Enig, this is not the case. Her group has analyzed the fat from countless deep fryers and has never found trans fats to have been formed. In order to make a trans fat, you've got to have nickel (or some other catalyst) along with the heat. The fact that you can't get trans fats from keeping oil at a high temperature doesn't mean, however, that you should eat deep-fried foods from restaurants, because the oils used for commercial frying often contain a significant amount of trans fats right from the start (i.e., they come out of the container that way). Moreover, restaurants often use deep fryers to reheat foods that have already been cooked once in trans fats. As these foods are reheated in the deep fryer, the trans fats come out of the foods and into the oil waiting to be picked up by the next food fried. We try never to eat fried food—unless we fry it ourselves in fresh, stable oil at relatively low temperatures, because unsaturated oils kept at high temperatures for a long time *can* oxidize and become lipid peroxides.

Because of the treacherous nature of trans fatty acids and lipid peroxides and their near universality in processed foods and oils, you need to be ever vigilant. You need to select your cooking and salad oils with care. (We've given you a complete list of oils and their uses in chapter 13, "*LifePlan* Nutrition.") Always purchase oils from health food stores, and get those that are in dark glass bottles. After you open them, refrigerate them. If you like the taste, use olive oil whenever possible. If you don't like the taste, learn to. And if you consume a lot of unsaturated oils, take a lot of vitamin E, the primary fat-soluble vitamin that gets into the lipid bilayer and keeps the fatty acids there from oxidizing (see chapter 5, "Antioxidant Use and Abuse").

The Fatty-Acid Game Plan

Eat only good-quality unprocessed fats. Make sure that you get plenty of good-quality, unperoxidized, essential-omega-3 fatty acids by eating sardines, cod-liver oil, flax seed oil, or by taking fish-oil capsules (don't forget to test them every two or three days). Take vitamin E to protect these fats without depleting your body's own vitamin E. Keep your insulin levels low in order to increase the activity of your desaturase enzymes, so that you can make all the unsaturated fats you need to keep your membranes supple and make everything work better. Watch your consumption of vegetable oils, even good-quality unprocessed ones, because most vegetable oils are high in omega-6 fats, and you need to keep your omega 6–to–omega 3 ratio as close to 2:1 as possible. It's difficult to do this by simply consuming more omega 3s, so you'll have to cut back on your omega 6s. Remember, our Paleolithic ancestors didn't have purified vegetable oils—they got their omega-6 fats in small amounts from the plants they ate, and so should you.

If you have neither the time nor the inclination to follow these steps, then just throw a wallaby on the barbee and eat it whole like the folks did at Arnheim Land. That's one sure way you'll get plenty of all the right kinds of fats that haven't been altered, and you'll get them in the correct proportion. *Bon appétit,* mate!

BOTTOM LINE

Humans and their prehuman ancestors have feasted off the "fat of the land" for at least three million years, but the fats our ancestors ate vary dramatically from what we consume today. Unlike most of us finicky modern humans, who eat only the muscle meats of animals (if we eat them at all), our ancestors at the whole carcass—the skin, the muscles, the organs, the brain, the intestinal fat, and even the marrow from the bones—all but the fur, horns, hooves, and bones. Doing so gave our ancient ancestors the sorts of fats they needed to thrive—and, therefore, the fats we're designed by the forces of nature to function best on. And so to reclaim our birthright of wellness, we must do likewise, at least within the context of our modern palate.

The shift to a different type of fat has occurred, really, only within the last hundred years or so—an eye blink in terms of the millennia of human existence. In 1910 we consumed 83 percent of our fat as animal fat and only 17 percent as vegetable fat, and practically all of that came from eating the actual vegetables. Now, we get three times the amount of vegetable fat—mostly from cheap vegetable cooking oils and shortening—and a little more than half the animal fat. And, unfortunately, we have added a new kind of fat, an unnatural, processed one called trans fat, to the mix. Trans fats, widely used for baking, turn up in all kinds of processed foods.

The fats and oils you eat are made a part of the cell membranes of every cell in your body. You must have high-quality ones of the right types for the cells to function properly: cholesterol and saturated fats give the membranes a defined structure and polyunsaturated fats give them flexibility. Both are important for their proper function. The artificially produced trans fats, formed by the process called partial hydrogenation, pollute the cell membranes and interfere with their function. Their toll on health is vast, including: lowering HDL (the good cholesterol), raising LDL (the bad cholesterol), raising overall cholesterol, decreasing reproductive functions, lowering the nutritional quality of breast milk, weakening the immune system, stiffening the cell membranes, interfering with the production of good essential fats from dietary fat, contributing to the development of obesity, and, most importantly, directly contributing to the development of insulin resistance and hyperinsulinemia. These fats occur in all sorts of prepackaged and processed foods, from margarine and salad and cooking oils to bakery goods, chips, crackers, and candies. Look for the words *partially hydrogenated* on the label and avoid any food containing these fats.

For health, we recommend that you increase your intake of the important fats our ancestors ate that are now deficient in the diets of most

Americans—the fats called omega 3s, which occur in cold-water fish (sardines, wild salmon, mackerel, herring, and tuna) and in the oils extracted from them, such as cod-liver oil, and in the fat of game animals. We also recommend that you increase your intake of the monounsaturated fats, found richly in olives, olive oil, avocados, canola oil, and true nuts and their oils. The saturated fats in your diet should come from quality sources, such as meat, poultry, dairy, and eggs.

Avoid using bottled vegetable oils, soy oil, other cheap cooking oils, margarine, and shortening, since these contain both trans fats and large amounts of omega-6 oils, which early humans only ate in the small amounts present in the plants themselves. To mimic our ancestral intake, keep the ratio of omega-6 to omega-3 oils about equal in your diet. For most people, that means eating more of the 3s and less of the 6s.

On page 320, you'll find a list of the best oils to use for salads, cooking, and supplementing your diet.

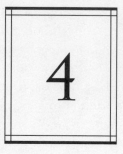

4

CHOLESTEROL: THE GOOD, THE BAD, AND THE UGLY

Half the modern drugs could well be thrown out of the
window, except that the birds might eat them.
—MARTIN H. FISCHER

Not since the witch trials of Salem has such an all-out cam-
paign been launched against the innocent based on so little
truth and so much misinformation as in the case of cholesterol.
The media and the medical-pharmaceutical complex has vilified
it, demonized it, and placed a bounty on its head as if it were a
serial ax murderer. And the government has spent many, many
millions of dollars to alert the public about this deadly killer
through its National Cholesterol Education Program (NCEP).
For years, people have been told that cholesterol is the villain
making the nation sick at heart. They've been told that if they cut
the cholesterol and fat from their diets and load up on complex
carbohydrates, they'll reduce their cholesterol readings. Unfortunately, most of the time it doesn't work, leading at best to frustration and at worst to a prescription for expensive drugs with
potentially dangerous side effects. As a nation, we're still in the
midst of the Cholesterol Madness that we wrote about in *Protein
Power*. Madness has given way to mania. Respected authorities

continue to sound the call to reduce blood cholesterol through adoption of the (largely ineffective) low-fat diet but now also insist that, based on revised lower numbers of what's a "safe" level of cholesterol, nearly 40 percent of the adult population of America should begin taking cholesterol-lowering medications forthwith or risk dire cardiovascular consequences. Such terror tactics justifiably alarm the public, but they must warm the cockles of the hearts of the drug companies that manufacture the cholesterol-lowering pills being pushed down that trusting public's throat. In this chapter you'll learn just what cholesterol is, why it can be good or bad, and how to use our plan to lower your cholesterol naturally without dangerous drugs. Why all this furor over a simple *naturally occurring* body chemical? What is this substance cholesterol that it should incite such fear in the hearts and minds of men?

Look Upon the Face of the Demon

Whether in dreams or in life, one way to conquer fear is to put a face on it and to look squarely into that face—in effect, to stare down the fear. So with that in mind, let's look into the face of this "demon" cholesterol and see what, if anything, we should fear.

Cholesterol, which most people call a fat, is actually a waxy alcohol—hence the similar endings to the two words cholester*ol* and alcoh*ol*—that gives structure to the cell membranes of every single one of the bizillion cells that make up any member of the animal kingdom. Were you able to extract every last molecule of cholesterol from your body—an event that we sometimes think some misguided nutritional authorities would find desirable—you'd disintegrate; you'd melt into a puddle like the Wicked Witch of the West did when Dorothy doused her with the bucket of water.

In fact, your body's need for cholesterol is so keen that virtually every single one of your bizillion cells can—and will—make it if necessary. Your skin and your intestinal tract make a fair amount, but the bulk of your body's cholesterol comes from the cholesterol-production factory in your liver. While your diet does provide some of this critical raw material, what you eat will account for *at most* about 20 percent of your blood cholesterol. The liver's cholesterol-production factory produces the other 80 percent, and in fact, the production line there monitors how much cholesterol comes in with the food you eat and can step up or slow down its production accordingly to keep the supply adequate to meet the body's daily and ongoing needs.

Without enough cholesterol, the body can't properly replace and renew its worn or damaged cells, since making a new cell requires the production of a new cell membrane, and making a new cell membrane requires cholesterol. Without new cells, the body will age and die. (That's not to say, of course, that that aging and death won't ultimately occur no matter how much cholesterol the body has to build new cells, but why hasten the process?) Without enough cholesterol, how can the body completely replace the lining of the intestine every four or five days (which it does), regularly renew hair, skin, and nails, repair the wear and tear on the skeleton and the muscles that occurs just from living, repair injured tissues, or continue to produce the many hormones—such as estrogen, testosterone, progesterone, DHEA, cortisol, and aldosterone—that the body builds on a cholesterol framework? The answer is that it can't. And pharmaceutically shutting down the natural production of this important substance in a mindless race to get the level of blood cholesterol down can only do harm in the long run.

We'll examine exactly what kind of damage the body can sustain from the use of these drugs shortly, but first it's important that you understand a little about the lingo of cholesterol, so that you'll be able to make sense of your own cholesterol numbers and the seemingly endless types of fat-consuming molecules in the blood. It's no longer sufficient to speak of just cholesterol; you must know its fractions—and now, even the fractions have fractions and subtypes that play crucial roles in what's becoming an increasingly complicated overall picture of cholesterol and cardiovascular health. Let's look at what all these fractions are and what they do.

Cholesterol, as we've said, is not a fat but a waxy alcohol. As such, it can't travel independently in the blood, because the blood is basically a water-based liquid, and quite simply, oil and water don't mix. To keep the waxy cholesterol suspended in the watery blood, the body developed water-soluble carrier proteins on which the cholesterol molecules (and for that matter the actual fats in the blood, the triglycerides) can safely ride from place to place. You're most likely already familiar with these carrier proteins, called lipoproteins, by their names: high-density lipoprotein (HDL), low-density lipoprotein (LDL), very low-density lipoprotein (VLDL), and a newer and less famous one, intermediate-density lipoprotein (IDL). Laboratories have long been able to separate the various fractions based upon their weights or, more correctly, their densities. When spun around vigorously in a centrifuge, the various molecules will arrange themselves in layers by density: the HDLs are the most dense, made almost entirely of scavenged cholesterol and protein; the LDLs are next dense, containing protein and cholesterol for transport to the tissues but some amount of triglyceride as well; the IDLs are less dense, sort of LDLs with more triglyceride molecules added on; the VLDLs, less dense still, are like IDLs with yet more added triglyceride; and finally, the least dense of all, the individual triglyceride molecules themselves (about which you'll learn more shortly).

You can think of these carriers as transport vehicles shuttling the cholesterol and triglycerides about. These two raw materials (one structural, cholesterol, and one a fuel, triglycerides) leave the liver packed onto VLDL carriers. As the transport vehicle makes its way through the bloodstream, it delivers triglycerides to the tissues that need them for energy. As it dumps its load, it transforms into an IDL molecule and continues on its journey, depositing yet more triglycerides into the places that have put in a hormonal order for them to burn for energy or to store as fat. When the IDL has delivered enough triglycerides, it becomes an LDL particle and begins to fill delivery orders for both cholesterol and triglycerides, being taken up by the special docking facilities (the LDL receptors) on the cell surfaces of cholesterol-dependent tissues throughout the body. With that background, let's look at the individual players in the typical lipid panel.

Total Cholesterol. This is the sum of the amounts of cholesterol contained in the blood attached to all the various carrier lipoproteins. As a measure—unless it's very, very high or very, very low—it doesn't really tell you much about your overall cardiovascular health.

HDL Cholesterol. This carrier protein primarily functions to pick up the cholesterol in the tissues throughout the body and ferry it back to the liver for recycling or elimination in the bile. Scavenging cholesterol out of the tissues earned HDL its reputation as the "good" cholesterol. It's the type you want to increase—and the more the merrier—which you can do by eating good-quality fats (especially the essential fats found in fish oils), exercising, and drinking wine. In short, by following the prescription we outline in the *Protein Power LifePlan,* most people will see a nice rise in HDL if it's low (below 30 mg/dl in men or 40 mg/dl in women), and it should remain in the healthy range (over 40 mg/dl for men and 50 mg/dl for women) if it's already there and may even go up considerably. Laboratories can now separate the total HDL into at least five subclasses, named, appropriately enough, HDL 1 through 5. At this point, there's still great debate in research circles about the minute interworkings of these various subtypes and their specific significance to your health, but they each appear to respond to different lifestyle manipulations. The HDL 2 subclass, for instance, has been shown to be especially involved in the cholesterol retrieval-and-disposal function, so it stands to reason that increasing this fraction should improve your ability to extract cholesterol and eliminate it. We now know that exercise will increase the HDL 2 fraction, and that red wine will improve the HDL 3 subclass, which may or may not be more important than HDL 2, depending on which research you read. So far, medical science has yet to clearly define the clinical significance of these various subclasses of HDL, and at least at this juncture—even though the technology now allows us to measure such fractionation—we have to say it's still the total HDL reading that matters most. We reserve the right to change that recommendation as medicine's understanding of the various roles of HDL subclasses becomes clearer, but for now, just try to keep your total HDL up as high as you can through diet and exercise.

LDL Cholesterol. LDL lipoproteins function to transport cholesterol to the tissues and deposit it there for use as a raw material.

In and of itself, this function isn't bad—in fact, it's quite necessary—but sometimes there's a glitch in the system and the LDL gets disoriented and attracted to the artery walls, and it deposits its cholesterol payload where it doesn't belong, in the lining of the blood vessels. But despite its rap sheet as the "bad" cholesterol that hardens your arteries, LDL becomes disoriented only if it becomes damaged, which chiefly occurs by being rusted by oxygen or caramelized by blood sugar. No matter how high the LDL levels in the blood, only that which is oxidized or glycated (altered by the attachment of blood sugar) will feed cholesterol to developing arterial plaques and promote the development of artherosclerosis. Still, the higher the amount of LDL that is floating around in the blood, the more likely that some of it will be damaged. So in general, we agree with keeping the LDL within reasonable limits, but, more important, we recommend you direct more effort toward preventing its damage than lowering its numbers. And that means stopping smoking (a potent generator of free radicals that could damage and disorient your LDL cholesterol), keeping your blood sugar stable and relatively low, and eating a diet high in antioxidant foods, one that provides plenty of vitamin E, vitamin C, coenzyme Q10, alpha-lipoic acid, and all the raw materials your body needs to make its own glutathione (see chapter 5, "Antioxidant Use and Abuse"). By doing these things—all of which play roles in the comprehensive health and wellness outlined in this book—you can substantially reduce the chances that damaged LDL will find its way into the walls of your arteries and plug them up.

Unlike HDL, however, a simple total LDL reading doesn't provide enough useful information to assess your heart disease risk. The subclasses of LDL clearly alter the clinical picture; in other words, the kind of LDL you have is more significant than the absolute amount in determining your risk for heart disease. Unfortunately, the LDL reading reported by most laboratory tests doesn't even actually measure the LDL itself. Instead it measures the total amount of cholesterol, the triglycerides, and the HDL fraction—all of which are inexpensive to measure—and then uses three parameters to derive the LDL reading by a mathematical calculation called the Freidewald equation:

$$LDL \text{ cholesterol} = \text{total cholesterol} - HDL \text{ cholesterol} - \text{triglycerides}/5$$

With that in mind, let's digress a moment here to address an issue related to LDL and cholesterol levels that has cropped up in the last few years and seems to cause great consternation for some of our readers.

Since the publication of *Protein Power* and the adoption of our dietary strategy by over two million people around the world, we've received countless letters, phone calls, and e-mail missives from people who have used it and reaped great health rewards. In the patients we've taken care of firsthand over the years, we've almost always seen dramatic improvement in all the lipid (blood fat) numbers. Only very rarely have we seen no change or a rise in total and LDL cholesterol, but once in a while, we'll run into a patient or get a letter from someone whose cholesterol has actually gone *up* following our plan. Their letters or calls usually run something like this:

"I've been following your plan for x-amount of time, to the letter, and I really expected that when my lab tests came back I'd see a big drop in my cholesterol and LDL—but look what happened! My cholesterol was 210 at the start, my HDL was 25, my LDL was 125, and my triglycerides were 300. Now, because of your diet, my cholesterol is 230, my HDL is 50, and my LDL has risen to 162! Oh yeah, and my triglycerides did fall to 90. Why didn't your diet work, and what are you going to do about this?" Our response would be to cheer—because the second laboratory picture has vastly improved in the parameters that really matter. Remember, the LDL reading done in this fashion isn't really a reading at all. It's a calculation based on other lipid readings, and it may or may not accurately reflect the actual amount of LDL present. But what this second set of lab results most certainly reveals is a doubling in HDL, the "good" cholesterol, and an even more dramatic drop in triglycerides (the two most important predictors of heart disease, as you'll soon see). It also reveals a sea change in the kind of LDL being made—a much more important factor than the absolute amount.

You see, the genes you inherit play a big role in determining the sort of LDL your body will naturally tend to make. The body can make particles of LDL that are small and dense, like little BB pellets, or it can make large, fluffy particles that are more analogous to, say, cotton balls. (It can actually make particles of every size and density between the BBs and the cotton balls, too, but for the purposes of this discussion, let's assume that there are only two types of LDL—small, dense BBs and large, fluffy cotton balls.) These two basic types of LDL particles have given rise to the identification of two different groups of people with two very different degrees of risk for heart disease. Those who make mostly the cotton ball LDL scientists label subclass A, and we speak of their having a type A LDL pattern; those who produce mainly dense LDL BBs science has dubbed subclass B (no relation to BB, just a happy coincidence), and we speak of their having a type B LDL pattern. While the difference may seem arcane, it's actually quite important because of the way these two different particles behave. The small, dense LDL BBs appear to be more easily oxidized and damaged and as a result are much more prone to enter the artery walls and thereby promote the development of rapidly enlarging, brittle atherosclerotic plaques that obstruct blood flow. The large, fluffy cotton ball LDL particles much more vigorously resist oxidative damage—in fact, some researchers have even suggested that they might actually have some anti-oxidant protective function, and in short might even be beneficial. Time will tell about that. But why is this distinction so important? Because lifestyle can change the pattern of LDL particle that you make. You can—with proper diet and exercise—coax your body into making cotton balls instead of BBs, and in the doing can radically alter your heart disease risk even at the same absolute LDL reading.

On a low-fat, high-carbohydrate diet, most people (especially men) will tend to produce small, dense LDL BBs; even if they manage to lower their LDL cholesterol reading, they're doing themselves little good, since they're packing their profile with these dense, dangerously atherogenic LDL particles. Conversely, on a higher-fat, lower-starch and lower-sugar diet (such as the *Protein Power LifePlan*), the vast majority of people will produce mainly the large, fluffy—and infinitely less harmful—cotton ball

LDLs. And even in those few people who don't drop their overall LDL level, that which they make becomes less dangerous and, according to some research, possibly even protective. Can you find out which type you make? Sure, with a relatively simple—but pretty expensive—blood test.

Although for years the laboratory test that measures the sub-classes of LDL—called an LDL gradient-gel electrophoresis (LDL-GGE)—was generally performed only in a research setting, it is now available through national reference laboratories in physicians' offices. The LDL-GGE can directly determine the LDL particle size and can tell you volumes about your real risk for heart disease and whether or not you should be alarmed about an LDL reading that's a little higher than recommended "normals" dictate. This test becomes especially important when we are making the case that a particular patient doesn't unequivocally need to go on cholesterol-lowering drugs despite an LDL in the 130 to 160 range. We find ourselves fighting this very battle all the time when, in trying to offer the best nutritional advice for total body wellness to the patients who consult us, we run counter to some other authority's dictate that the total cholesterol and LDL levels must fall by medicinal means, regardless of the damage that medicine may do to the body as a whole.

A strong connection exists between triglycerides and LDL subclass: when the triglycerides fall, the body generally makes mostly large, fluffy LDL cotton balls; when the triglycerides rise, the body makes LDL BBs. That means that just knowing your triglyceride reading gives you some insight into your LDL pattern. And it also explains why we would cheer that "rise" in LDL described in the example above. Low triglycerides equate with an improvement in LDL subclass and a reduction in heart disease risk.

Triglycerides. These molecules, composed of three fatty acids attached to a sugar-based (glycerol) backbone, are the transport-and-storage form of fat in the body. The body uses triglycerides as a high-octane fuel for energy production in the cellular furnaces (the mitochondria) throughout its tissues. In fact, they're the very best fuel for the muscles and heart to run on and the fuel the body prefers to use when the metabolism is running smoothly.

When the burning pathways aren't operating because insulin is too high, for example, the body stores them away. The cellulite on hips and thighs, the spare tire roll around the middle, the beer gut, and the love handles all represent energy stored as triglycerides in the fat tissue depots there.

The body also stores triglycerides in and around the organs and in between the layers of muscle tissue—in a steak, you'd call it fat marbling and pay a premium for it—but in your own muscles, it's not such a good sign. Incoming dietary triglycerides, as well as those we pull from these storage depots, ride around on the VLDL, IDL, and to some degree on the LDL lipoproteins as they make their way through the blood. When things are running smoothly, the flux of incoming triglycerides and those retrieved from storage remains in balance with the amount we're burning for energy, and the baseline levels of triglycerides, VLDL, and IDL in the blood are low. When things get out of kilter metabolically speaking—such as when insulin resistance rears its ugly head—the levels of triglycerides and triglyceride-rich lipoproteins rises in the blood. And the risk for heart disease rises right along with them.

Although people are all too familiar with the supposed risks of high cholesterol, many people are unaware of the newer research that has shown that a high triglyceride level puts you at the highest risk of all for having a heart attack. For that reason, we're far more concerned with our patients' triglyceride readings than with what their cholesterol is. A triglyceride measurement—an easy and relatively inexpensive test to do—gives a reasonable reflection of cardiovascular risk, since, as we've already mentioned, low triglyceride readings, in general, correlate with large, fluffy, less harmful cotton ball LDLs. We like to keep the triglyceride readings of our patients below 100 mg/dl if possible—and in most cases the dietary changes alone will accomplish that goal. But a recently published study by a Harvard medical research team led by J. Michael Gaziano places even more importance on the triglyceride reading as a predictor of heart disease.

The Harvard group undertook a study to uncover exactly which of the many lipid parameters would not just predict risk for heart disease but also pinpoint as closely as possible who would actually go on to have a heart attack. The researchers took blood samples from a large group of people, both men and women, with no previous history of heart disease, froze their blood specimens, and waited to see which people would later have a heart attack. They then went back to perform a detailed analysis on the blood specimens to determine which blood tests would have most accurately predicted the risk. Their conclusion was that the triglycerides and the HDL cholesterol tests were the most sensitive indicators of who was at risk and who was not. Specifically, they felt that a ratio derived by dividing the triglyceride reading by the HDL reading predicted most accurately of all who would have a heart attack. When they divided their study groups into quartiles (25 percent of the group), they found that those people with the highest triglyceride-to-HDL ratios were sixteen times more likely to have a heart attack than those with the lowest ratios. In simple terms what that means is that by keeping your triglycerides low and raising your HDL levels, you can join that happy group that's not very likely to have a heart attack.

This data is borne out nicely by an Italian study known as a centenarian study.[1] In this investigation, the researchers collected data from healthy people who had reached at least one hundred years of age and were still mentally and physically fit. Their purpose was to examine them, their lifestyle, and their laboratory values to try to determine whether they had some factor in common that would predict their longevity and health. After their search, they came up with three factors: a low level of fasting insulin, low serum triglycerides, and moderately high levels of HDL. Sounds like what we advocate in the *Protein Power LifePlan*—and what most of our patients and readers achieve. Maybe we should have named it the Centenarian Plan instead.

Lipoprotein(a). Abbreviated Lp(a) and called by most everyone "L-P-little-a," this carrier molecule is a variant of LDL with an extra apoprotein A attached to it. In structure it's similar enough to one of the body's chief clot-dissolving substances, called plasminogen, that some researchers think it increases heart attack risk

---

1. V. Marigliano et al., "Normal Values in Extreme Old Age," *Annals of the NY Academy of Sciences,* December 22, 1992, vol. 673; pp. 23–28.

by interfering with the body's clot formation–clot dissolving balance, tipping the scales in favor of clot formation. As such, it's been strongly implicated as an instigator in the development of obstructive clots in the coronary arteries and the resultant heart attacks.

While everybody makes some amount of Lp(a), most of us don't make much, with average "normal" values usually falling around 4 mg/dl. The tendency to make too much Lp(a) passes from parent to child as a dominant genetic trait, meaning that one-half of the children of a person with the tendency will inherit it. These people may have Lp(a) levels as high as 25 or 30 mg/dl, which can be quite dangerous because of its untoward influence on blood clotting. Producing Lp(a) at these levels may increase the risk for heart disease by three times or even more if coupled with low HDL levels. For that reason, people who have had a parent with premature heart disease or stroke or who developed these problems themselves prematurely should have blood tests done to determine whether they make too much of this altered lipoprotein. If so, it's even more critical that they control other risk factors, such as lowering their triglyceride levels, raising their HDL cholesterol, and lowering and stabilizing their blood sugar through proper diet and exercise. Interestingly—and this is the dirty little secret that the low-fat establishment doesn't want you to know—eating saturated fat actually lowers Lp(a) levels. Although you can't change your genetic blueprint, you can modify other factors that will determine whether it will cause you harm or not.

Fibrinogen. This component of the body's blood-clotting system is not related to cholesterol or its carriers. Fibrinogen forms the strands of the framework onto which the clot forms. The higher the amount of fibrinogen in the blood, the greater the tendency to form clots and, therefore, the greater the risk for heart attack or stroke. When the body sustains an injury of any kind, fibrinogen rushes to the site to begin to patch the damage with a clot, snaring the solid components of blood (the red blood cells, white blood cells, and platelets) in a web of fibrous strands. For this reason, it's difficult to get an accurate measure of fibrinogen if you've been sick, injured (even a minor injury), had surgery, or even been under major psychological stress, because the levels skyrocket in these circumstances. Levels taken in the absence of such traumas that rise above 335 μM/l can signal an increased clotting risk. Smoking also drastically increases fibrinogen levels, and in anyone with a high reading, stopping smoking is of paramount life-saving importance.

If you suffer from any of the many insulin-resistance disorders—diabetes, high tryglycerides, low HDL, excess weight—you should ask your physician to check your fibrinogen level, since it tends to run higher in the presence of these disorders. The good news is that eating a diet lower in carbohydrate, partaking of a little wine or alcohol, and exercising will help to lower your fibrinogen.

Homocysteine. This amino acid, which, like fibrinogen, is not related to cholesterol, occurs naturally in everyone's blood. The body normally metabolizes it effortlessly in a process that depends on the vitamins folic acid, B_6, and B_{12}, as well as magnesium. However, some people inherit a genetic tendency for faulty homocysteine metabolism, allowing high levels of it to build up in the blood. High levels of the amino acid damage the cells lining the blood vessels, paving the way for atherosclerotic plaque, a theory of heart disease championed by Kilmer McCully.[2] While only about 1 percent of the general population has the condition, it occurs in about 25 percent of people with heart disease. A simple blood test will usually tell the tale—values higher than 10 μM/l spell increased risk—and anyone with a family history for heart disease should have the measurement made. Fortunately, treatment is quite straightforward: simply ensure that your diet (or supplemental intake) provides at least 400 *micro*grams of folic acid, 3 mg of B_6, and 100 *micro*grams of B_{12} every day.

Does cholesterol itself cause heart disease? As you'll soon discover, the issue is far from settled. But if you were to ask one hundred people at random on the street whether reducing cholesterol to as low a level as possible is healthy, the overwhelming majority would answer yes, and they would answer incorrectly. As

---

2. K. S. McCully, *The Homocysteine Revolution: Medicine for the New Millennium* (New Canaan, Conn.: Keats Publishing, 1997).

research continues to accumulate, it clearly demonstrates that the level of cholesterol per se has precious little to do with predicting who will have a heart attack and who won't; even people with low cholesterol levels have heart attacks, and people with high cholesterol readings escape them. To be sure, if you display the data cleverly, you can see the familiar trend that shows the higher the cholesterol level, the higher the risk for death from heart disease, as shown in figure 4.1. It would appear from this graph that there's a steady rise in the death rate as the cholesterol increases, implying that the lower the cholesterol the better. What such data don't reveal is what happens to people with cholesterol readings below 180 mg/dl. Let's add that data into the picture and we'll get figure 4.2. Look at how the mortality curve shoots sharply up

FIGURE 4.1

Heart Disease vs. Serum Cholesterol

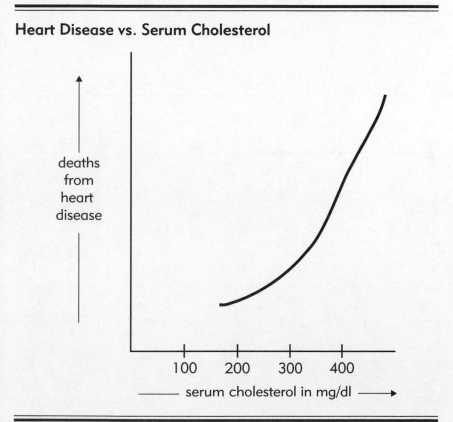

FIGURE 4.2

Total Mortality vs. Serum Cholesterol

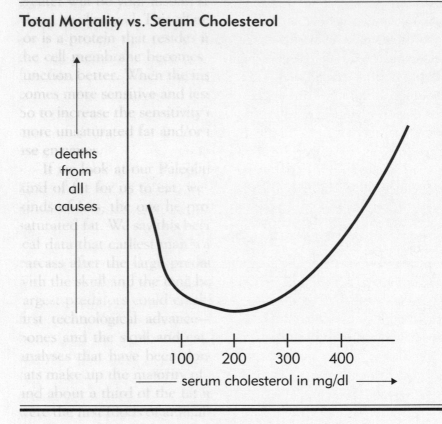

---

as cholesterol falls below 160 mg/dl. It climbs even more steeply at the low end of cholesterol levels than at the high end, meaning that having a cholesterol reading below 140 mg/dl is as bad as or worse than having one above 240 as far as risk of dying goes. At the lower end of the scale, deaths don't occur from heart disease and stroke; rather people in that group die from cancer, suicide, homicide, and vehicular trauma (which quite often is disguised suicide). Research suggests that these mortality risks increase whether you push your cholesterol to these low levels using an ultra-low-fat diet or drugs. Just a quick glance at this U-shaped line shows where you want to be—down there in the flat part of the bottom, where the incidence of deaths of all kinds is lowest. That means your best bet would be to keep your cholesterol in the 160 to 220 range, and, interestingly, that's where most of our patients naturally land following our plan.

Is the race to push cholesterol ever lower by any means—even the use of exceedingly costly and toxic drugs—justified? Our unequivocal position is no, but let's examine the issue in a bit more depth and see what the research tells us. Let's go right to the source of the terror and look at the "evidence" from the many cholesterol-lowering trials and see what we can learn from them.

If You Torture the Data Enough, They Will Confess

Since the failed cholesterol-lowering Veteran's Administration trial of 1969, the proponents of the cholesterol-is-killing-you theory have continued to beat a dead horse in the righteous certainty that their assumption is correct despite the facts to the contrary. Study after study has failed to demonstrate that lowering cholesterol with the low-fat diet (the only one ever really studied as a therapy in such trials, since, for gosh sakes, everyone *knows* it's the healthiest one) or with medication has prevented death either from heart disease or from other causes. In fact, many of them have shown an *excess* number of deaths among the intervention groups (those receiving the treatment being studied). The Minnesota coronary survey of 1989 failed. The MRFIT study in 1982 failed. The WHO mulifactor study of 1983 failed. The Gothenburg study of 1986 failed. The WHO clofibrate study, a dismal and embarrassing failure, actually caused 29 percent more deaths in the study group who received the drug, than in the control group who didn't. Place that figure against the backdrop: physicians prescribed clofibrate to more than 3.5 million people in 1978. How many excess deaths did the drug cause that year?

Have there been no successful cholesterol-intervention trials? Not unequivocally. Although cholesterol-lowering proponents often cite it as a success, even the Finnish mental hospital study—which did show a fall in the rate of heart disease both by reducing smoking and by changing diet—was flawed in its design, since it was simply an intensive community-based program without a control group. Who's to say if the fall in heart disease rates correlated with decreased smoking or change in diet? We'd put our money on their tossing the smokes, but there's simply no way to tell from that kind of data. Even the ongoing and highly publicized Framingham study has failed to show any clearly demonstrable correlation between cholesterol levels and the development of heart disease. To illustrate our point—that drug intervention to lower cholesterol is a fool's bargain—we're going to look more closely at two of the studies which purported to show benefit, and let you in on the real results—whatever their propagandized "spin" to the contrary.

The Helsinki Heart Trial. This study of more than five years' duration examined the effects of the drug gemfibrozil (Lopid) in the prevention of coronary events (heart attacks) in more than two thousand men who took it compared to another two thousand who did not. It's important to note that the study included only middle-aged men, offering absolutely no clinical evidence of any sort that women, younger men, or the elderly would benefit from taking it at all—and in our opinion, for these groups the risks of taking gemfibrozil clearly outweigh any small benefits.

Those men who took the drug did achieve a 10 percent reduction in cholesterol, and the proponents equated that with a 34 percent reduction in their risk of heart attack. And, indeed, during the five-year period of the study, seventy-nine people in the control group suffered nonfatal heart attacks, whereas only fifty-one of those receiving the drug did. Twenty-eight fewer heart attacks sounds great, right? But let's look a little deeper. How many people died in each group? You'd think that far more of the control group would have, since twenty-eight more of them had heart attacks, but you'd be wrong. Only forty-two of those *not* on the study drug died during the five years, while forty-five in the group who took gemfibrozil died. So although taking the drug resulted a "34 percent reduction in risk," in absolute numbers that meant just under 1.4 percent fewer "serious cardiac events." Overall, more men died who took the drug than those who received no drug at all. But, more important, look at the side effects the men suffered from taking this drug: those men who took the drug experienced a 55 percent excess in the development of gallstones. In other words, as one researcher put it, gemfibrozil proved a more effective method of causing gallstones than of preventing heart attacks. To our way of thinking, it makes no sense to take a drug to reduce your risk of having a nonfatal heart attack if by doing so you increase your odds of dying of something else. Dead's dead, whatever the cause.

The Finnish Multifactor Trial. This trial focused on lowering both cholesterol and high blood pressure in a long-term study involving 612 middle-aged businessmen (again only men) who took prescription medications (clofibrate and probucol to lower cholesterol and beta blockers and thiazide diuretics for blood pressure) for five years and 610 matched controls who did not. The drug trial—hailed as a tremendous success—claimed to have achieved a 64 percent heart disease risk reduction for those who took it. However, when the investigators looked more closely at the data, the death rates during the study showed, to their horror, that substantially more men in the intervention group (that is, those who took the drugs and achieved the tremendous benefit of lower cholesterol and lower blood pressure) died than in the group that received no treatment. They followed these two groups for another ten years after the study ended, and guess what? The trend continued: more men died in the intervention group than in the control group. As the years passed, it became clear that using the drugs—just for that five-year period—to control cholesterol and blood pressure continued to *decrease* the life expectancy for many years to come.

We've been treating cholesterol and triglyceride problems in our patients (and we've personally treated thousands and thousands of them—many more, we'd dare say, than virtually any one of the major-drug-company-funded cholesterol-lowering trials[3]) for over a decade using our nutritional strategy and doing quite well in the vast majority of cases. For example, we recently requested an independent statistical analysis of the laboratory results of our patients and discovered to our delight and vindication that on average, our program reduces cholesterol levels by 44.4 mg/dl within the first twelve weeks, triglycerides by 137.1

---

3. With the exception of the MRFIT trial, which, while huge, like virtually all of the other such studies, ultimately failed to show any real reduction in all-cause mortality among those who received the cholesterol-lowering intervention.

mg/dl, and blood sugar by 36.7 mg/dl; and drops the all-important triglyceride-to-HDL ratio by 2.5! From what we've seen over the years we've been doing this, the majority of people—probably 80 to 85 percent—substantially lower their cholesterol using our program. Those who begin with an already normal or even slightly low cholesterol—or those whose cholesterol was artificially lowered by cholesterol-lowering medications—sometimes will see a transient rise in both total and LDL cholesterol. The average person, and in some cases, even their physician, may find any cholesterol rise—even a temporary one—worrisome, but this temporary bump isn't of great concern to us, because we've come to understand what's going on and what it means: the pattern of LDL particle type has shifted.

By eating according to the *Protein Power LifePlan,* a diet that more closely mimics the one nature designed for our use, most people will make more LDL cotton balls and fewer dense LDL BBs, drop their triglycerides and raise their HDL, and lower their fibrinogen and their homocysteine—and all of these changes will have a major and lasting impact on their risk for having a heart attack—without the use of toxic drugs.

That Way Danger Lies

Finally, let's take a look at the dangers of cholesterol-lowering drugs—especially the statin drugs, which currently include lovastatin, simvastatin, pravastatin, fluvastatin, and atrovastatin. These drugs all work by the same method—they slow down the cholesterol-manufacturing process in the liver by interfering with the helper enzyme that controls the rate of production—a substance with the unwieldy name HMG-CoA reductase; the higher the activity of this enzyme, the more cholesterol gets made and vice versa. And that may sound like a really fine thing—if your cholesterol's high, you just take a pill and reduce the amount that you make. But taking that pill isn't without a price, both in terms of dollars and in terms of damage to your overall health. Once again, you have to ask the basic question: What good does it do to lower your cholesterol if you increase your risk of something worse? What kind of something? Try these on for size:

- *Severe liver damage.* As quoted from one company's published circular, the drug caused "marked persistent increases (to more than 3 times the upper limit of normal) in serum tranaminases [liver enzymes] . . . in 1.9% of adult patients who received lovastatin for at least one year."
- *Skeletal muscle destruction (rhabdomyolysis).* Again quoting from the company's circular, "Rhabdomyolysis has been associated with lovastatin therapy alone . . . and when combined . . . with either gemfibrozil or lipid-lowering doses (>1 gram/day) of nicotinic acid [niacin]." The circular goes on to warn that similar muscle destruction has also been seen in combining lovastatin with anti-cancer drugs, antifungal drugs (ketoconozole), and one of the calcium-channel-blocking drugs (mibefradil).
- *Acute renal (kidney) failure.* Combining gemfibrozil and lovastatin (or any other statin drug) increases the likelihood that the damaged muscle tissue that makes its way into the bloodstream and ultimately to the kidneys will cause damage there sufficient to make them fail. The treatment for such failure—if it persists—is dialysis.

One of the most damaging common side effects of the statins doesn't even merit mention by this drug manufacturer in its information circular: taking statin drugs depletes the body of coenzyme Q10, a critical antioxidant for the heart. Because the body's production of coQ10 also depends on HMG-CoA reductase, when the drugs interfere with its activity—thoughout the body—the levels fall. CoQ10, an over-the-counter supplement in the United States but a prescription drug in other parts of the world, has been shown to improve the provision of energy to the heart muscle cells and has been used in large doses, administered by vein, to treat congestive heart failure. CoQ10 provides antioxidant protection all over the body (see chapter 5, "Antioxidant Use and Abuse," for more details), and its depletion, therefore, seriously increases the risk of oxidative damage to tissues bodywide.

As a last recommendation here, we strongly recommend that anyone who has previously taken or currently takes statin drugs for cholesterol lowering should immediately begin taking coQ10. Don't even wait until tomorrow—go get some today. You should take at least 300 mg of an oil-based formulation of coQ10 every day as long as you're bound to take these drugs (which we hope with the help of your physician won't be long) and at least 100 mg every day thereafter. It's very important that the coQ10 you purchase be suspended in oil in a gel cap; a dry powder in a gelatin capsule simply won't do much good and you'll be wasting your money.

In a very few cases, cholesterol and LDL levels may remain somewhat elevated even on the *Protein Power LifePlan* regimen— after all, a large genetic component and many other lifestyle factors also exert influence on LDL production. Unless the numbers run really high—cholesterol readings over 250 or LDLs above 190—we usually don't get too excited, but sometimes patients and their physicians do. In these instances, we recommend using the only "drug" ever shown in clinical testing to reduce all-cause mortality (that is, to save more lives than it costs): niacin.

In those rare cases where our patients require LDL and cholesterol lowering beyond that which our nutritional program delivers, we usually use this simple, inexpensive, and relatively side effect–free vitamin. Testing long ago showed that niacin will effectively lower LDL and cholesterol, but the high doses needed to make it work also made some people flush—in effect, it gave them a terrible hot flash. In an effort to prevent that unpleasant (but pretty harmless) side effect, manufacturers produced a sustained-release form of the vitamin that indeed prevented the flushing sensations but, unfortunately, also caused severe liver damage, which limited its use as a therapy. (We find it interesting that the same effects and worse ones haven't prevented the continued prescription and use of gemfibrozil or the statin drugs.) But necessity, the mother of invention, led to ingenuity and the development of a product marketed as "No-Flush Niacin." This vitamin—and that's really all it is, a vitamin—is the hybrid of a single molecule of inositol and six niacin molecules. This blending of two vitamins provides the cholesterol-lowering benefits of niacin but prevents the flushing side effect. For our patients we recommend beginning at a dose of 500 mg No-Flush Niacin three times a day, but that dose can be pushed up to 1,500 mg three times a day without problems if needed. In our experience, that's rarely the case.

The Safest Alternative

How do we help our patients reduce lipid levels without routinely prescribing incredibly toxic drugs? Well, we aim our sights at the hormone insulin, which plays a critical role here; high levels of insulin spur the HMG-CoA reductase enzyme, causing the liver to make more cholesterol. Reducing insulin levels reduces the activity of this enzyme, and production slows down, naturally. Certainly, the high-carbohydrate, low-fat diet can't do this—that's been clearly shown—since such a diet *raises* insulin. But the regimen that we prescribe—one that includes plenty of protein, plenty of folic acid and B vitamins, plenty of natural antioxidants, and plenty of good-quality fats and that eliminates or sharply reduces the insulin-raising sugars and starches—will almost always reduce lipid levels and improve lipid ratios without the risk of such dire side effects as these drugs can cause. So eat, drink, and play, and you'll keep your lipids in line naturally!

BOTTOM LINE

Over the last decade, the medical-pharmaceutical-media complex has demonized and vilified cholesterol as if it were a serial killer and not the *naturally occurring* and *necessary* substance that it is. The press to drive cholesterol readings ever lower has resulted in revised "safe" normal readings that will place upward of 40 percent of adult Americans in need of powerful and potentially dangerous prescription cholesterol-lowering medications to "protect" them from the risk of cardiovascular disease from elevated cholesterol.

What is cholesterol? Far from villain, this waxy alcohol (not a fat at all) occurs in every cell of every organ and tissue in your body. It functions there in many ways, among them, giving shape and structure to the cell membranes and providing the raw materials to produce the sex hormones, "youth" hormones, and the hormones that help us to withstand stress and reduce inflammation. Without enough cholesterol, the body can't properly replace and renew its worn or damaged cells, since making a new cell requires the production of a new cell membrane, and making a new cell membrane requires cholesterol. Without new cells, the body will age and die.

The vast bulk of the cholesterol in your blood (about 80 percent, in fact) is produced by your own liver. Only about 20 percent bears any relation to the cholesterol you eat. In fact, the body can sense how much you eat and step up or slow down its production of this critical substance according to your need. And getting a sufficient amount of cholesterol from the food you eat is critical to maintaining a stable mood. Without it, both animals and people become depressed, in part because the brain contains an enormous amount of it. When cholesterol in the blood falls too low, it's as dangerous to health as rising too high. The mortality risk is lowest in people with total cholesterol levels between 160 and 220, and here's where we suggest it should stay and where people following our nutritional regimen generally wind up *naturally*.

Taking potent cholesterol-lowering medications to achieve a "risk reduction" has never been shown in clinical research to actually improve mortality. In fact, in the biggest trials, significantly more people who took the drug died than those who did not. They didn't die of heart attacks, but dead is dead whatever the cause. And the drugs aren't without risk of serious side effects, such as muscle and liver destruction. The statin class of drugs, in particular, shuts down the production of one of the body's most essential coenzymes (coenzyme Q10), which has been clinically shown to improve the heart muscle's ability to regenerate energy and which serves as an antioxidant to protect the heart from damage. (In Japan, coQ10 is a prescription drug, used to treat congestive heart failure, which it will quite effectively do at higher doses.) People who take or have taken any of the statin drugs should supplement their diets with at least 100 to 300 mg per day of an oil-based formulation of coQ10 to replace the depletion.

The measuring of cholesterol's components has increased by leaps and bounds in the last five years. Where there was once only total cholesterol, then "good" and "bad" cholesterol, laboratory tests can now differentiate dozens of subtypes within the categories. But while these may be useful in the research lab, what's important to people in the real world is being able to know from their readings what puts them at greater risk for having a heart attack and what reduces that risk. Recently published research has shown that the two readings most predictive of who will have a heart attack are not the amount of cholesterol or even the amount of the "bad" LDL. Instead, your best assessment of risk comes from your triglycerides and your "good" HDL cholesterol. The lower the triglyceride-to-HDL ratio, the lower your risk for heart disease. A reading of 5 is set as the break point; above 5, there's risk, and the farther above 5, the more risk. Conversely, below 5, risk decreases, and the farther below, the better. On our nutritional regimen, we usually see this ratio drop substantially below 5 and quite often below 2.

Rarely, we see levels of "bad" LDL rise slightly on the plan, which can be alarming to patients. Research has now shown, however, that even this slight increase isn't a danger. Two types of LDL particles have been identified: a small, dense type and a larger, fluffy type. Studies have shown the dense type promotes atherosclerosis (hardening of the arteries), while the fluffy type does not. On a low-fat, high-carbohydrate diet (the very one most often prescribed to lower cholesterol), levels of this dangerous, dense form of "bad" LDL rise, offsetting any benefit from the modest lowering in cholesterol the diet may cause. However, on our regimen, a lower-carbohydrate, higher-fat diet, the body mainly produces the harmless large, fluffy LDL, further reducing heart disease risk.

By simply changing the way you eat to a diet lower in starch and sugar and higher in good-quality fats, you can reduce elevated cholesterol, lower your triglycerides, alter the type of "bad" LDL you produce, increase your "good" HDL levels, and reduce your risk for heart disease—without resorting to expensive and potentially damaging medications.

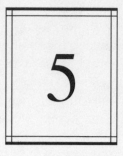

ANTIOXIDANT
USE AND ABUSE

When iron is oxidized, we generally call the end result
rust. When bronze is oxidized, we call the green film
produced a patina. When we are oxidized, we call it aging.
—STEVEN N. AUSTAD, PH.D.,
Anti-aging Scientist

Not only did our Paleolithic ancestors consume more meat and more fat than we do, they ate a much, much wider range of foods all around. Experts estimate the Stone Age peoples as well as many contemporary hunter-gatherer peoples dined on as many as 100 to 150 different foods. Compare this to the fifteen to twenty-five or so foods that most of us eat today. You don't believe that you only eat fifteen to twenty-five different foods? Neither did we until we started really looking at what we ate.[1] Most of us stick with the same few individual foods and dishes. When we go to restaurant we typically find ourselves ordering the same thing again and again, using the rationale that if we are going to spend good money for restaurant food, we are going to make

---

1. Keeping an accurate food diary is an enlightening experience because you discover that not only do you not eat as many different foods as you imagined but also you eat a lot more than you thought.

110

sure we get something we like. Our predecessors had no such restraints; their only restraint was seasonal availability.

The rich variety of plant foods available to them gave our ancient ancestors enormous amounts of widely different antioxidants that we don't really get today eating our routine fifteen to twenty-five different foods, many of which have been purged of all antioxidants by processing. Many of us try to replace these lost antioxidants by taking them in supplement form, but it's not the same. In the health food store we get single antioxidants, or we may even get a sort of multi-antioxidant with maybe a dozen different antioxidants combined. Compare this to the 150 or so compounds, many of them antioxidants, that are in any fruit or vegetable. And if you eat a wide variety of fruits and vegetables, you get many, many more than the 150 compounds you would get in just a single one. In fact, experts have estimated that a wide range of fruits and vegetables contain more than four thousand flavonoids, only one of the many kinds of antioxidants. In addition to antioxidants, plants contain hundreds, or even thousands, of compounds that haven't been identified and that work in ways unknown. Because of the wide variety of these disease-fighting substances that can't possibly be replicated in a pill, we encourage our patients to get as many of their antioxidants from food as they can. There are a few specific antioxidants that we do use in larger, medicinal doses, but before we discuss them let's look at the antioxidant big picture, because unbeknownst to many people there can be a downside to taking large amounts of specific antioxidants indiscriminately.

The Fire Within

In order to understand *anti*oxidants, we must first understand the oxidants against which they work. The process of existing, of simply drawing breath, involves the burning of metabolic fuels—fats, carbohydrates, and proteins—for the energy necessary for life. Most of the fuel burned in the body is done so in small sausage-shaped furnaces inside the cells called mitochondria. As fuels burn in the mitochondria, negatively charged particles (electrons) travel from these fuels down the electron-transport chain, passed hand to hand, much like a bucket brigade, to oxygen molecules, which accept them to ultimately form water. As the electrons make the jumps down this chain, they release energy that the cell captures and uses for all its cellular processes. Desite its fairly tight control of the energy-transfer process, the electron-transport chain sometimes springs a leak and allows electrons to escape. These escaping electrons then attach themselves to other atoms or molecules and convert them into free radicals.

Free radicals are unstable molecules or atoms in seach of stability. They ultimately achieve stability by either transferring their extra electron to another atom or molecule or by grabbing an electron from another atom or molecule. In either case, the free radical achieves stability only at the expense of creating another free radical, which then prowls the body seeking rest from its torment. It attacks another stable atom or molecule, feeds on its electrons, and creates yet another free radical perpetuating the chain reaction, which can have disastrous consequences if not halted. William A. Pryor, Ph.D., author of the standard scientific textbook on free radicals, calculated that a single free radical could damage about twenty-six molecules of a polyunsaturated fat before the chain reaction finally lost steam and played itself out. (As we shall see, the destruction of unsaturated fats is one of the most damaging effects of free radicals.)

Antioxidants step in and stop this chain reaction by sacrificing themselves and taking a free radical–electron bullet for the good of the body. When the antioxidant molecule accepts the renegade electron from the free radical, it more or less removes the curse from it and, just like in the vampire movies, takes the free-radical curse upon itself, but with a difference. The antioxidant molecule becomes a benign free radical by hiding the extra electron away and rendering it harmless. Then another member of the antioxidant family comes along and takes away the fugitive electron, restoring the molecule to its previous full antioxidant glory. The newly restored antioxidant then returns to the field of free-radical battle and starts the cycle again.

Free radicals and antioxidants are not single gladiators engaging in hand-to-hand combat on a lonely field of battle. Free radicals are made by and escape the metabolic process by the billions; exposure to ultraviolet light (sunlight) generates free radicals; common chemicals and other toxins we are exposed to daily add to the load; and even our own immune systems contribute to the total. Bruce Ames, Ph.D., a biochemist at Berkeley and a legend in the field of free-radical research, estimates that oxygen free radicals (from the air we breathe) actually reach and damage the DNA inside each of the cells in the body in the neighborhood of some ten thousand times per day. If you multiply ten thousand times the one hundred or so trillion cells in the body, you're talking about an enormous number of free radicals—and those are just the ones that got through the defenses. Barry Halliwell, Ph.D., Professor of Medical Biochemistry at the University of London's King's College, estimates that the adult body at rest produces almost 4 pounds of oxygen free radicals each year. That's at rest; exertion would produce a tenfold increase in this amount. It's reasonable to assume, then, that a normal active human produces 10 to 20 pounds of oxygen free radicals per year. And that's just one kind of free radical; there are many others that add to the total that could easily exceed 100 pounds per year.

With these kinds of numbers it's a wonder that we aren't totally subsumed by free-radical damage. Since we aren't, it's obvious that we muster a pretty evenly matched free-radical defense. Free radicals do get through, however, and the damage they cause has inspired a whole theory of aging called, appropriately enough, the free radical–damage theory of aging. Proponents of this theory believe that the cumulative damage we sustain from years of free-radical bombardment ultimately takes its toll and defeats us. And while it is true that our bodies do incur a lot of damage from free-radical hits, there are literally hundreds of other compelling theories of aging. Looking at the big picture, however, it's probably safe to assume that free radicals do indeed wreak their havoc, but other forces are at work as well that drive us relentlessly to our senescence and beyond.

Before we consider the defenses we have against free-radical attack, let's look at a couple of specific forms of free-radical treachery. When most people think of free-radical damage, it's the damage to DNA, the genetic material of the cells, that they have in mind. We saw earlier that the DNA of each cell gets a damaging free-radical hit about ten thousand times per day. And remember, that's in *each* cell. Since DNA controls the replication of cells, damage to the right area of the DNA chain could cause a mutation and possibly the formation of a cancerous cell. The resultant rogue cell could begin to reproduce pell-mell and ultimately become a deadly tumor. In fact, this is exactly what happens in many cases. What's amazing, however, given the ten thousand hits per cell per day, is that it happens as infrequently as it does. The fact that we all don't come down with cancer right and left is a testament to our free-radical defenses and to our bodies' abilities to undo the DNA damage that free radicals cause. Fortunately, we have a damage-control team of enzymes that scurry along the DNA chains locating and clipping out the damaged segments and replacing them with normal segments, preventing the altered DNA from having a chance to mutate the cell. But without our free-radical defense team—antioxidants—many more than the already enormous ten thousand damaging free radicals would get through to the DNA and probably overwhelm the DNA repair team's ability to control the damage.

A second, less well known type of free-radical damage (but probably more contributory to the aging process) is that to the lipid membrane. As you learned in chapter 3, "The Fat of the Land," the more supple and fluid the lipid bilayer that makes up the cell membranes, the better all the physiological processes work. Anything that stiffens these membranes, such as the incorporation of trans fatty acids or the loss of the body's ability to desaturate fatty acids, restricts the activity of the normally fluid membranes and brings about a decline in health. If normal, unsaturated fats that compose the cell membranes suffer a free-radical attack, they become damaged and lose their ability to keep the membrane supple.

Although the cell membrane has to be supple to work properly, it also has to have some structural rigidity to keep it from collapsing. This rigidity is supplied by cholesterol, which fits in between the fatty-acid molecules in the membrane and gives them structural support. We need just the right balance between suppleness and rigidity for the membrane to work perfectly; as we age, however, our cell membranes become increasingly more rigid. For years scientists believed that this increasing age-related rigidity of the cell membrane resulted from an ever enlarging amount of cholesterol being continuously incorporated into it. This rationale made sense, because as people age they usually find their cholesterol levels slowly increasing, and this increased level of cholesterol in the blood, so the theory goes, makes its way into the cell membranes, causing them to stiffen. Besides, it's always politically correct among scientific groups to blame cholesterol for everything. But in this case, as in many others, it's the wrong answer.

Of Damaged Fats and Rancid Fish

In a number of clever experiments, researchers at the University of Texas Health Science Center in San Antonio fingered lipid peroxides, not cholesterol, as the culprit causing our membranes to stiffen as we get older. What are lipid peroxides? Fatty-acid molecules that have been attacked by free radicals. Anytime a fatty acid reacts with oxygen it undergoes a process called peroxidation that converts it to a lipid peroxide. A fat or an oil composed of many lipid peroxides is a rancid fat. The more unsaturated the fat, the more prone it is to peroxidation, which explains why fish spoil so quickly: they are loaded with highly unsaturated fats.

Since we have multiple millions of free-radical attacks on our cell membranes daily, how come we don't just resolve ourselves into a rancid dew? Just as the body protects and repairs DNA, so it does with the fatty acids in the cell membrane. Antioxidants prowl the lipid bilayer, sacrificing themselves to disarm free radicals and prevent their attack on a fatty acid. When free radicals do make it through this antioxidant Maginot Line and attack fatty acids, converting them to chain-reacting lipid peroxides, enzymes called peroxidases spring to the fore and neutralize them. With the one-two combo of antioxidant protection and lipid-peroxidase cleanup, our fatty-acid membranes are able to maintain their fluidity despite the constant exposure to free-radical bombardment. But this unremitting free-radical exposure does take its toll over a lifetime. One of the unfortunate side effects of aging is that we are unable to produce enzymes such as peroxidase as efficiently, and we are unable to produce and recycle our antioxidant forces as readily as when we were young. Consequently, the free radicals, which, sadly, we continue to produce in full force, begin to wear us down, attacking our lipid membranes and converting unsaturated fatty acids to stiffer, less functional lipid peroxides that we are unable to neutralize quickly. Do we just stand by and wring our hands as this process grinds on? Is there anything we can do? Fortunately there is a lot we can do, and the arena of free-radical combat is one place where the basics of the Paleolithic diet and the advances of modern medicine join forces. But before we move on to that how-to part of the chapter, let's take a look at another problem free radicals cause: the peroxidation of cholesterol.

LDL cholesterol—a particle composed of cholesterol, triglycerides, and specific carrier proteins—is the chief villain in the cholesterol theory of heart disease. But that's really an unfair indictment because *normal* LDL doesn't cause any problems. The problems start when the LDL somehow gets altered and stimulates certain cells of the immune system to surround it and gobble it up. Most scientists believe that the process responsible for altering the LDL particle is oxidation, or attack by free radicals. When free radicals attack the LDL particle, they can hit the unsaturated fats in the triglyceride molecule and peroxidize them and/or they can go after the cholesterol portion and peroxidize it. (Cholesterol peroxides are nasty compounds that can cause us a lot of grief, and we'll discuss how to avoid them later in this chapter.) The oxidized LDL particle filled with its cargo of lipid and cholesterol peroxides is ripe for capture by the immune system and incorporation into the arterial wall. If we can somehow prevent this alteration of the normal LDL, we should be able to prevent the development of heart disease. As it turns out, vitamin E is the primary antioxidant responsible for protecting the LDL particle, and numerous studies have shown that individuals who regularly take vitamin E supplements have greatly reduced rates of heart disease.

So, Can We Pop a Few Vitamin Pills and Live Forever?

Unfortunately, as with almost all things in medicine, it's never as simple as that. As H. L. Mencken noted, for every complex problem, there is always a simple solution; and it's almost always wrong. This has never been demonstrated more aptly than with the CARET study—the infamous beta carotene and retinol efficacy trial designed to test whether taking beta carotene and vitamin A would prevent lung cancer. First, a little background.

Cigarette smoke contains countless numbers of damaging free radicals that usually overwhelm the antioxidant capacity of the smoker's body. And, as you might imagine, smokers have not only lowered blood levels of most antioxidants, particularly vitamin A, but an increased incidence of a number of malignancies, particularly lung cancer. When researchers looked at the diets of smokers and found that those smokers who ate diets high in colorful fruits and vegetables were much less likely to develop cancer the stage was set for a controlled scientific evaluation of beta carotene and vitamin A as a simple solution to lung cancer. As it turned out, this simple solution to a complex problem was not just wrong but deadly.

The CARET Study: Too Much of a Good Thing?

In the CARET study researchers studied both men and women who had greatly increased risk of developing lung cancer due to heavy smoking, asbestos exposure, or both to see if supplementation with either beta carotene or vitamin A would reduce their risk. More than eighteen thousand subjects were given 30 milligrams of beta carotene or 25,000 IU of vitamin A or both or a placebo. Researchers expected that the subjects taking both beta carotene and vitamin A would have the greatest cancer-fighting antioxidation intake and would develop fewer lung cancers. Unfortunately, that's not how it worked out.

As the study progressed, the researchers noticed that the subjects taking both the vitamin A and the beta carotene were developing and dying of lung cancer at much higher rates than expected. Partway through the study a statistical analysis revealed that the participants taking the beta carotene and the vitamin A had a *28 percent greater* rate of death from lung cancer than those taking the placebo and a 17 percent increase in deaths from all causes. The results were so horrendous that for ethical reasons the study was discontinued almost two years ahead of schedule.

What went wrong? It was clear from previous research that beta carotene and vitamin A were protective against lung cancer, so why didn't the supplements protect these study subjects? The failure of the CARET study has been the subject of great speculation and continuing debate. The manufacturers of vitamin supplements have come up with dozens of reasons why the beta carotene and vitamin A didn't help (it was too little too late; the vitamin A was synthetic, not natural; the dose was too low; the dose was too high, and so on). Some scientists have speculated that the cancers were already in place and that the vitamin A and beta carotene simply accelerated their development under the theory that whatever is good for you is also good for the cancer. Other scientists have theorized that when beta carotene is broken down in the body, some of the resultant compounds could possibly be carcinogenic when combined with some of the chemicals in cigarette smoke.

Another possibility is that the antioxidant supplements compromised the smokers' immune systems. So far we've dealt only with the harmful actions of free radicals, but free radicals do have their benefits. For example, the immune system is able to harness the destructive power of free radicals and turn it on the body's enemies. In simple terms, certain cells of the immune system capture foreign or potentially harmful pathogens, such as bacteria, viruses, and cancer cells, hold them still, and execute them with blasts of free radicals. These immune soldiers then clean up the battlefield by consuming their victims. Perhaps the immune systems of the smokers in these studies were barely holding their own against the toxins in the cigarette smoke, the infectious bacteria that chronically infect smokers' lungs, and the cells in the lungs that mutate at high rates after tobacco smoke exposure, when along came a single antioxidant in supplement form that quenched the very free radicals needed to combat these dangerous forces.

No one knows for sure the actual cause or causes of the greatly increased rates of lung cancer in the group of subjects taking the vitamin A and beta carotene supplements. What we do know, however, is that a *diet* rich in the fruits and vegetables containing beta carotene *does* protect smokers against lung cancer. It's only when we try to tease out the specific agent that we think is protective and give that in relatively large amounts without the combined efforts of the thousands of other phytochemicals in the actual plants themselves that we get into trouble. It's almost always better to pop the plant than to pop the pill.

Supply the Raw Materials and Let the Body Do the Rest

Our philosophy on antioxidants (with certain exceptions that we'll get to later) is to give the body all the raw materials it needs to make its own antioxidants and let it go to work. If we make our own, we most likely won't overdo it and hobble our immune system with too much free-radical quenching.[2] Many of the raw materials are found in plants, and we advise our patients to eat a wide variety of colorful fruits and vegetables, nuts, and green, leafy vegetables. We've endured a fair amount of criticism over our recommendation to our patients and readers to avoid or at least limit their consumption of cereal grains, potatoes, bananas, and other starchy and carbohydrate-laden plant foods, because these foods do contain their share of antioxidants and other beneficial substances. While it is true that these foods offer some vitamin and antioxidant benefits, it is also true that they stimulate a rise in insulin levels and all the consequent metabolic changes that accompany that rise, which, in our opinion, negates the positive

---

2. A number of studies have appeared in the medical literature that correlate the consumption of large doses of antioxidant supplements with an increased risk for the development of certain cancers.

effects of the nutrients these foods contain. We would be in a real mess if the only way we could get these nutrients was via these starchy foods, but fortunately it isn't. We can get all the antioxidants we could ever need without a single cereal grain or potato ever passing our lips by sticking to the fruits and vegetables that are green and colorful and that have very little effect on our insulin levels (see chapter 13, "*LifePlan* Nutrition," for more details).

While we're on the subject of the antioxidants and phytochemicals found in plants, here's a little secret that the makers of no-fat products and the promoters of low-fat diets are not likely to tell you: many of the most potent cancer-fighting nutrients in plants can't be absorbed well without some fat accompanying them. Specifically, carotenoids, found in colorful fruits and vegetables, and lycopene, found in tomatoes, require fat for their absorption.[3] If you make a salad loaded with various greens, slices of cucumber and tomato, and diced bits of carrots and other colorful vegetables, then top it with one of the zillions of no-fat dressings available to the low-fat conscious, you will be missing out not only on taste but on many of the nutrients in the salad that you simply won't be able to absorb without fat. Make sure that when you eat a salad, you dress it with a real oil-based dressing, made with virgin or extra-virgin olive oil, canola oil, or nut oil, all of which contain a whole host of valuable nutrients and antioxidants. If you eat steamed vegetables, drizzle them with olive oil or melted butter, so that the fat-soluble nutrients don't go unabsorbed.

YOU DESERVE ORAC TODAY

Scientists have recently developed a method to measure the ability of whole foods, blood, and just about any substance to neutralize oxygen free radicals in the test tube. The results of this test are termed the Oxygen Radical Absorbance Capacity—the ORAC—of the substance. Although a relatively new research tool

---

3. Lycopene is the latest single nutrient to be fawned over by the nutritional establishment since a recent study appeared showing that men who consumed large amounts of tomato-based products suffered much lower rates of prostate cancer than those who didn't. There is little doubt that the shelves of health food stores everywhere will soon be laden with multiple brands of lycopene supplements—but eat tomatoes!

that hasn't had the chance yet to be put to a huge amount of work, the ORAC evaluation is already paying dividends. Scientists have shown that getting plenty of foods with a high ORAC value:

- raises the antioxidant power of human blood;
- prevents loss of long-term memory and learning ability in middle-aged rats;
- protects capillaries—the tiniest blood vessels, and the ones most prone to damage—against free-radical injury.

When scientists evaluated foods for their total antioxidant capacity by adding up the capacities of the known antioxidants in the foods, such as vitamin C, vitamin E, and the various carotenoids, the total fell far short of the measured ORAC, indicating that either unknown substances are contributing to the free-radical quenching effect or the combination of antioxidants is greater than the sum of the individual components. This whole-is-greater-than-the-parts phenomenon advances our argument for choosing the whole food over one, or a few, of the individual antioxidant components.

Although researchers haven't had time to evalute every food in existence for overall antioxidant ability, the foods they have analyzed stack up just as we would expect given our knowledge of the Paleolithic diet. Aside from meat, what did our Paleolithic ancestors eat? Probably not a lot that we would recognize as food today—roots, shoots, certain types of leaves—but there is little doubt that they ate berries when they could find them. Berries are a terrific source of nutrients and a great carbohydrate bargain to boot—in fact, they are about the best carbohydrate bargain you can find in the fruit family. And guess what? They are at the top of the list of foods so far analyzed for ORAC units.[4] (See table 5.1.)

A great way to add berries to your diet and boost your body's levels of antioxidants tremendously is to have a glass of Paleolithic

---

4. Actually prunes and raisins are at the very top of the list, but these are fruits with the water removed, making them denser (i.e., more fruit and sugar for a given weight). When plums and grapes—the fruits that make prunes and raisins—are ranked, they come in below all the berries in ORAC units per weight.

TABLE 5.1

Foods Highest in ORAC (units per 100 grams [3.5 ounces])

FRUITS		VEGETABLES	
Prunes	5770	Kale	1770
Raisins	2830	Spinach	1260
Blueberries	2400	Brussels sprouts	980
Blackberries	2036	Alfalfa sprouts	930
Strawberries	1540	Broccoli florets	890
Raspberries	1220	Beets	840
Plums	949	Red bell pepper	710
Oranges	750	Onion	450
Grapes, red	739	Corn	400
Cherries	670	Eggplant	390

Punch (see the recipe on page 366) with your breakfast. We usually make our daily Paleolithic Punch (or, more descriptively, Paleolithic Slurpy) with frozen blueberries, raspberries, and strawberries, which provides us with almost 3,000 ORAC units each day—as much as or more than many Americans may get in an entire week of eating the typical American diet—and we get it each day just at breakfast. Our glass of Paleolithic Punch gives us not only all this antioxidant capacity but also about 6 grams of dietary fiber, one-half of what is in the typical American diet for an entire day. And we get all this nutrition for only about 7 or 8 usable grams of carbohydrate, an amount well within the per-meal guidelines for even the strictest level of rehabilitation on the *Protein Power LifePlan*. Paleolithic Punch solves another problem that has bedeviled patients and readers alike: What replaces orange juice at breakfast? While one small glass of orange juice contains almost 30 grams of usable carbohydrate, it provides only a fraction of the ORAC units found in a same size glass of Paleolithic Punch. So, if you're talking about nutritional bang for your buck, Paleolithic Punch has it all over orange juice; it has more fiber, more ORAC, fewer carbs, and, we think, a far superior taste. And, you're getting the whole food with all its other phyto-chemicals besides just the antioxidant power. Go for it!

GLUTATHIONE: WE CAN'T TAKE IT, SO WE'VE GOT TO MAKE IT

Although plants contain a generous quantity of antioxidant and antioxidantlike substances, the most abundant antioxidant we have in our bodies we make ourselves. It's called glutathione, and we make it from three amino acids, one of which is cysteine, a sulfur-containing amino acid. Since sulfur-containing amino acids are found primarily in meat, a meat-based diet gives us plenty of the raw materials needed for the production of this most impor-tant antioxidant. (And, since sulfur-containing amino acids are for the most part lacking in foods of plant origin, we have an explanation for the immune-system suppression that typically ac-companies a true vegetarian, or vegan, diet.)[5] Glutathione is a multifunctional antioxidant and a whole lot more. One of its main antioxidant functions is to recycle vitamin C. You'll recall that whenever an antioxidant takes an electron from a free radical, the antioxidant itself becomes a benign free radical unable to harm but also unable to act as an antioxidant. When a Vitamin C mole-cule neutralizes a free radical, it must pass this extra electron along to another substance to regenerate its full vitamin C antioxi-dant capacity. Glutathione performs this task and takes the elec-tron from the vitamin C molecule, recycling it back into action. As long as we have plenty of glutathione we don't need to take megadoses of vitamin C because our glutathione continues to re-cycle the vitamin C we already have along with whatever we get from the fruits and vegetable that we eat.

Glutathione also gets rid of hydrogen peroxide. How do we get hydrogen peroxide? When free radicals damage fats, lipid per-oxides result. These peroxides, while not actually free radicals

---

5. Occasionally we see patients who, for ideological reasons, are vegans, but who, for health reasons, want to adopt a vegan version of our program. We simply add indi-vidual sulfur-containing amino acid supplements to their diets along with regular injec-tions of vitamin B_{12}. (Plants contain no B_{12}; it must be gotten from foods of animal origin and can't be absorbed well without another component found only in animal foods.) See Micronutrient Roundup in the appendix for supplementation details.

themselves, can react with other substances—iron, for instance—to produce the hydroxyl radical, the most dangerous and most unstoppable free radical of all. Glutatione gobbles up these peroxides before they have a chance to convert to the hydroxyl radical.

Glutathione acts as a detoxifying molecule. In the liver, the sulfur portion of the glutathione molecule combines with many toxic substances, rendering them harmless and carting them out of the body via the kidneys. Just as many drugs are capable of doing, both alcohol and acetaminophen (the common painkiller found in Tylenol) can damage the liver if consumed in excessive amounts. This damage occurs because these substances—especially when taken together—deplete the liver of its protective glutathione, allowing a buildup of liver-poisoning toxins.

Strenuous exercise also drains the body of glutathione. Any type of exercise increases the metabolic rate and, as a consequence, the production of free radicals. Vigorous exercise dramatically increases the production of free radicals and just as dramatically reduces the levels of glutathione. Colds, sore throats, and other respiratory infections are endemic among long-distance runners, especially those who eschew a meat-based diet in the mistaken notion that a low-fat, vegetarian diet is more healthful for them. If you are a long-distance runner or involved in any other form of strenuous exercise of long duration, you must make sure that you maintain your glutathione levels by consuming plenty of sulfur-containing amino acids and by taking alpha-lipoic acid supplements, which recycle your glutathione.

Why can't we just take glutathione supplements and be done with it? Well, we can, sort of, but we have to take them intravenously. You can find glutathione on the shelves of your local health food store, but don't buy it. Save your money. Glutathione is made of three amino acids connected together, and since digestive enzymes break these amino acid bonds, it doesn't survive the digestive process intact. So any glutathione supplement you take won't get from your mouth into your bloodstream intact. Like many other physicians, we sometimes give glutathione intravenously in our clinic for a variety of conditions, but this glutathione goes directly into the blood and doesn't have to traverse the digestive system, where it would surely be destroyed.

Although you can't boost your glutathione levels by taking glutathione supplements, there are steps you can take to increase and maintain your stores of this important molecule:

- *Eat meat*—or other animal proteins, such as fish, poultry, or eggs—which contains an abundance of the sulfur-containing amino acids necessary for the production of glutathione.
- *Take alpha-lipoic acid,* a unique antioxidant that we'll discuss in some detail later. Lipoic acid recycles and regenerates glutathione. Lipoic acid is found mainly in red meat but is actually one of those compounds that we can benefit from taking in much larger doses than we could ever get from food alone. We routinely give our patients 100 to 300 mg of lipoic acid daily.
- *Make sure that you get enough selenium.* Selenium, an element that is found in meat, seafood, egg yolks, and, depending upon the soil in which they're grown, certain plants—especially garlic, onions, and broccoli—is a key cofactor that assists the enzyme that makes glutathione. Since most of our patients get plenty of meat, we recommend that they take only 100 *micro*grams of a selenium supplement two or three times per week. In addition to its role in the production of glutathione, selenium is a cancer-fighting element in its own right. A number of studies have shown selenium's effectiveness in preventing malignancies of all sorts. If you don't eat meat, make sure you take 200 *micro*grams of selenium daily. Don't take more, however, because selenium can be toxic in excess doses, causing hair loss, fingernail changes, and neurological symptoms.
- *Avoid eating lipid peroxides and cholesterol peroxides.* Remember, one of glutathione's primary jobs is to destroy peroxides before they can cause any damage, and whenever a peroxide is destroyed, a glutathione molecule is neutralized. We produce plenty of our own peroxides that require destruction without bringing any on board via our diet. Those that we do consume deplete our glutathione. Where do we

get lipid peroxides in the diet? All kinds of places, some obvious, some not so obvious. One common source is scrambled eggs. Egg yolks contain a large amount of cholesterol that is easily oxidized when subjected to heat and air. When we scramble eggs we break the yolks and expose the cholesterol within to both heat and air, producing a slurry of cholesterol peroxides. Although for Hedonists and Dilettantes the occasional omelet will do little harm, we recommend that most of the time you adopt a Purist's approach and eat your eggs poached, boiled, or fried in such a way that the yolks remain intact, protecting their cholesterol contents from peroxidation. A not-so-obvious source of lipid peroxides is powdered eggs; and, unfortunately, they're used routinely in commercially prepared foods requiring eggs, especially bakery goods. Commercial bakery goods are loaded with both trans fatty acids *and* lipid peroxides, so do yourself a favor and avoid them. Once you're reached your health goals and are into the Maintenance phase of your rehabilitation, you may wish to occasionally indulge in a serving of pastry, pie, or cake. If so, it's better if you make them yourself from wholesome ingredients. You'll not escape the insulin-raising consequences of the sugar and the flour when you so indulge, but you can at least avoid lipid peroxides and trans fatty acids. And remember, the emphasis here is on the word *occasional.* If you intend to maintain your health goals, it's really okay to treat yourself to such goodies only now and again.

- *Avoid excessive exercise of long duration without periods of rest and recuperation.* If you are a long-distance runner, however, make sure you follow the above suggestions and take some time off for rest and other types of less strenuous activities. Give yourself time to recuperate and your glutathione time to regenerate.

Nutrient Supplements:
The Fruits of Modern Technology

Although we can get plenty of nutrients from the Paleolithic diet—antioxidants and other phytochemicals from plants and all the raw materials for glutathione and countless other nutrients from meat—we don't have to stop there. Our goal is to use whatever means we have at hand to make the most of our genetic potential. And the fruits of modern technology can help us greatly. A vast amount of medical literature and our own clinical experience have shown us that supplementing our diet with a few individual nutrients can improve our health tremendously. We routinely give our patients and take ourselves a few supplements that, with the exception of vitamin E, you may never have heard of. All these nutrients are found in food and, in fact, in larger amounts in the Paleolithic diet than in any other type of diet. But modern research has shown that taking these supplements in amounts exceeding that which can be gotten from food alone will pay huge health benefits.

Vitamin E

If we could give only one vitamin supplement it would have to be vitamin E, the powerful antioxidant found in oils, nuts, nut butters, seeds, meat, and in small amounts in green, leafy vegetables. With food alone, you would have to really work hard to get much more than about 10 or 15 mg of vitamin E a day, which would give you the USDA Recommended Daily Allowance but not even close to the 500 mg or so that it takes to really maximize beneficial effects of this hardworking nutrient.

Nutrients can be either fat soluble or water soluble or, in the case of lipoic acid, both. Fat-soluble nutrients can make their way into and through the fatty cell membranes; water-soluble nutrients do their work in the blood or in the cell fluid inside the cells. Vitamin E falls into the fat-soluble category. Its main job is to prowl the lipid bilayer, the cell membrane, for free radicals, quenching them before they can damage the fatty acids and convert them to lipid peroxides. Having plenty of vitamin E on board ensures that your cell membranes will be fluid and supple, allowing all the protein structures located therein to work properly.

One of the protein structures located in the cell membrane is the insulin receptor. It seems reasonable to suppose that vitamin E would make the insulin receptor work better and actually increase insulin sensitivity, and that's precisely what happens. As we discussed in chapter 2, studies have shown that patients taking vitamin E supplements have improved insulin sensitivity even without changing their diets. If you take vitamin E along with an insulin-lowering diet, your insulin sensitivity will improve even more rapidly.

Although vitamin E performs a multitude of valuable tasks from preventing wrinkles (see chapter 10, "Sunshine Superman") to protecting against cancers, its real claim to fame is preventing heart disease. Several large studies involving tens of thousands of subjects have shown that individuals who take vitamin E supplements have about a 40 percent lower risk for developing heart disease than those who don't. How does vitamin E work to prevent heart disease? No one knows for sure, but it is known that vitamin E prevents the oxidation of the lipids in the LDL particle. Remember, the LDL particle is composed of fatty acids and cholesterol, neither of which is soluble in water, bound to a carrier protein that transports them through the blood. Vitamin E, like cholesterol and fatty acids, is not water soluble, so it hitches a ride on the LDL particle to get from the digestive system through the blood and to the tissues. While traveling along, vitamin E roams the fatty-acid and cholesterol structure of the LDL particle, searching for free radicals and neutralizing them, thereby preventing free-radical damage. A recent study found that the low levels of vitamin E in the LDL were correlated with the development of heart disease, and that the lower the levels, the worse was the disease. By taking plenty of vitamin E, we take major steps against the oxidation and damage of our LDL particles and the resultant development of the number one killer in this country.

Vitamin E is so important and is found in such small amounts in the diet that nature has devised a recycling scheme to make the best possible use of the small amount we have. Vitamin C, lipoic acid, and glutathione all recycle vitamin E. The nutrient-dense foods you eat on the *Protein Power LifePlan* along with the accompanying supplements will ensure that your protective levels of vitamin E remain high and fully active.

Vitamin E is actually a conglomerate made up of eight similar but different molecules: four *tocopherols* and four *tocotrienols*.

Most of the studies in the past have been done with *alpha*-tocopherol, but that doesn't mean that it's the only important component of vitamin E. Far from it. Because of the multitude of studies demonstrating the virtues of alpha-tocopherol, however, most of the vitamin E supplements you find are composed entirely of this form. Don't buy these. Look for supplements that contain natural vitamin E as mixed tocopherols and tocotrienols. The ones with the tocotrienols may be difficult to find, but they are available; ask someone at your health food store to order them for you. We take at least 400 to 500 mg daily of a tocopherol/tocotrienol mix and recommend that dose to most of our patients. Since vitamin E is a fat-soluble vitamin, taking it with a little fat or with a fatty meal ensures its absorption. We usually take ours with our daily dose of fish oil.

Vitamin C

Thanks to the efforts of Linus Pauling, just about everyone has heard of vitamin C and its effect on the common cold. But vitamin C is much, much more than just a cold remedy. The long list of vitamin C's tasks in the body include regenerating vitamin E; strengthening the immune system; acting as a cofactor in the production of collagen, the connective tissue that holds the body together; assisting vitamin E in preventing the oxidation of LDL; preventing mutations leading to cancer by guarding DNA against free-radical attack; and even preventing free-radical damage of sperm.

Dr. Pauling recommended exceedingly large doses of vitamin C and took them himself as part of his daily regimen. We believe that the USDA's Recommended Daily Allowance for vitamin C (60 grams) is way too low, but we balk at giving megadoses because of its effect on iron storage. Vitamin C enhances the absorption of dietary iron, and most of us today already have too much iron in our bodies as it is. People who have too much iron stored away can develop serious heart problems if they take large doses of vitamin C. If our patients are drinking their Paleolithic Punch regularly, we recommend that they take a 200-mg vitamin C supplement daily. If they don't drink the Paleolithic Punch, we usually have them supplement with 250 mg of vitamin C twice daily.[6]

COENZYME Q10

Coenzyme Q10 (CoQ10), like the last supplemental nutrient on our list, is less well known than vitamin E and vitamin C but no less important. Although this important nutrient has been used throughout the world for many years to treat a variety of disorders, it is just starting to receive the attention it deserves in this country. We use it in our practice extensively and recommend it in varying amounts to every patient we have, particularly those patients with diabetes or cardiovascular disease.

CoQ10 is a coenzyme, meaning that it works with, or helps, an enzyme that catalyzes important reactions. In addition to being a potent fat-soluble antioxidant, coQ10 is also intimately involved in the energy-production processes in the body and is found in highest concentrations in the mitochondria, the energy-producing furnaces found in all the cells. CoQ10 assists in the production of ATP (adenosine triphosphate), the energy currency of the body. Since it is so important, the body produces its own coQ10, and in the early years of life it is found in abundant quantities in all the cells. As the body ages, however, the quantities of coQ10 diminish. This nutrient is found in meat, especially red meat and organ meats, but in fairly small quantities compared to the amounts needed to replace that lost through aging.

Since coQ10 is involved so closely with the energy-production processes in the body, you might guess that it would be found in large quantities in the heart muscle, the hardest-working muscle we have. You would be right. CoQ10 is an essential nutrient for proper functioning of the heart. Japanese physicians have used coQ10 almost since its discovery in the late 1950s to successfully treat congestive heart failure (poor heart pumping caused by a weakening of the heart muscle). Over the past few years a number

---

6. If you want to take the mega multiple-gram doses of vitamin C as per Dr. Pauling, please get your ferritin levels checked before you do to make sure that you don't have any traces of an iron-storage problem. See chapter 8, "The Modern Iron Age."

of forward-thinking physicians have been using coQ10 for the same thing in this country with phenomenal results.

Along with its energy-production functions, coQ10 is also a potent antioxidant. Since it is oil soluble, it gets into the lipid bilayer of the cell membrane and, like vitamin E, roots out and destroys free radicals before they can damage the fatty acids and peroxidize them. CoQ10 also rides along with vitamin E in the LDL particle and helps protect the LDL from oxidation by both neutralizing free radicals itself and by regenerating vitamin E.

Physicians have used coQ10 both as a preventive against the development of breast cancer and as a treatment once the cancer has been established. Researchers in Denmark have shown that cancer patients have lower blood levels of coQ10 than do control subjects and that breast cancer patients specifically demonstrate great improvement when a small dose of coQ10 is added to their other therapies.

American dentists have recently discovered that coQ10 is an effective treatment for periodontal (gum) disease. Japanese dentists have been using coQ10 to both treat and prevent periodontal disease for years. In fact, many Japanese brands of toothpaste, mouthwash, and other oral hygiene products contain coQ10. We recommend that our patients with gum disease chew coQ10 gel caps along with taking it orally.

Since coQ10 is an oil-soluble substance, it needs to be taken with a fatty meal for maximal absorption. We take ours along with our vitamin E when we take our fish oil. Many brands of coQ10 are available at health food stores, but you've got to make sure to get one that is dissolved in oil—otherwise, you're wasting your money. Many coQ10 supplements are in powdered form in a capsule; these won't absorb at all if you don't take them with a fatty meal or a dose of oil. Save your money. Look for coQ10 in oil-filled gel caps—they are more expensive but well worth the money.

If our patients are in good health (which is usually not the case or they wouldn't be our patients), we give them 90 to 100 mg of coQ10 per day, the same amount we ourselves take daily. When medical problems are present, especially heart problems, we increase the dosage of coQ10 to as much as 300 mg per day.

If any of our patients have been taking any of the statin types of cholesterol-lowering medications before they come to see us, we always prescribe at least 300 mg per day of coQ10 for a month or so. The enzyme that the statin drugs inhibit is involved in the body's production of coQ10, and patients who have been on the drugs for a while invariably have a coQ10 deficiency that needs to be remedied.

ALPHA-LIPOIC ACID

Although the last of the supplements on our list is the least known of all, it is the real workhorse of the bunch. Like coenzyme Q10 alpha-lipoic acid has been used throughout the world to treat a variety of disorders but is just beginning to receive attention in the U.S. We use it extensively in our practice in varying amounts. Sometimes called thioctic acid, it is, like coQ10, a coenzyme used in the energy-producing processes, especially those using glucose. Unlike the other antioxidants we've discussed that are either fat or water soluble, lipoic acid is both: it penetrates both the cell membrane and other fatty areas and is at home in the watery contents of the cell also. Lipoic acid also recycles or regenerates vitamin C, vitamin E, coQ10, and even glutathione. In fact, assuming you have plenty of sulfur-containing amino acids on board, the very best way to boost your glutathione levels is to take lipoic acid.

Since lipoic acid acts to help burn glucose for energy, it is an effective agent for diabetics, who often have trouble getting glucose into their cells. German physicians have used lipoic acid for decades to treat many of the side effects of diabetes, especially diabetic neuropathy (the degenerative nerve disease that often accompanies diabetes and causes tingling and loss of feeling, especially in the lower legs). We always give plenty of lipoic acid—both intravenously and orally—to our diabetic patients.

Lipoic acid, via a number of biochemical mechanisms, protects against heart disease and stroke, improves memory, and slows brain aging. Lipoic acid also delays the development of cataracts, the age-related clouding of the lens of the eye that can progress to blindness. Free radicals from sunlight and other sources damage proteins in the fluid in the lens, causing it to go from clear to opaque over time. Glutathione is the major antioxidant that protects the lens of the eye, but studies have shown that lipoic acid stimulates glutathione production in the eye, protecting the lens and preventing the development of cataracts.

We routinely give our patients 100 to 200 mg of lipoic acid daily—the same amount we usually take ourselves. To patients with diabetes we usually give 300 mg twice per day. You can find lipoic acid at any health food store, and since it is both water and fat soluble it can be taken with meals or alone.

If you eat a variety of fresh foods, drink your Paleolithic Punch, and supplement your diet with vitamin C, vitamin E, coQ10, and lipoic acid in the doses recommended, you will be able to mount a formidable defense against free-radical attack while at the same time not hindering your immune system from doing its job. The variety of the Paleolithic diet combined with just these few supplements gives you 98 percent of all the best that antioxidant nutrition has to offer.

BOTTOM LINE

Our Paleolithic ancestors not only consumed more meat and more fat than we do, they ate a much, much wider range of foods all around. Experts estimate that Stone Age peoples as well as many contemporary hunter-gatherer peoples dined on as many as 100 to 150 different foods. Compare this to the fifteen to twenty-five or so foods that most of us eat today. The rich variety of plant foods available gave our ancient ancestors enormous amounts of widely different antioxidants that we don't get today eating our routine fifteen to twenty-five different foods, often purged of them by processing. Many of us try to replace these lost antioxidants by taking them in supplement form, but it's not the same thing. In pill form, we can get single antioxidants or sometimes a multi-antioxidant with maybe a dozen different antioxidants combined. Compare this to the 150 or so compounds, many of them antioxidants, that are in any fruit or vegetable. And if you eat a wide variety of fruits and vegetables, you get many more than the 150 compounds that you would get in just a single one. In fact, experts have estimated that a wide range of fruits and vegetables contains more than four thousand flavonoids, only one of the many kinds of antioxidants. In addition to antioxidants, plants contain hundreds or even thousands of compounds that haven't been identified and that work in ways unknown. Because of the wide variety of these disease-fighting substances that can't possibly be replicated in a pill, we encourage our patients to get as many of their antioxidants from food as they can. There are a few specific antioxidants that we do use in larger, medicinal doses, including vitamin E, alpha-lipoic acid, vitamin C, and coenzyme Q10.

What do antioxidants do? They defend your body against the damage caused by free radicals. Where do the free radicals that attack us come from? Free radicals are made by the billions within our bodies in the production of energy within our cells; we produce them when we exercise; exposure to ultraviolet light (sunlight) generates free radicals; common chemicals and other toxins we are exposed to daily add to the load; and even our own immune systems contribute to the total, producing free radicals as weapons to destroy invading microbes. Researchers estimate that oxygen free radicals (from the air we breathe) actually reach and damage the DNA inside each of the cells in the body in the neighborhood of some ten thousand times per day. Free radicals damage the delicate fats contained within the membranes of every cell in the body, hampering their flexibility. We depend upon our antioxidant network to defend us from this damage by neutralizing the free radicals that can at best age us and at worst lead to the development of more ominous disorders, such as insulin resistance or even cancers.

The body makes its own potent antioxidant to neutralize free radicals, a substance called glutathione, from sulfur-containing amino acids (richly found in meat, fish, poultry, eggs, garlic, onions, and broccoli), the mineral selenium (found in highest amounts in seafood, shellfish, liver, and meats), and vitamin E (found in nuts and seeds). For health, we must eat a diet such as we describe in the *Protein Power LifePlan* that provides the body with the raw materials to continually manufacture this critical defender. The antioxidants function as a team: when one neutralizes a free radical it passes it to an antioxidant team member and becomes renewed and ready to return to the front lines of defense. For that reason, taking individual antioxidants in large doses may prove counterproductive—as was borne out in the famous CARET study, in which long-term smokers were given large doses of beta carotene and vitamin A to see if these would prevent cancer. In fact, so many *more* cancers occurred in the group taking these individual vitamins that the researchers had to end the study early. Wholesale gobbling of individual antioxidants without the full network of their helping comrades may be counterproductive. For that reason, we encourage you to use your carbohydrate allotment to eat the fruits, vegetables, nuts, and seeds richest in antioxidants and all the thousands of related compounds that may regulate and mold their actions: colorful vegetables (peppers, squashes, tomatoes), salad greens, asparagus, cruciferous vegetables (broccoli, brussels sprouts, cabbage, cauliflower), onions, garlic, mushrooms, berries, and melons. For an antioxidant-filled treat, try our Paleolithic Punch (see page 366), which will greatly enhance your ability to fend off free-radical damage for fewer than 10 grams of usable carb.

If you eat a variety of fresh fruits and vegetables, drink your Paleolithic Punch, and supplement your diet with vitamin C, vitamin E, coQ10, and lipoic acid in the doses recommended (see the Micronutrient Roundup in the appendix), you will be able to mount a formidable defense against free-radical attack while at the same time not hindering your immune system from doing its job. The variety of the Paleolithic diet combined with just these few supplements gives you 98 percent of all the best antioxidants nutrition has to offer.

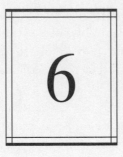

THE LEAKY GUT: DIET AND THE AUTOIMMUNE RESPONSE

*I have finally kum to the konklusion that a good reliable sett ov
bowels iz wurth more tu a man than enny quantity ov brains.*
—JOSH BILLINGS (1818–1885)

Sometime about 8 millennia B.C., as the vast glacial expanses
began to melt and recede, our ancient ancestors in the Near
Eastern parts of the world, where the land was warmer and fertile,
took notice of the wild grains that grew around them. It's not hard
to envision one member of a band of early humans out gathering,
plucking the stalks and tentatively giving the grain a chew to see
if it was fit to eat—and being disappointed, because grains in their
native state don't offer much in the way of food for humans. Our
intestinal tracts—unlike those of our herbivorous friends who
have multichambered stomachs to digest and redigest such matter—don't have the capacity to break down the tough protective
coatings of raw grain. But curiosity and necessity often breed per-
severance, so at some point an enterprising human discovered
how to dry the grain and pulverize it. Processing the grain in such

136

a manner sort of takes the place of the multichambered digestive scheme of ruminants such as bison, cattle, deer, and mammoths and does render food that humans can digest—at least if it's cooked. Once early humans learned that they could eat grain if they processed and cooked it, the paleohistorians tell us, they soon began to include wild grains among the foods that they gathered; not long after that, they began to sow it and reap it. And the rest, as they say, is history.

But simply being able to make use of a particular plant for sustenance—through our own clever manufacturing process—doesn't automatically mean that it's a food ideally fit for human consumption. Such is the case with most grains: although most of us tolerate them to a point, they pose a definite health risk for some people. And even those of us who appear to tolerate them may not really be escaping unscathed. Just because eating grains isn't overtly poisoning us or causing visible disease symptoms doesn't mean it's not causing subclinical problems. Our "modern diet"—and by that we refer to the dietary change that occurred with the advent of agriculture—has put a chink in our digestive-system armor and as a result has left us vulnerable to a wide variety of serious health problems ranging from inflammatory diseases of the bowel itself to such seemingly disparate disorders as rheumatoid arthritis (as well as other arthritic conditions) and multiple sclerosis. Not all of us develop the severe and well-documented intestines-damaging intolerance to wheat gluten, but it does occur quite commonly. Moreover, research has demonstrated that less obvious degrees of wheat intolerance may occur in much larger segments of the population.

With that in mind, let's turn our attention to an examination of just what kind of Faustian bargain we made for ourselves when we hammered our spears into plowshares.

Skin Tight

The body has two external surfaces to defend: the one that everyone is familiar with, the skin surface, and the other, which few people recognize as external to the body, the lining of the intestinal tract. What may seem to you to be deep, deep within your body—the contents of your very guts—is actually very carefully kept on the outside. So the body, as we think of it, has a tunnel, an external passageway, right through the middle of it, beginning with the mouth, extending down the esophagus, the stomach, the small intestine, the colon, and the rectum, and finally emerging at the far end. What's inside that tunnel isn't technically inside your body, even though it goes right through the middle of it. Initially, that may seem a difficult concept to grasp, but it can also be a valuable one, as we've found many times with our kids when they expressed doubt about some food they were eating. We'd tell them, "Just keep reminding yourself it's not really inside your body; it's just passing through." The barrier to entry of what passes through the portal of this exterior tunnel is quite high. The body normally screens what it lets in with exceptional care—after all, who knows what's on it or where it's been? Let's see how this works.

Our skin is composed of superficial covering cells called epithelial cells that adhere tightly together and act as a barricade against outside agents trying to get it. These epithelial cells serve as our first line of defense against infection and toxic exposures from without. Similarly, enterocytes, specialized "skin" cells that line our gastrointestinal tract, provide the same protection from within. Within each portion of this tunnel that goes through us, the cells modify themselves to withstand the environment to which they're normally exposed. For example, within the mouth, the lining cells toughen to withstand variances in the temperature and consistency of the foods and beverages we consume. The stomach's lining cells toughen in a different way; they must be able to withstand the strong acid secretions that turn what we eat into a homogenous liquid. Neither the lining of the esophagus nor that of the oral cavity could withstand this acid, but fortunately they don't have to as long as the muscular valve separating the stomach from the esophagus (called the lower esophageal sphincter) works properly to keep the acid contents of the stomach contained. When the sphincter fails in its job, however, acid reflux and heartburn—which would be better called esophagus burn—result. (If you've ever been afflicted with these maladies, you'll be pleased to know that the *Protein Power LifePlan* nutritional regimen almost always eliminates them within just a few weeks. Then it's not only good-bye to the burn but also to the daily use of antacid liquids and tablets and acid blockers. But we digress.)

The lining of the gut beyond the stomach changes dramatically, because here—in the approximately 22 feet of small intestine—the business of digestion takes place. The "skin" here has again been modified to its dual special purposes, which is first to break down the incoming food into the smallest basic units and then to absorb these nutrients into the body. (Remember, at this point, the food—along with the bacteria, dirt, toxins, or whatever else came in for the ride—is technically still "outside.") The lining along this 22 feet of intestine folds up into tight gathers or folds called villi to increase the digestive and absorptive work surface. In fact, the folds are so tightly packed that if you were to flatten them into a sheet, a single centimeter (less than half an inch) of intestinal lining would cover a doubles tennis court—an astounding bit of origami.

These tiny villi themselves pinch up into still tinier folds—called microvilli—forming a bristly surface called the brush border. It's actually here, at the brush border, that the digestive enzymes chop incoming proteins into individual amino acids and starches into simple sugars, because the lining cells will admit and deliver to the bloodstream only those nutrients that have been reduced to their simplest form. (The intestine handles fats a little differently. The cells of the brush border will admit individual fatty-acid molecules inside, where they're repackaged into triglyceride molecules and swept up with the fluid that bathes the cells—the lymph—for transport first through the lymphatic system, then through the blood to the liver for further processing.) The intestinal barrier, when it's functioning normally, should admit only nutrients and serve as a barrier to keep out anything else that might prove harmful to the body. And here's how it does it.

The War Without and Within

When we were in medical school, one of our microbiology professors used to delight in enlightening his students each year with this factoid: Each year, every American eats about 9 pounds of fecal matter. As disgusting as it may be, that indeed is the statistic—9 pounds per person per year. Unfortunately, there's a lot more in our food supply than we would like to imagine, and some of it is downright unpleasant. (This is the part where it's good to remind yourself that what you eat isn't really inside your body until you digest and absorb it!) We depend on the lining of the gut to defend us from such contamination—not just the dirt and bacterial contaminants that might come with this 9 pounds of fecal matter, but the toxins, protozoa, and other parasites as well. To rise to the job, the "skin" of the gut lining has modified itself in yet another way by the creation of specially constructed junctions—called tight junctions—between each cell, which serve to prevent the contents of the intestines from slipping between the enterocytes and gaining access to the bloodstream. Normally, nothing except water, small ions, and cleanly reduced simple nutrients should pass through or between the cells.

The tight-junction system should effectively screen out large molecules—such as incompletely digested starches or proteins or fiber that would otherwise slip between the cells—leaving them inside the passageway of the intestine to be carried with the contents on through into the colon and finally out. As long as these millions of tiny seals remain tight, the system works as it should. But sometimes the tight seals malfunction and leak, and when they do, all manner of problems can result.

But first, let's get back to the problem of those 9 unpleasant pounds we ingest and, more specifically, to the millions of bacteria that enter our intestinal tracts yearly in the relatively contaminated food we eat. How can it be that in spite of a frontal assault by these millions of friendly and not-so-friendly bacteria in what we eat and drink we only rarely fall prey to food-borne bacterial diseases? What stops them? The ever vigilant intestinal defense system, and here's how.

For bacteria (or other living creatures, such as parasites) to do us harm internally, they must first attach to and then breach the gut wall. In the stomach, a thick mucus gel that coats the surface to protect it from acid also repels the attachment of bacteria. But within the small intestine, an intricate, mobile, absorbent surface can't be gummed up with such a gel and still function, so here the body has adapted in several different ways: The tight junctions provide a barrier to the entry of bacteria between cells; the waves of contraction that propel the intestinal contents along prevent bacteria from staying in one spot long enough to attach; and the surface cells continually slough away, carrying along with them any recently attached bacteria that may have managed to elude all the other defenses so far. This sloughing-and-renewal process completely replaces the lining of the intestine every four or five days (illustrating, we might add, yet another reason for an adequate daily protein intake: to be able to maintain this spectacular renewal process and keep the gut healthy).

If a crafty or lucky bacterial invader successfully attaches to a lining cell, the game's still not over, because the immune surveillance of the gut fights back. Special cells in the lining attract the invader and take it prisoner. These cells engulf the bacterium in a protective bubble and hand it over to local immune defenders (called macrophages) that patrol the area, which, in turn, present their prisoner to yet other specialized white blood cells (called lymphocytes) that then manufacture specific weapons (called secretory IgA antibodies) designed to kill that bacterium and any others like it. These armed lymphocytes return to the intestinal front lines, carrying their bacterial death potions carefully packaged in sealed bubbles that they smuggle through the gut's lining cells and dump on the surface. Any bacterium still in the area similar to their prisoner will perish, and not only that, the armed lymphocytes will remember the face of the invader forever, so that if one like it ever dares to show up again, the immune response will be swift and sure. When everything works as it should, the entire operation effectively eliminates unwelcome bacterial invasion and creates a rapid response system without alarming the locals—that is, the gut defends itself without inflaming the surrounding tissues, a process unique in the body's immune wars. Usually, immune-defense skirmishes result in redness, swelling, and pain; for proof, you need only think of the pain caused by boils, gouty attacks, and pinkeye. But the gut carries out this stealth operation without inciting such misery, and by virtue of its chronic assault by incoming bacteria, it must wage the battle constantly. In fact, by some research estimates, over two-thirds of all immune-defense activity within the body occurs in the gut. When you recognize its importance in immune defense, it's easy to see how critical a properly functioning gut is to your overall health and well-being. But as important as it is for our health, a hypervigilant immune-defense system can cut both ways, and in the process that which would help us can do us harm.

A Chink in the Armor

When all works well, nothing slips through the defenses of the intestine that shouldn't; unfortunately, all doesn't always work as we'd like. Occasionally, hostile bacteria infect the intestine—for instance, such terrors as cholera, amebic dysentery, and typhoid, along with viruses and other more mundane agents of gastrointestinal distress. By their sheer numbers or the action of poisons they produce, they can alter intestinal function, overwhelm the natural bacterial balance, and undercut the gut defenses. Mechanical problems can arise as well to disrupt the delicate healthy balance, for example, the temporary paralysis or sluggishness of the small intestine following surgery (especially abdominal surgery) interrupts the natural waves of motion that keep the bacteria swimming in the soup. Unmoving bowel contents invite infection, which can sometimes be fatal. But the converse, forced movement, also proves troublesome; the chronic use of harsh laxatives or frequent "cleansing" enemas can damage the bowel lining and weaken its natural defenses as well. But while these situations certainly occur, their frequency pales in comparison to another common cause of bowel dysfunction: cereal grain intolerance.

We mentioned previously that grains weren't fit for human consumption without first being processed by drying, pulverizing, and cooking. And even then they may not be ideally suited for us, because grains, and in fact many plants as you'll recall from chapter 1, "Man the Hunter," contain numerous anti-nutrients designed to discourage their consumption by any plant predator who would destroy their chances for propagation. Even pulverizing and cooking doesn't eliminate the anti-nutrients and potentially harmful substances contained in grains, legumes, and other plants or render them incapable of damaging the human intestine.

A diet heavy in starches and sugars can overwhelm the absorptive capacity of the gut and send unprocessed nutrients downstream into the colon, which, unlike the protected environment of the small intestine, houses zillions of hungry microbes—some friendly, some potentially hostile—waiting to digest what comes in. The bacteria in the colon, at least the "good" ones, live there in symbiosis with us, trading their digestive services for a safe place to live and plenty to eat. When the friendly bacteria that should inhabit the colon digest incoming fiber, they liberate a fatty-acid byproduct (butyric acid) that nourishes the "skin" lining of the colon. It is, in fact, the preferred nutrient for these colonocytes. When loads of incompletely digested starch and sugar come in, it's a veritable bacterial picnic; they set to work fermenting the incoming bounty in a process identical to the fermenting of grape juice to make wine or of barley to make beer and with much the same result: the production of various alcohols and gasses.

Sometimes, the products of this overactive fermentation process flush backward, reentering the small intestine. The unaccustomed exposure to what ought to be in the colon inflames the lining of the small intestine, blunts its bristly microvilli, impairs proper digestion and absorption, and, in the beginnings of a vicious cycle, sends even more incompletely digested foods downstream. But, even more important, the inflammation weakens the tight junctions, which open wider, permitting larger molcules—such as incompletely digested plant proteins—to slip between the cells.

These plant proteins—called lectins—can cause serious trouble once they breach the protective barrier of the gut wall because the bloodstream on the other side is swimming with immune cells on the prowl for any substance they recognize as foreign to the body and, therefore, potentially harmful to it.[1] If this immune patrol detects such a substance—and the plant proteins qualify—it

1. Technically, lectins are glyco-protein complexes, not just plant proteins, and some plant proteins that are not truly lectins cause problems, too. For simplicity, we're calling them *all* lectins here.

attacks, surrounding the offender and releasing chemicals that raise the alarm for more defenders to join the fray. In response, the body produces and dispatches masses of immune cells to the scene to destroy the intruder. After the kill, however, all's not quiet on the intestinal front. These immune defense cells, like their brethren we spoke of before, never forget a face. They remain on alert to attack any similar intruder, potentially forever. And that sounds great—but there's a catch.

A Dangerous Case of Mistaken Identity

Many of these plant proteins that can slip through the leaky junctions of an inflamed intestinal tract may share common characteristics with certain body proteins. For example, the lectin in wheat, called wheat germ agglutinin, or WGA, contains chains of amino acids in a nearly identical arrangement to those found in the joint cartilage or joint-lining tissues of some people and identical, as well, to segments of the myelin proteins in the nerve-covering layers in others; the lectin in kidney beans, called phyto-hemagglutinin, or PHA, resembles segments of a part of the filtering apparatus of the kidney in some people, as well as other tissues throughout the body. Some lectins have a similarity to the insulin-producing cells of the pancreas, cells in the gut lining, or the retina of the eye. The list goes on and on. And unfortunately, these similarities in appearance can give rise to errors in identification or mistaken identity—in other words, in an effort to rid the body of all foreign invaders, the immune system may mistake its own tissues for the enemy they resemble and attack. Sort of a shoot-first-and-ask-questions-later phenomenon in which the body turns its destructive power on itself, causing a variety of disease processes collectively termed autoimmune disorders. This disparate group of medical maladies includes such illnesses as Crohn's disease of the bowel, ulcerative colitis, rheumatoid arthritis, ankylosing sponydlitis, systemic lupus erythematosus, psoriasis, type I diabetes mellitus, glomerulonephritis (a kidney inflammation), multiple sclerosis, and potentially many others as well—from thyroid inflammation to allergies to skin rashes to asthma. What's the basis for making such connections? Let's take a look.

Epidemiologists have shown, for example, that multiple sclerosis occurs much more commonly in areas where the populations rely primarily on wheat and rye, and much less frequently in regions that depend on other staple grains (such as rice, corn, and millet). And to take the hypothesis back considerably further, paleopathologists (scientists studying diseases of ancient populations) tell us that these autoimmune disorders do not seem to have plagued humans prior to the adoption of an agricultural way of life. In fact, paleopathological researchers have been able to track the appearance of rheumatoid arthritis—which leaves its characteristic fingerprints on the bones that remain—as it followed the spread of wheat and maize cultivation around the globe. Prior to the adoption of these grains as food, there is no evidence of rheumatoid arthritis in the fossil record; after their introduction, rheumatoid arthritis appears. It's at the very least a case of guilt by association.

Interestingly, many cases of inflammatory or autoimmune arthritis also involve inflammation of the intestine. And here's the rub: Which came first? Research seems to indicate that the development of a leaky gut that would expose the immune system to look-alike molecules (whether plant lectins, bacteria, or viruses) may be the instigating event for the development of these diseases in genetically or physically susceptible people.

It is for this reason that we recommend that people with a family history of any of the autoimmune disorders we've been discussing should adopt at the very least the Dilettante's approach to their *Protein Power LifePlan* nutritional regimen. By doing so, they'll eliminate the biggest offenders—the lectins of wheat and corn—and thereby reduce their risk for developing these problems themselves. But our advice to reduce or avoid grains isn't just for those with a known family history of these specific autoimmune disorders. Lectin mimicry is a lot like Russian roulette: any of us might be at risk, and if you indulge in a diet heavy in grains and weaken your tight junctions, you never know when the lectin with your name on it might get through. Those people who already suffer from one of these autoimmune disorders will respond best if they eliminate all avenues of immune-system stimulation that the lectins found in grains and beans can cause. We recommend they adhere—at least the majority of the time—to the Purist's version of the plan if they wish to maximally alleviate their symptoms. But everyone on the *Protein Power LifePlan* will benefit from at least a *reduction* in these potentially harmful foods.

Healing the Breach—Plugging the Leaks

Once assaulted and inflamed, the debilitated intestinal tract requires rest and proper nourishment to heal. Its recuperative powers can astound—remember that under normal circumstances it sheds and replaces its lining completely every four or five days—given a conducive environment and the right nutrients. But healing the body nutritionally requires a functional, intact, and healthy intestine. It's the only route (at least in the world outside a hospital) by which we can replenish the nutrients necessary for wellness and a major avenue through which we eliminate the toxins and other wastes of living.

When we undertake the care of patients for metabolic disturbances—whether that means elevated triglycerides or cholesterol, high blood pressure, diabetes, or obesity—we must first be sure their gut is up to the task. If it is, we begin the nutritional rehabilitation with one version or another (depending on their willingness to change dietary habits) of the *Protein Power LifePlan* as outlined in this book. If it's not, we must set about to heal the bowel first. And here's how we go about it. (We want to stress that almost everyone—probably 90 percent of people—will be able to begin with regular food and achieve all the health benefits of the plan; only those with true intestinal malfunction need the more stringent nutritional measures that follow.)

In all cases, we begin by eliminating from the diet those things that the gut *doesn't* need, such as potentially inflaming substances—most especially the lectins of grains and beans—in order to rapidly halt the immune-system confusion and reduce its activity. That's step number one. Then we focus on what the gut *does* need in the way of nourishment. In the small intestine (and to a degree in the colon as well) the lining cells depend on a particular

amino acid richly present in meat called glutamine as their chief
nutrient source. An assaulted, traumatized bowel needs substantially more of this nutrient than a healthy bowel does—and more
than can be obtained by food alone. So step number two is to
provide the cells with the "food" they need most during their
healing process—about 20 to 40 grams of glutamine a day. We've
seen patients with inflammatory bowel disease of many years' duration experience marked reduction of their symptoms with just
these two simple steps.

The colon's lining cells can also use glutamine as a nutrient;
although they prefer short-chain fatty acids such as butyric acid
that their friendly bacteria inhabitants normally provide for them
from fiber digestion, they have to make do with glutamine for a
week or so. It's more important initially to allow the bowel to rest
and to reduce the hotbed of bacterial fermentation that can back-
flow into the small intestine and continue to inflame it, so at first,
we don't complicate matters with added fiber in a really sick gut.[2]
Later, when the digestive processes of the small intestine are
working better, and healing has restored the tightness to the leaky
junctions, we add the fiber back in to keep the resident bacterial
butyric-acid factories busy churning out nutrients for the colon.

But while all this gut healing is going on, there's still a body to
maintain, so even during the intestinal healing process, we try to
replace the nutrients critical to the body's overall health and well-
being in a way that takes it easy on the injured and beleaguered
intestine. That means the protein and essential fats the body must
have need to be replaced in as easily absorbable a form as possible. For our clinic patients who need it (and we hasten to repeat
that most people will not need to go to this trouble) we construct
a supplemental "gut-rehab" meal replacement, which helps to rest
and nourish their intestinal tract. For people with severely disordered intestinal tracts—for instance, those afflicted with Crohn's

---

2. If something such as abdominal surgery or the use of large doses of broad-
spectrum antibiotics has killed off most or all of the friendly bacteria in your colon, that
ecological balance may have to ultimately be restored as well. After all, one can hardly
expect a colon full of dead bacteria to cooperate in their task of turning fiber into
nourishment for the colonocytes, but that's not an issue of paramount importance at
this stage of the game.

disease, ulcerative colitis, severe irritable bowel syndrome with cramping and chronic diarrhea, or those who have suffered severe trauma that disabled their bowel for a time—we recommend the use of this kind of meal replacement (or a reasonable facsimile) for a short time before they begin the food plan. The gut-rehab meal provides them with a healing dose of glutamine, plenty of readily absorbable protein, important essential fats, and the micronutrients the body as a whole requires. In most cases, we keep patients on the rehab formula for less than a week, and that usually allows their gut to begin to recover. Then it's on to a Purist version of the diet—at least at first—and the road to better overall health and wellness through nutrition.

Although we don't know of any commercially available product quite like the one we give our patients, you can approximate it from items available at most health food stores. You'll want a source of complete and easily digested protein—preferably a cross-flow microfiltered whey powder—that contains no more than a few grams of carbohydrate per serving. It should be fortified with vitamins and minerals and, if possible, *should not* contain added iron; in no circumstance should it contain aspartame. To each serving of protein powder (the exact size of which will depend on your personal minimum protein per-meal requirement as specified in tables 13.1 and 13.2 in chapter 13, "*LifePlan* Nutrition") add about 10 grams of L-glutamine powder and 8 ounces of cold water. In addition, once a day you'll need to take at least two other supplements: a couple of over-the-counter magnesium-potassium tablets (such as the 300mg/99mg magnesium-potassium aspartate) and a couple of tablespoons of cod-liver oil. For taste and palatability, we recommend Carlson's Cod Liver Oil in the lemon flavor. Keep it in the refrigerator at all times. (This home-made version will work just fine; it's just a little more trouble. However, if you or your physician prefer to use the product we developed for our clinic patients, please feel free to contact the office at the address listed in the appendix.)

Whether you use our meal or your own version, drink four or five servings per day on the gut-rehab protocol as outlined above. Remain on it *for just a few days,* eating no solid food but drinking plenty of clear, calorie-free fluids, such as water or herbal tea. You cannot and absolutely should not remain on this very low-calorie regimen as your sole nutritional source for more than a week. (*Warning: If you currently take medication for your heart, your blood pressure, or blood sugar—especially if you take insulin—do not use this protocol without the express permission of and under the watchful guidance of your personal physician.*) It's only to be used briefly for the rehabilitation of a very sick bowel.

Following the brief gut-rehab protocol, you should commence the Purist version of the plan for a few weeks at least and then decide which level of commitment you feel suits you best for the long haul. Although the choice is always yours, if you suffer from a chronic intestinal problem or autoimmune disorder, we urge you to be mindful of the dangers of resuming even a small intake of the grain products that probably got you in the health fix in the first place. Does that mean you'll never be able to enjoy pasta or bread or chips again? No, but if you're a person who's intolerant or sensitive to grains, never for an instant believe that your gut won't pay a price of some kind when you put a load of wheat or corn into it. Some people are so sensitive that even a tiny bit of wheat gluten, for instance, will—as they say—get their bowels in an uproar. Others won't have obvious symptoms unless they really overdo it and can get away with a small dose of grain-based food now and again. We both fall into that latter category; it takes a pretty good fall off the grain wagon to cause us to develop notable gut symptons (although a Monday-night-football party with gua-camole and far too many baked lentil chips comes to mind). But we're not so foolish as to believe we can get away with it for long without consequences, and neither should you be. Not from an insulin-sensitivity standpoint, not from an autoimmune-risk standpoint, and not from a gut-health standpoint. Grains simply aren't good food for humans—even for those who *appear* on the surface to tolerate them.

Remember that your earliest ancestors subsisted for many thousands of generations without grain products of any sort—no bread, no linguine, no tortillas, not even any rice. Their intestinal architecture is yours, their gut physiology is yours, their immune defenses worked in 30,000 B.C. in just the same way as yours do today. And if you suffer from intestinal or autoimmune disorders at the dawning of the twenty-first century, it may just be that your Fred Flintstone gut doesn't know what to do with George Jetson's grains.

BOTTOM LINE

Humans turned to the use of grain as a food only about eight to ten thousand years ago. Wild grain is virtually inedible as a food for humans, but by learning to dry and grind the grain, humans can make use of it for food. Doing so allowed us to build great civilizations but at a price. Simply *being able* to make use of a particular plant for sustenance doesn't mean that it's good for us. Such is the case for most grains, and here's why.

The human intestinal tract is designed to break down the foods we eat and to absorb the nutrients from them. Its lining provides a barrier that permits certain necessary substances to pass through and prevents all else from getting in. A diet high in grains can cause a fermentation in the intestine (after all, fermented wheat and hops produces beer and bubbles) that can, in turn, cause inflammation that weakens the tight junctions between the cells that line the tract. From this damage, "leaks" develop that allow prohibited substances—such as incompletely digested plant proteins—through the barrier.

These plant proteins, called lectins, cause trouble once absorbed into the bloodstream because their structure is so similar to the structure of body proteins; some of them are like the proteins in joint surface tissues, others like the filtering apparatus of the kidneys, and still others like the covering of nerves. Because they are the same but foreign, the lectins attract the attention of the immune-defense system, which attacks them; unfortunately, once stimulated, the immune system may then mistakenly attack the body tissues they resemble, causing a host of disorders ranging from readily identifiable diseases (such as arthritis, inflammatory bowel diseases, multiple sclerosis, and autoimmune kidney disorders) to less obvious problems ranging from rashes to allergies to asthma.

All plants have proteins that can behave as lectins, but most are not overtly harmful. The worst offenders are the lectins from grains, especially wheat and corn, but also problematic are those from dried beans, such as kidney beans. Removal of these foods from the diet may be important to us all, but it is especially important for people at risk for autoimmune disorders (rheumatoid arthritis, ankylosing spondylitis, psoriasis, type I diabetes mellitus, multiple sclerosis, Crohn's disease, ulcerative colitis, glomerulonephritis, and, potentially, others).

In our patients who have these disorders (or a strong inherited risk for them) we begin with a gut-rehabilitation regimen that eliminates all grains. In addition, we supplement their diet with a daily dose of 20 to 40 grams of glutamine (an amino acid that nourishes the cells that line the intestinal tract) and we make sure they get enough good-quality protein and essential fat to sustain their needs in an easy-to-absorb form. To make this easier, we use a supplemental food product (a shake) to meet their nutritional and medical needs *for the first few days to a week* of their treatment to allow the intestine to heal, and then we move them to the Purist's version of the plan. You can make an approximation of our supplemental product with items available in your grocery or health food store; see the instructions on page 148 of the chapter. *(Warning: If you currently take medication for your heart, your blood pressure, or blood sugar—especially if you take insulin—do not use this protocol without the express permission of and under the watchful guidance of your personal physician.)*

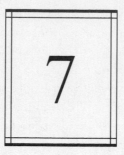

7

How Sweet It Is... Not!

Things sweet to taste prove in digestion sour.
—*Richard II,* ACT I, SCENE 3

We modern humans love our sugar; we love that sweet taste. When the sweet taste buds on our tongues start firing, we know we're in for a delicious, intoxicating treat—and our whole physiology gets ready to handle what's coming—or, at the very least, tries to. Doubtless our ancient ancestors must have also relished the sweet sensation, since they surely had the same taste receptors for sweet. When they stumbled upon a cache of wild honey—if accounts of modern hunter-gatherer groups compare—they had a veritable honey fest. So what could be wrong with our enjoying something sweet now and again just as they did? Absolutely nothing—*now and again.* Where our situation differs from that of the hundred thousand or so generations of humans that went before us is in accessibility. After all, how much honey could a Paleolithic human eat at a sitting while fending off angry bees? So, for our earliest ancestors, a honey find would have been a rare treasure, not a daily occurrence.

Contrast the rarity of wild honey in the lives of ancient humans with these modern statistics. The most recent estimates peg the intake of sugar (and other caloric sweeteners, such as corn syrup, honey, and fructose) in the United States at 150 pounds per person per year. With 365 days in a year, that's about half a pound of sugar per day for every man, woman, and child in this country. Compare that figure with the 2 pounds per person per year we consumed at the turn of this century. Even since 1970 our annual sugar intake has leaped another 24 pounds per person, a skyrocketing trend. It's frightening to think where that average yearly intake of sugar may be hovering twenty years from now. And who is consuming the most sugar of all? Far and away it's kids, and especially young men between fifteen and twenty-four. In this group, sugar (along with the other nutritionally empty, high-calorie sweeteners) makes up a bigger share of their dietary calorie intake than any other category—meat, milk, or fruits and vegetables combined. This addiction to empty sweetness represents an enormous departure from the diet of our ancient ancestors, and one that will create a health-care crisis in the not-too-distant future as this generation of sugar babies grows to adulthood. In fact, it already is.

Look around at the youth of today; obesity among children is escalating at an alarming rate—*doubling* in just the last decade. It's reaching epidemic proportions, not just among American kids but around the world, as we continue to export our very American habit of swilling enormous containers of colas, chomping super-large orders of fries, and gobbling bags of sugar-laden carbo junk all day.

Research has proven that fat kids turn into fat adults, and that's bad enough because statistics bear out that fat adults frequently become sick adults. But what's worse is that fat kids are now turning into sick kids. The disease that we once called adult-onset diabetes has now begun to turn up in kids as young as eight and ten. And the rising incidence of such a disease among so young a group has set the epidemiological and nutritional researchers into a twirl of trying to figure out why. First, of course, these wizards of nutrition looked to blame that usual suspect, dietary fat. Surely, they reasoned, all these obese kids are simply eating too much fat, and that's the problem. But when they looked at the real data, what they found was that, amazingly, kids—like all Americans—have been eating less fat in recent years. And even more amazing, the kids that ate the least fat were the fattest! Positively puzzling—unless, of course, you understand a little about human metabolism and biochemistry and don't have an anti-fat bias already built into your thinking. So, if it wasn't fat, what then *could* it be? And the answer came to them: exercise. It must be that kids today don't get enough exercise. That's what's making the rates of obesity skyrocket and type II diabetes appear in second-graders. And while kids may indeed not be getting enough exercise, that's simply not going to adequately explain the explosion of these disorders.

Only recently have some researchers turned their attention to what we feel is the real culprit: sugar. A study published in the March 1999 issue of the journal *Pediatrics,* for example, showed that what you feed kids for breakfast and/or lunch will set the tone for their desire to eat for the rest of the day. Feed them quickly absorbable carbohydrate junk, and they'll eat nearly twice as much later. According to U.S. Secretary of Agriculture Dan Glickman, "These findings provide the first solid evidence that carbohydrates are one piece of the puzzle in determining what makes some people overeat." We agree—but it's one heck of an enormous piece. Sugar in all its forms is causing this epidemic in both kids and adults, and restriction of sugar *in all its forms* will end it. Let's explore that notion in more detail.

White Powders in All Forms

For quite a long time now we've maintained that white powders are addictive. Whether the powder in question is flour, sugar, crystalline fructose, heroin, or cocaine, all of them are detrimental to your health and all of them make you want more. As you'll recall from chapter 1, "Man the Hunter," one quite serious theory about the origin of agriculture involves the addictive nature of grain. Human beings—at least the great majority of them—seem to have traded in their autonomy and domesticated *themselves* in order to have ready access to the designer drug of the day: *flour* and the products made from it. Plainly put, grains stimulate the brain and affect its chemistry in much the same way that narcotic drugs do, and therein lies their strong draw and addictive potential. As civilizations grew, largely fueled by the growing of grains, a system arose whereby he who ruled the wheat field ruled the world. All the great kings and powerful pharaohs of antiquity ascended to their lofty positions on what amounted to a sort of drug trade—only in this instance, the drug was wheat—with their vast holdings and incredible wealth dependent on controlling the production, distribution, and storage of the product. We, modern humans, inherited the great civilizations that were born out of this primitive "drug" culture, but along with them, we fell heir as well to the diseases that consuming grains brought. (Recall the damaging effects of grains—beyond their simple carbohydrate consequences—from chapter 6, "The Leaky Gut.") But at this point, let's continue to examine the carbohydrate-equals-sugar angle.

A Rose by Any Other Name . . .

Many people are of the opinion that there are good and bad carbohydrates, when in actuality there are barely tolerable and awful sugars. We say *sugars* because all carbohydrates are sugars in one form or another. Whether it's a whole wheat bagel or a jelly bean, all carbohydrates are either simple sugars themselves or a number of simple sugars hooked together. In medical parlance, the number of individual sugar molecules hooked into the chain dictates what they're called. For example, those that are but a single sugar molecule we call a simple sugar; glucose (blood sugar) and fructose fall into this category. Two simple sugars hooked together make a *di*saccharide; an example is sucrose, common table sugar. Three hooked together form a *tri*saccharide, and many sugars linked into a long chain are a *poly*saccharide. Starches such as wheat, oats, corn, rice, beans, and potatoes are examples of polysaccharide sugars. The term *starches*—or the newest nutritional euphemism, *complex carbohydrates*—sounds so much more noble and healthy and downright American. But in fact they're just sugars, too. Our human intestinal tract has no means to absorb these big starch molecules. In order for them to get into the body, they've got to be broken down into their individual simple sugars by the digestive system. So whether it began life as a fat-free bagel, a quarter cup of sugar from the sugar bowl, a canned soft drink, a bowl of fettucine, a baked potato, or a handful of jelly beans, by the time your intestinal tract gets finished snipping the links of those starch and sugar chains, it's all been reduced to . . . sugar. Specifically, to glucose. And in the end there's very little metabolic difference between your eating a medium baked potato or drinking a 12-ounce can of soda pop. Each contains about 50 grams of easily digestible and rapidly available glucose. It may surprise you to know that the potato might even be slightly worse in terms of the rise in blood sugar that follows it.

That's not to say that there aren't some differences in the metabolic impact of various foods; there are. And that notion has given birth to a whole new nutritional dogma—and a couple of best-selling diet books—built around a measurement called the glycemic index. Let's examine this little jewel under the high-powered loupe and see if it's paste or real.

The Perils and Pitfalls of the Glycemic Index

Since excess blood sugar clearly exerts untoward metabolic effects, researchers have studied the rates at which different types of carbohydrates make their way from the mouth through the digestive tract and into the blood. The fruit of these researchers' labor is the glycemic index, a measure of how quickly and how much various dietary starches and sugars raise the blood sugar. The standard against which all carbohydrates were measured was once glucose, but in recent years that standard has been replaced with something more commonly eaten: white bread. In developing this carbohydrate rating scale—that is, the glycemic index—researchers had their subjects consume 50 grams of starch in the form of white bread and then measured their blood sugar levels over a several-hour period to see how high they rose. They then calculated an average value based on those levels. The scale considers this computed average for white bread to have a glycemic index value of 100. Once that was determined, the subjects then consumed 50 grams of other carbohydrate foods (for example, apples, bananas, carrots, rice cakes, and so on) to see how the blood sugar rise they caused compared to the white bread standard. For example, if the food in question caused a rise in blood sugar one-half as high as that caused by white bread, it received a rating of 50; if it caused a rise in blood sugar 20 percent higher than that caused by white bread, it was rated 120 on the glycemic index scale, and so on.

In the last couple of years several new dietary regimes have become popular—through such books as *Sugar Busters!* (Ballantine, 1998) and *Enter the Zone* (HarperCollins, 1996)—based on the concept of limiting carbohydrate foods with a high glycemic index and relying chiefly on foods that rate low on this scale. The benefit of this strategy lies in curbing the blood sugar rise caused by foods high on the index in order to limit the rise in blood insulin that follows. Because of this documented effect, we're frequently asked in interviews about how the concept relates to our *Protein Power* strategy. And that's not so easy to answer as it may seem.

Certainly we applaud the concept of reducing blood sugar and keeping a tighter rein on insulin levels, both of which eating foods lower on the glycemic index will generally do. However, strictly focusing on the glycemic index can lead you astray. In the first place, although we feel that the index offers some broadly applicable principles, we also feel that it contains some flaws that render it useless as a helpful tool to guide a nutrition-conscious general public. For example, the scale derives its values really only for individual foods, and few of us begin with a completely empty stomach, eat a single food at a sitting, and wait two hours for its digestion and absorption before eating another food. We eat mixed meals, and the mixing of foods with varying index values alters the combined value, and, more important, the rate at which the sugars absorb. It would be impossible to devise a rating scale for every meal combination that every person might select or for a person to make any sort of determination about the glycemic average of the meal he'd just eaten. So where's the utility in the scale? How can it really help guide choices? Even considering just a single food, the index value can vary all over the map, depending on the food's ripeness and how it's prepared. A ripe banana, for instance, can have up to double the glycemic index of a greener one, and who decides just how ripe or how green a banana is? Another common example: a serving of mashed potatoes can have a 25 percent higher glycemic index value than the same amount of potato simply boiled and cut into small cubes. And beyond the potential for error introduced by these kinds of variances, values within the same individual eating the same food prepared the same way aren't fully reproducible from one day to the next.

In the application of very broad strokes of the scale, we do find some use. In general, a given food eaten raw will rate lower on the glycemic scale than if it's cooked; quick-cooked foods will be lower than those subjected to prolonged cooking; greener ones will rate lower than riper ones; and less processed (potatoes cut into large chunks, for instance) will be lower than more highly processed (mashed or pureed). Beyond those generalities and the knowledge that some foods rate generally high and some rate generally low, we don't see a lot to get worked up over, preferring instead to focus on the absolute amount of effective carbohydrate in the foods, not the glycemic index per se.

But in addition to its lack of accuracy that would allow a person to make an informed nutritional decision, there's yet another glaring problem with relying on the glycemic index as a carbohydrate guidebook. Although the scale implies that foods with lower ratings are preferred to those with higher ones, being lower on the glycemic index doesn't necessarily mean that a given food is especially healthier than one with a higher value. For example, the simple sugar fructose, found naturally in honey, many fruits, and some vegetables, carries a very low glycemic rating of 32. It would, therefore, seem to make good nutritional and metabolic sense to eat fructose in preference to foods containing mainly glucose (index 137) or starchy foods, such as potatoes (index 121) or white bread (index 100) that the body quickly breaks down into glucose. But this simplistic approach points up another critical flaw in the whole glycemic index concept. Let's examine the effects fructose has on the body in more detail.

The Trouble with Fructose

The body handles fructose in a different manner than it does the other main dietary simple sugar, glucose. Because fructose doesn't require the assistance of insulin to get into the cells, fructose itself occasions no immediate insulin rise. Some nutritional gurus have touted that feature as a plus—a fact that has not escaped food manufacturers, who now stuff this sugar into most of their junk—but in the long run we don't agree. In fact, we lay blame for much of the epidemic rise in diabetes and obesity in this country on the high consumption of fructose, which represents a major departure from our ancestral diet. While many people equate fructose with "fruit sugar," the amounts of it contained in fruit or honey (sources occasionally available to our prehistoric ancestors) are minuscule compared to the quantities of *added* fructose now found in many commercially prepared foods and soft drinks. More on that subject in a bit, but first let's look at what happens to fructose when it's absorbed.

Once in the bloodstream, fructose moves quickly into the liver to be, among other things, processed into glycerol, a component of the triglyceride molecule. As a consequence of this transformation, eating significant amounts of fructose will usually cause a substantial increase in the levels of VLDL (very low-density lipoprotein) cholesterol and triglycerides in the blood and, not only that, will promote the peroxidation of those fats and others within the body into dangerous compounds. (Research has shown that extra vitamin E will help to offset the damage done by fructose in peroxidizing fats; this is yet another reason we recommend eating foods that contain vitamin E and even supplementing the vitamin daily.)

Studies of both rats and people have also shown that regularly consuming large amounts of fructose impairs the body's ability to properly handle glucose and ultimately leads to hyperinsulinemia and the development of insulin resistance. (In fact, fructose feeding has become a standard method in research labs to cause lab rats to become insulin resistant as well as to develop high blood pressure.) Furthermore, elevating blood lipids and promoting their peroxidation and the development of insulin resistance and hypertension are not the only detrimental effects of this low-glycemic food; fructose is also instrumental in damaging and aging our tissues by a process called fructation or fructosylation.

You see, simple sugars, such as fructose and glucose, can attach to various body proteins and initiate a reaction (called fructation or glycation depending on the sugar involved) that alters and damages the protein forever in a process not entirely unlike the combination of dairy protein and fat with sugar and heat to make caramel. The process occurs with such predictable regularity that physicians can use the product of the reaction of glucose with the proteins of red blood cells—called glycated hemoglobin—to determine a patient's average blood sugar reading over the last couple of months. The attachment of glucose to blood cells, while not beneficial, does little permanent harm, since the life of a red blood cell is a mere 120 days before it's recycled and replaced with a new one. But this same caramelizing process goes on in virtually all tissues throughout the body, many of which aren't as quickly replaced as blood cells. What's more, the tendency for glucose to attach to proteins and damage them pales in comparison to the power of fructose to do it. By some estimates, fructose attaches to body proteins ten to fifteen times more readily than glucose does—and the presence of iron in the tissues fans the flames of the "caramel" production (see chapter 8, "The Modern Iron Age"). Year in and year out, from the time we're born, this damage wrought by the caramelization process accumulates in our bodies; over a lifetime it wreaks the most havoc in long-lived proteins, including elastin, the protein that gives youthful elasticity to the skin; crystallin, the special protein that forms the lens of the eye; DNA, the genetic blueprint present in all cells; and collagen, the structural protein that accounts for over 30 percent of the body's protein mass, occurring in tissues all over the body, including the hair, skin, and nails, the walls of all arteries and veins, and the framework of bones and organs. Damage to these critical protein structures results not only in such cosmetic maladies as wrinkles and age spots, but in serious health problems ranging from cataracts to failure of major organs, such as the kidneys and the heart.

What's worse is that the consumption of fructose is on the rise—and our kids are at the greatest risk of all. The most recent figures estimate that, on average, every man, woman, and child in America swills 54 gallons of regular soft drinks each year. While the consumption of diet soft drinks (also not a good choice, as you'll see in a bit) has remained pretty steady in the last decade at 10 gallons per person per year, the figures for regular soft drink consumption began a steep climb in about 1992, from just over 30 gallons a year to the current 54 gallons. Why? We can't say with certainty, but we feel that the introduction of the practice of upsizing has played a big part. By that we mean that people probably aren't buying nearly twice as many individual sodas; they're simply buying the same number of sodas but getting—and no doubt drinking—two or three times as big a serving at a whack. And what's in that super-large serving has changed over the years as well.

Not too many years ago, sucrose—common table sugar—sweetened most sweet foods, both at home and away. Since sucrose is a disaccharide composed of a molecule of glucose attached to a molecule of fructose, anytime you ate or drank anything sweetened with it, you got one half of your sugar dose as glucose and the other half as fructose. Now more and more food manufacturers have turned to the use of high-fructose corn syrup because it's cheaper and sweeter than sucrose. In fact, the whole New Coke versus Coke Classic debate originated when the Coca-Cola Company decided to switch a few years back from the sucrose in the classic recipe to the cheaper (and sweeter) high-fructose corn syrup that (rumor has it) their chief competition, Pepsi, had always used. Now virtually every can of regular soda of any stripe contains mainly high-fructose corn syrup and/or sucrose as a sweetener—including brands we've spotted in health food stores labeled all natural as though they're nutritious. Thanks to this widespread switch, soda pop drinkers around the globe now consume not only more sugar from their super-duper-size servings, but also vastly more fructose than ever before in the history of man. Think of the teenagers you see hanging out at the fast-food establishments, chug-a-lugging not 12-ounce cans of soda, but quart-size cups of flavored high-fructose-corn-syrup carbonated water one after another day after day. They're practically becoming insulin-resistant wrecks right in front of your eyes. Many of them already have begun to develop "middle-aged" diseases: they're fat, they're soft, they're becoming diabetic, and their triglyceride and cholesterol levels have already begun to rise. And the fructose is already busily at work making "caramel" in the arteries of their hearts and their kidneys and in the lenses of their eyes. If something doesn't stop it, history may well record the Great Diabetes and Heart Disease Pandemic of the 2020s, when all these fructose-fed kids start moving into their thirties.

But what's the alternative to sugars? If eating these things causes such serious health problems—and make no mistake, in the vast quantities of Americans who currently consume them, they do—what should you use in place of the sucrose, fructose, and corn syrup you currently use to sweeten your foods? Would artificial sweeteners be any better? In the great scheme of things, probably not.

Fool's Gold? The Artificial Sweeteners

We humans are a clever bunch, always exploring, inventing, building, trying to come up with some improvements on Mother Nature's bounty. And our quest for the perfect artificial sweetener fits into this scheme. We keep hoping that the wizards of food chemistry will uncover some wondrous powder that looks like sugar, tastes like sugar, sweetens like sugar, cooks like sugar, behaves like sugar, but has no calories or adverse health consequences. So far, it's a no go. But science forges on undaunted. Let's take a look at what's out there now and try to get to the bottom line. What are the potential problems you'll be signing up for if you pick up a chunk of this fool's gold?

Saccharin. Americans have been consuming this calorie-free substance for over a hundred years, since its discovery in 1879 at Johns Hopkins University. Produced from petroleum-based substances by the Sherwin-Williams Company (yes, the paint people), saccharin was first used as a food preservative and antiseptic, but with a sweetening power three hundred times greater than sugar and found to be stable in liquids and in cooking, those roles soon gave way to its use as a sweetening agent in the wake of sugar shortages created during the two world wars.

Concerns about its safety as a food additive arose in the late 1960s, culminating in FDA-sponsored testing to refute or verify the claims. In these tests, investigators fed high doses of saccharin to laboratory rats throughout their lives and noted a significant increase in the incidence of bladder tumors in the test animals. Doubts were cast on the cancer-causing conclusions that were reached because they were based on saccharin intakes that in humans would have equaled eight hundred diet drinks per day. Because of these doubts as well as saccharin's usefulness as a sugar substitute for the many diabetics in the country (and there were ten times fewer of them then than now) and enormous public protest, the FDA finally decided not to ban the sweetener but rather to insist that labels of products containing it must carry the warning about the potential to cause bladder cancer in lab animals. And so they do to this day.

Does saccharin in modest doses cause cancer? Probably not. In fact, a large study conducted in Copenhagen between 1979 and 1981 and published in the *International Journal of Cancer* in 1983 showed no increased risk for bladder cancer in either men or women—humans, not rats—who regularly used artificial sweeteners (specifically saccharin and cyclamate). But does that mean that saccharin is totally without problems? Unfortunately, it doesn't. In a study published in November 1998, a group of Belgian researchers demonstrated that saccharin (as well as other bitter-tasting artificial and herbal sweeteners) stimulates the pancreas to release insulin, not a particularly beneficial effect for people trying to keep their insulin levels controlled.

So where does that leave us in relation to how saccharin might fit into our nutritional regimen? In a Purist approach to *Protein Power LifePlan* nutrition (see chapter 13, "*LifePlan* Nutrition"), saccharin or any other artificial sweetener has no place. However, in small doses, used occasionally, it's probably not too dangerous for those people willing to accept a bit of risk for a bit of sweet. The watchwords are *occasional* and *small doses*. If you stick to those parameters when you need some additional sweetness, you'll fare pretty well with saccharin.

Acesulfame K. In the same general chemical family as saccharin, acesulfame potassium (or, as it's usually called, acesulfame K) is potentially fraught with the same problems relative to cancer causation and the stimulation of insulin release. Thus far no human data has emerged (just as in the case of saccharin) to indict the sweetener as carcinogenic. Like saccharin, it's noncaloric and stable in liquids and in cooking. Is it safe to use? In small amounts infrequently, probably so. But once again, our advice to *Protein Power LifePlan* Dilettantes and Hedonists who might choose to use acesulfame K is to use it sparingly!

Cyclamate. Cyclamate was discovered in 1937 at the University of Illinois by accident (like so many other scientific discoveries over the years) when a scientist inadvertently laid his cigarette near a pile of powdery residue and discovered on putting it back into his mouth that it tasted sweet. What he found was a noncaloric artificial sweetener about thirty times sweeter than sugar that was stable in liquids and in cooking. It first began to appear in foods and beverages in the 1950s, dominating the market throughout most of the 1960s until—as happened at about the same time with saccharin—questions arose about its potential for causing bladder and other cancers and the safety of its long-term use. Although these questions persist, cyclamate has remained in use in the United Kingdom and Canada throughout the years without any evidence of an upswing in the rates of the cancers it supposedly can cause. In the United States, however, the FDA banned its use in 1970 despite the vociferous protests of those who felt it unfair to the diabetic population to withdraw it from the market. Despite hundreds of tests and numerous appeals by its manufacturer over the last thirty years, the United States ban remains in effect today. In 1985 a panel of scientists from the National Academy of Sciences reviewed all the testing and issued a pronouncement that there was not substantial data to indict the sweetener as a carcinogen itself, but their report fell short of exonerating it entirely, leaving doubts that it might behave as a tumor promoter. And so the debate about the safety of cyclamate goes on, and for now, in the United States, so does the ban against its use. Is this sweetener safe? Probably so for those who would accept a bit of possible risk for a bit of sweet. But just as with saccharin, the safety hinges on small doses used occasionally.

Aspartame. With aspartame, once again science stumbled into a sweet discovery. This time while looking for a drug to treat ulcers, G.D. Searle & Co. found a sweetener two hundred times sweeter than sugar without the bitter aftertaste of the artificial sweeteners that preceded it. The developers must have shouted "Eureka!" thinking they'd found the perfect sugar substitute. But the portrait of aspartame wasn't so perfect. To begin with, it isn't noncaloric; aspartame has the same 4-calories-per-gram burden as table sugar, although, admittedly, it takes a lot fewer grams of aspartame to sweeten something. And even though it's stable in liquids, such as diet drinks, it isn't heat stable and consequently has limited usefulness in cooking. But we, and millions of others, willingly accepted these drawbacks for something that tasted cleanly sweet (not bitter) but didn't raise insulin levels measurably. Very soon, saccharin disappeared in diet drinks in the United States to be totally replaced by aspartame. Diners in restaurants became accustomed to the little blue packets of Equal alongside the pink packets of Sweet'N Low on their tables, and Americans converted.

Then, as with all artificial sweeteners that preceded it, serious challenges to aspartame's safety began to surface. First were claims that because the body breaks down the dipeptide molecule (a linkage of two amino acids) into methanol (wood alcohol), a known toxin that can cause blindness, and formaldehyde, a known cancer-causing agent, the product posed significant safety risks to the public. The FDA evaluated these charges and concluded that the levels of these substances that occurred from the metabolism of aspartame did not reach toxic levels, and in fact, fruits, vegetables, and fruit juices exposed people to higher levels of methanol than aspartame did. And the furor died down somewhat and allayed our concerns about recommending its use.

Subsequent to the publication of *Protein Power,* however, scientific papers came to our attention, followed by a thoughtfully written book by Russell L. Blaylock, M.D., called *Excitotoxins: The Taste That Kills* (Health Press, 1996) that caused us to review and ultimately to reverse our stance on this sweetener. (See Resources in the appendix for related readings on this subject.) We now feel that aspartame may pose significant hazards to the brain and nervous system and we no longer recommend its use. As a wise old Greek once said, "To admit that you were wrong is merely to admit that you're wiser today than you were yesterday." Here's why we no longer recommend this sweetener and, furthermore, actively discourage its use.

Aspartame differs from other types of artificial sweeteners in that it is a dipeptide, a molecule made by joining two amino acids together; in other words, it's a tiny protein fragment. It can enter the bloodstream intact and find its way through the circulation to a vulnerable area of the brain called the bare area, where it can gain entry to the brain. Why is that a problem? The brain is quite picky about what it lets in and what it keeps out. Surrounding virtually the entire brain, a structure called the blood-brain barrier shields the brain from direct bloodstream access, allowing only certain ions and nutrients to pass. In the bare area, however, the barrier skips a spot, and here the brain can be vulnerable to entry of unwanted substances that once inside may stimulate the brain abnormally, an effect called excitotoxicity. Such is the case for aspartame; this sweetener—along with other similar molecules, most notably MSG (monosodium glutamate), the food additive and flavor enhancer so pervasive in processed foods—behaves as a brain excitotoxin. Its chemical structure allows it to fit into a receptor within the brain called the NMDA (N-methyl-d-aspartate) receptor, triggering such overstimulation in the nerve cell that it dies. In other words, the brain cell literally becomes excited to death. Certainly we use only a small percentage of our brain in thinking and functioning, but shouldn't we want to keep all of it that we can? And besides, certain areas of the brain, such as the hippocampal area, which is involved in memory, are quite sensitive to these kinds of toxic insults. Interestingly, the toxic effects are made worse by low levels of magnesium within the cells (see chapter 9, "The Magnesium Miracle"), a condition that afflicts the vast majority of people with insulin-related diseases, such as diabetes, obesity, and hypertension—the very population relying the most on diet foods artificially sweetened with aspartame.

Reports in the medical literature suggest that in susceptible people, consuming aspartame may result in such symptoms as mood disturbances, sleep disturbances, headaches, dizziness, short-term memory loss, fuzzy thinking, and inability to concentrate. And what's more, the concern on the part of some clinicians and researchers is that the excitotoxic effect may permanently damage the brain and nervous system. Thus far, the FDA has failed to be swayed by the scientific evidence that there may be some serious problems with this sweetener, relying instead on other data that indicate that aspartame is safe, and aspartame is still sweetening everything from diet sodas to pudding cups in America. Even so, we urge you to avoid its use. The possible risks to your brain simply aren't worth it. Our advice—if you must have more sweetness than a tiny amount of honey, the natural sweetener stevia (see below), or sucrose provides—is to sparingly use other artificial sweeteners less fraught with risk until something better comes along.

Sucralose. This sweetener has been on the market in Canada for more than ten years. It, not aspartame, sweetens the diet sodas there and also comes in a sprinkle-on form called Splenda™. This substance, six hundred times sweeter than sugar, actually derives its chemical nature from the sucrose molecule. Sucralose manufacturers replace two of the components of sucrose (the hydroxyl groups) with chlorine molecules. Making this simple substitution not only enhances its sweetness manyfold but also makes the altered sucrose molecule unrecognizable to the digestive machinery that would normally break it down and absorb it. That means that even though the taste buds perceive its intense sweet taste, the body can't absorb sucralose; therefore, it can't cause the rise in blood sugar and insulin that would follow a similarly sweet dose of sucrose. Sucralose remains stable, withstands heat in cooking, measures like sugar, to most people tastes remarkably like sugar with no detectable aftertaste, and contains no absorbable calories—so it looks perfect. But is it? It's tempting to say so, but based on the track record of its forerunners, we'd have to say let's wait and see. To date, it looks like the most promising sugar substitute yet formulated, and it's the one we currently use ourselves when we occasionally need an extra bit of sweetness (which is actually a pretty rare occurrence for us).

The FDA took this sweetener under advisement about ten years ago and finally in 1998 approved it for use in the United States, but it's still not readily available on shelves across America or in American diet soft drinks. However, if we can make any comparisons with the market experience of our friends in Canada, it will soon replace aspartame in soft drinks in this country as well. Already market testing of a diet RC cola with sucralose has reached some areas of the country, and from the reports we've received, it's quite good. At this point—subject, of course, to a change in our position based on any new information that may come to light—we can recommend sucralose as a reasonably safe alternative sweetener to sugar, but we still add that you should use all sweeteners responsibly—that is, in small doses and only occasionally.

Stevia. This natural sweetener, made from an extract of the leaves of the South American plant *Stevia rebaudiana,* has been widely used in Asia for quite some time. It has appeared on the American market in recent years and is sold primarily in health food stores, where it is widely recognized as a sweetener. To date, although it may be added supplementally to foods, the FDA does not permit it to be labeled as a sweetener. Testing performed so far does not indicate any cancer-causing potential, though only time will tell. The extract products, which come in drops, refined powders, and the raw ground stevia leaves, sweeten quite potently and, like saccharin, cyclamate, and acesulfame K, can turn bitter if you use even a touch too much. Its bitter characteristics place it in the same group as those sweeteners that can stimulate the release of insulin, and for that reason, as with the others, we recommend using it only sparingly. It remains stable in liquid, making it useful for sweetening tea or coffee, and in heat, so it can, in theory, be used in cooking, although few recipes have been adapted for its use to our knowledge. All in all, it's not a bad alternative sweetener.

Sugar Alcohols. These products, such as xylitol, sorbitol, and maltitol, retain the sweet-taste-bud stimulating properties of sugars, but their altered structure prevents their absorption from the intestinal tract. As a consequence, eating them won't make your blood sugar rise or spur a release of insulin. Their lack of effect on the blood sugar and insulin metabolism has placed them in the forefront as sweeteners for "diabetic" products, such as candies and chewing gum. In small doses, they appear to be harmless and in some studies have even proven helpful in reducing the frequency of middle-ear infections in children who chew gum sweetened with them or take a syrup containing them. As is our usual recommendation with artificial sweetening agents, the bywords are *small doses* and *used occasionally,* and for very practical reasons: since they're not absorbed and pass through with the intestinal contents, they can cause what's termed an osmotic diarrhea if consumed in large quantities. Use sparingly!

The Taming of the Sweet Tooth

In fact, the words *use sparingly* could apply to intense sweetness of any kind, natural or artificial. As always, if we look to our Paleolithic nutritional past for guidance in what we should be doing today, we'll quickly find that our ancient ancestors didn't have access to either the amount or the regularity of consumption of the intense sweet treats we've become accustomed to in modern times. Seasonal fruits and the occasional honey tree treasure were all that our physiology knew for more than a hundred thousand generations. And while we're not advocating that you should never enjoy luscious desserts or fine Belgian chocolates, we do urge you not to make these treats an everyday occurrence.

By constantly bathing your sweet receptors with intense—albeit artificial and noncaloric—sweetness, you dull them and blunt them. It's exactly what happens with the insulin receptors when they're continually bathed in high levels of insulin. They become sluggish and unresponsive to the point that it takes much more insulin to make them work. So, too, with your taste buds: if they're constantly bombarded with diet soda after diet soda, with artificially sweetened whipping cream, with "sugar-free" pudding and ice cream and gelatin, they'll simply quit sensing those things as sweet and increase your desire for even more intense sweetness.

During the first two or three weeks of changing over to a *Protein Power LifePlan* regimen, the craving for sweets can be very strong—remember the addictive/narcotic nature of sugar and starch. For some people, eliminating large servings of carbohydrates can prove daunting, which can make the diet a challenge to stick to at first. We know it's not easy (we've done it ourselves), but if you can manage to cut back your intake of intensely sweet foods and drinks for a month or two, you'll find that your desire for them lessens and finally disappears.

For a lightly sweet treat when you feel that sweet urge to splurge, add 2 ounces of Tazo Brambleberry or Wild Sweet Orange beverage to 8 ounces of sparkling mineral water.[1] Pour over ice, mix, and enjoy. This naturally sweet spritzer contains only about 3.5 grams of effective carbohydrate, no high-fructose corn syrup, and no added sugar.

After you've rehabilitated your insulin system, you may even find that you feel a little ill when you fall off the wagon and indulge excessively in sweets. Amazingly, in time you'll begin to appreciate the natural sweetness of snap peas, green beans, squash, and unsweetened fruits. Your sweet receptors will recover their sensitivity, just as your insulin receptors will recover theirs.

BOTTOM LINE

O ur ancient ancestors probably shared with us a love of sweetness. Written accounts of modern tribes of hunter-gatherers attest that they greet the finding of a wild honey tree with great joy and eat until they're quite drunk on sugar, and it must have been much the same fifty thousand years ago. Where our modern lives differ is not in our love of sweets but in our access to them. As a result, our consumption of sweetened foods continues to climb.

At the turn of the twentieth century, the consumption of sugar was about 2 pounds per person per year; at the start of the twenty-first, that number will exceed 150 pounds per year for every man, woman, and child in America. Quite a rise in our intake, not just of table sugar but of the other sweetening substances, too, including honey, fructose, corn

---

1. Tazo bottled products contain no high-fructose corn syrup or sugar. They're sweetened just with fruit. See Resources in the appendix.

syrup, and the cheaper and sweeter high-fructose corn syrup that now sweetens almost all regular soft drinks, "juice" drinks, and prepackaged sweet foods, such as ice cream, cookies, pastries, "nutrition" bars, and sweet cereals. Young people consume the most sugar and sweetening syrups—particularly young men between the ages of fifteen and twenty-four—who may eat more of their calories as sugar and sweetening syrups than as meat, milk, fruits, or vegetables. The consequences of their overworking their insulin systems in this way will very soon begin to show up in a health-care crisis of enormous proportions. In fact, it's beginning already: childhood obesity has doubled in the last decade, and type II diabetes (once called adult-onset variety) has begun to afflict eight- and ten-year-old children. What will become of this generation of sugar babies as they reach adulthood?

Dire health consequences are not just the result of increased consumption of sugar but of refined starches in general, since, after all, starches are simply sugars in disguise. Starches are sugar molecules hooked into long chains. It is the business of the digestive system to break those chains and turn all carbohydrates—whether table sugar, bread, potatoes, corn, bagels, rice, or pasta—into simple sugars, such as glucose; only then can the body absorb them. Some foods cause a quicker rise in blood sugar than others. Such differences in how the body processes different kinds of carbohydrate gave rise to the glycemic index—an interesting, but to our thinking not especially useful scale that rates how much various individual foods increase blood sugar. The main problem with such a scale is that in the real world people rarely eat a single food and the scale doesn't account for the changes in absorption that result from combining two or more foods.

Beyond just eating more sugar, however, in the last several decades, there's been a shift in food manufacturing away from sucrose (table sugar) to high-fructose corn syrup, which is cheaper and sweeter. This change to more fructose in the American diet is a critical one, since this particular simple sugar has been shown to promote the production of fat and to much more readily attach to body proteins and irreversibly damage and age them, leading to such serious disorders as kidney disease and cataracts as well as cosmetic ones, such as wrinkles. Some people have suggested that fructose would be a good sweetener for diabetics, since, unlike glucose, it doesn't require insulin to enter the cells; therefore, eating fructose doesn't cause a rise in insulin levels. But studies have shown that fructose promotes insulin resistance by other means. We recommend avoiding fructose except as it occurs in small amounts naturally in fruit and sharply reducing the amount of sugars of all types to a level at which insulin remains controlled.

Although sugar substitutes don't cause a blood sugar or significant insulin rise, they're still far from an ideal solution. Their intense sweetness continues the sugar habit by blunting the sweet receptors (taste buds) and creates the need for more sweetness. Some of them—especially aspartame (Equal, NutraSweet)—we strongly oppose. We are now aware of enough credible scientific research detailing the dangers to memory, sleep, and mood, and much more that may be suffered by some people using this sweetener that we discourage its use—particularly in conjunction with our program. When extra sweetness seems necessary, Hedonists and Dilettantes can use sparing amounts of saccharin or the newly approved sucralose (in Canada marketed as Splenda), neither of which appears to cause the toxic effects in the brain that may occur from aspartame. The better course is to avoid intense sweeteners as a general rule—our physiology simply was not designed to handle it on a regular basis—and to allow our taste for what's sweet to resensitize so that we can enjoy the natural sweetness of foods from ripe fruit to green beans, snap peas, and almonds. For a quick, lightly sweet treat, see page 170.

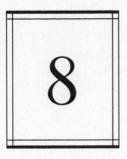

THE MODERN IRON AGE

*It remains now to discuss . . . iron, a metal which we
may well say is both the best and the worst.*
—PLINY THE ELDER

About twenty years ago a friend of ours who leads a fairly exotic life staggered into our clinic and flopped onto an exam table. He was as sick as a dog. He had been involved in a tempestuous relationship with a young woman who had recently acquired a small pig as a pet; shortly after its acquisition, our friend fell ill. His fever was over 103, he had been vomiting violently, and he had horrendous diarrhea—and he was convinced that somehow his girlfriend's pig was at the bottom of his misery. We drew blood for a comprehensive lab evaluation, and when the results came back they showed the classic signs of a viral illness, with everything else looking pretty much normal except his serum iron (actual blood levels of iron), which was so low that it was almost nonexistent. We scratched our heads over this low blood iron value and turned to the medical books to see if we could find any reason for this strange lab result. We didn't find anything about a low iron level associated with a viral infection, but we did find a mention of a transmissible virus of baby pigs that had symptoms much like those of our friend, confirming his suspicions. Our patient didn't have any of the other symptoms of iron deficiency, his red blood cell counts were all okay, so we did as all physicians should do when confronted with a lab value that doesn't make sense: we repeated it. It was almost a month later that we were able to corral our friend to come in for his blood draw. (By that time, he had made a complete recovery and had abandoned his former heartthrob—whom he took to calling the "pig woman"—to search for an inamorata with less agricultural inclination in her choice of pets.) This time when his lab result came back, everything was perfectly normal, including his serum iron. In the intervening years, we've learned why our friend's iron levels plummeted while he was under pig virus attack; it turns out that his prehistoric immune system was fighting back. Shortly you'll see how, but first let's look at iron itself.

Iron is absolutely essential for life. Without it we couldn't make the red blood cells necessary to transfer oxygen to the tissues or assemble the proteins we need to repair the wear and tear of daily living. We wouldn't be able to make functional enzymes, and many of our hormones wouldn't work properly. We couldn't synthesize DNA, and cell replication would be impossible. Our immune systems would be severely compromised, leaving us vulnerable to all kinds of infections. Even our fat-burning ability would be slowed because iron is required for the synthesis of carnitine, the molecule that ferries fat into the mitochondria for burning.

As essential as iron is to us, it is every bit as crucial to the rest of the earth's living creatures, including the microbes that sometimes make our lives miserable. Bacteria, for example, require iron to reproduce, and unless they can multiply, bacteria are harmless. As a first line of defense most living creatures have evolved the ability to withdraw iron from the circulation and sequester it away, making it unavailable to these microscopic invaders. For example, all the iron in an egg (more, by the way, than is in a piece of steak of equivalent weight) is contained in the yolk, where it can nourish the growing and developing chick. Although the shell seems solid, it is actually somewhat porous and doesn't effectively prevent the penetration of bacteria. But eggs stay fresh for a long time because the egg white contains no iron and is loaded with a substance called conalbumin that binds iron tightly and withholds it from any bacteria that might make it through the shell. Robbed of a ready source of the iron crucial to their survival, the bacteria die.

Compared to cow's milk, human breast milk contains ten times the amount of an iron-binding protein called lactoferrin and about one-half the amount of iron. The iron binding of lactoferrin coupled with the reduced iron content of breast milk wards off infections by denying the bacteria their crucial iron supply.[1] As a consequence, breast-fed babies have a lower incidence of infection than do bottle-fed babies, particularly those placed on iron-fortified formulas, both because of the lower iron content and added iron-binding capacity of breast milk and the protective antibodies and essential fats that pass to the infant in the mother's milk. And studies have shown that babies living under conditions of poor sanitation who are fed cow's milk from a bottle have a five times greater rate of mortality than breast-fed babies living under the same conditions. Even bottle-fed infants raised in areas with good sanitation have greater rates of mortality than those fed at the breast.

Since invading microbes need iron to replicate, one way the body can defend against infection is by lowering iron levels in the blood. Scientists have demonstrated that the presence of any rapidly dividing cell—whether bacteria, virus, cancer cell (we will address iron and cancer in due course), or parasite—causes the body to pull iron out of the circulation and hide it away. Although we didn't realize it at the time, this is what happened to our friend. His severe viral infection drove his body to sequester his iron in an effort to prevent the viruses from multiplying, accounting for the greatly lowered iron levels we found in his blood.[2]

The tendency for the body to sequester iron when under at-

1. Some infant formula preparations contain up to thirty times more iron than breast milk, without the added protection of more iron-binding protein.

2. A classic study (G. Cartwright and G. R. Lee, "The Anaemia of Chronic Disorders," *British Journal of Haematology* 21 [1971]: 147–152) published almost thirty years ago showed that the average iron values in healthy subjects were over three times as high as the average values in individuals with active infection.

tack has been overlooked with disastrous consequences by well-meaning health workers in underdeveloped areas. People—especially children—in Third World countries are often found to have lower serum iron levels, which on a superficial evaluation can appear to be iron-deficiency anemia. But appearances can be misleading. Often, because of their lack of proper sanitation and clean food and water, these individuals are riddled with parasites and bacterial infections, and their bodies have hidden away much of their iron in an effort to defend themselves. In addition, their protein-deficient diet makes it difficult for them to transport iron safely in their blood because the body must have sufficient protein to make the molecule called transferrin that keeps iron in the bloodstream hidden from microbes. In the past, physicians, nurses, and other health-care personnel have treated these individuals for what appeared to be severe iron-deficiency anemia[3] by giving them injections of iron (the proper treatment for severe iron deficiency) only to see their patients develop overwhelming infections and in some cases even die. Because they didn't have sufficient protein to make the transferrin necessary to safely bind the injected iron, it could then circulate free in their blood, providing a nutrient bounty for the rapidly multiplying parasites and/or bacteria that subsequently sickened or killed them.

Ideally, as far as our immunity is concerned, we would like to have enough iron to permit optimal functioning of our own immune system, yet not enough to be readily accessible to invading microorganisms. But the role of iron as an immune enhancer and a sort of antibiotic–anti-parasitic agent is not the whole story. Iron has a Goldilocks-and-the-Three-Bears quality in other areas of health. You don't want to have too much and you don't want to have too little. You want to have just the right amount. Let's look at what happens when you don't have enough and you have iron-deficiency anemia or, as the old Geritol commercials used to say, "iron-poor blood."

---

3. Third World residents often do have anemia because of their parasitic disease. On the one hand they are losing blood to the parasites, while on the other they are sequestering iron to ward off the parasites. The best way to treat these individuals is to treat their parasites and improve their sanitation. With a good diet their iron will take care of itself.

The Myth of Iron-Poor Blood

Anyone who grew up in the 1950s and 1960s as we did re-members well the commercials for Geritol that inundated the television airwaves. Recall this one for example:

A smiling husband enters his home, where he is dismayed by the sight of his wife. She is in curlers, tired-looking and leaning against the doorway. Moreover, the kitchen appears to have been untouched for some time, being strewn with unwashed pots and pans. The husband, feigning anger, draws a pistol from his jacket and fires it at his now apprehensive wife. From the pistol emerges a flag reading "Iron-poor tired blood? Try Geri-tol." A card reading "later" appears on the television screen, followed by the same setting but with remarkable differences. The household is spotless. The haggard-looking woman seen at the beginning of the commercial now is attractively coiffed and made up, and in the wording of the script for this commercial, "garbed in a slinky gown." Her husband enters to find her so attired and posing against the piano with a "come hither" look and a rose in her mouth. She literally sweeps her husband off his feet by embracing him passionately and enthusiastically, as the commercial ends with his saying, "My wife . . . I think I'll keep her!" The words "Feel stronger fast" appeared on the screen, and the audio portion of the commercial advised the viewer, "If you're tired because of iron-poor blood, Geritol can help *you* feel stronger fast. Maybe not *this* fast. But fast.[4]

Iron-deficiency anemia, or iron-poor blood, is the "not enough" part of the iron story. Millions of people go to their doc-tors each year with the complaint of fatigue, and a large portion of these millions of people go away with a prescription for an iron supplement. The first diagnosis that leaps to the minds of most physicians when presented with a patient complaining of tiredness

---

4. A description of a television commercial in the court records of a false-advertis-ing suit brought by the Federal Trade Commission against the J. B. Williams Company, the makers of Geritol, as quoted in *Iron and Your Heart,* by Randall B. Lauffer, Ph.D. (New York: St. Martin's Press, 1991).

and fatigue, especially if that patient is a female, is iron-deficiency anemia. Most doctors will draw some blood and check for a hemoglobin level, a measure of iron in the red blood cells. If the hemoglobin comes back a little low, or sometimes even on the slightly low side of normal, many physicians prescribe iron supplements in one of the many varieties available. Although most physicians don't routinely prescribe medications without justification, a less cautious approach is often the norm with iron, because their thinking is that even if the problem isn't really anemia, it won't do any harm to give a little iron and see what happens. But as we shall see, this isn't always the case. Once you understand how the body handles iron, you'll easily see the folly and sometimes downright danger of this approach.

The Iron We Eat

Iron is present in the diet in two forms: as heme iron and nonheme iron. Heme iron represents about 40 percent of the iron in meat, especially red meat, whereas virtually all of the iron in foods of plant origin is the nonheme variety. A typical mixed American meal contains around 10 to 20 mg of total iron, of which about 10 percent is heme iron. In normal circumstances, we absorb only about 10 percent of this iron from our food as it makes its way through the small intestine. Enterocytes, which are the cells lining the inside of the intestinal tract, absorb the iron from the digesting food as it passes by. These enterocytes function basically as way stations for the iron, which is either going to go on through the enterocytes and into the body or back into the intestine, depending upon the body's need at the moment. If the body is short on iron, then the enterocytes package the iron into storage molecules called ferritin and ship them into the circulation. If the body has plenty of iron on board, then most of the iron just hangs around in the enterocyte until it sloughs off into the interior of the intestine which happens about every four or five days or so, and makes its way out with the stool. The body can regulate its iron content by adjusting how much it takes in through the intestine, but it's not a totally foolproof method.

Various components of the foods we eat can in some measure

override the control exerted by the intestinal lining, and the two types of iron themselves make a difference. For instance, the body absorbs heme iron much more readily than nonheme iron, and some components of the heme iron even enhance the absorption of the nonheme iron as well. Vitamin C increases the absorption of nonheme iron by a factor of four; fructose and certain amino acids do, too. Oxalates, phytates, and tannates—all from plant sources—inhibit iron absorption. Most of the enhancers and inhibitors affect the nonheme iron, making absorption of iron unpredictable. The actual amount of iron absorbed can vary as much as tenfold, and it's often easy to absorb more iron than we really need to keep in balance. It's normal to lose about 1 to 2 mg or so of iron a day through sweat, urine, the sloughing of skin, nails, and hair, and the loss of the intestinal cells that shed back into the bowel, so if the system worked flawlessly and we absorbed 10 percent of the 10 to 20 mg we take in through the diet, we would stay in iron balance, neither gaining or losing. But, what if the system doesn't always work flawlessly? What if we absorb too much?

How does the body get rid of excess iron? The short answer is it doesn't. If we absorb more from our diets than we get rid of in our normal daily minuscule losses, we begin to accumulate iron. Other than by trying to slow down the absorption, we don't have a mechanism to limit the amount of iron we can store in our tissues. And to make matters worse, the human body is a real tightwad where iron is concerned. We recycle all our old iron and reuse it again and again. Most of our iron is the hemoglobin of the red blood cells, where it binds with oxygen and, in essence, allows us to breathe, and when these red blood cells wear out, which they do every 120 days or so, the body carefully extracts the iron that is in them and recycles it for making new red blood cells or stores it away for later use. None of it is gotten rid of. Even if more iron keeps on coming in, the body just keeps packing it away. It doesn't even *try* to get rid of it; rather, it stuffs and crams it away into the tissues, especially into glandular tissues, where it can cause significant problems, sometimes with disastrous consequences.

Why would nature have endowed us with the ability to store,

store, store iron but not the ability to ditch it when we get too much? No one knows for sure, but we have a pretty good theory. And guess what? It involves looking through the lens of human evolution at the lives of our prehistoric ancestors.

The Ancestral Iron Wars

During our evolution as humans we got plenty of meat to eat. Meat contains about 40 percent heme iron, which is the easiest iron to absorb, and it contains the amino acids that help the absorption of the other 60 percent of nonheme iron. The roots, shoots, berries, and nuts that supplemented the ancient diet contain vitamin C, which enhances the absorption of the nonheme iron in these foods and in the nonheme portion of meat. Early humans didn't have to worry about the many inhibitors of iron absorption because grains hadn't come on the nutritional scene yet, loaded with their phytates that prevent absorption; nor was there coffee or tea, containing iron-absorption-inhibiting tannins. In other words, back then iron was plentiful and easy to absorb. Given these circumstances it would seem that the Paleolithic life was one guaranteed to cause iron overload and that through the millennia our ancestors must have evolved a strategy to get rid of it. But they didn't. Why not?

After spending a lot of time thinking about this paradox and about the differences between life then and life now, the answer finally dawned on us: our ancestors all had parasites, and it was the blood-draining parasites that prevented iron overload. We rushed to the medical library and started doing searches for articles on contemporary hunter-gatherer societies. We found a couple of dozen studies of diverse populations varying in their geographic locations from Arctic Eskimos to tribes deep in South America and Africa, and voilà!—each and every one of these groups of people was infested with parasites, from malaria to ringworm to amebae to tapeworms. If these populations living a hunter-gatherer existence today all have parasites, then it stands to reason that our ancestors thousands of years ago had them, too.

The world teems with a wide variety of parasites, most of them

disgusting, and all of them needing iron to live and reproduce—
and the only place they can get it is from their hosts. It doesn't
matter if they are flukes (worms living in the blood) or worms
attached to the walls of the intestines or worms crawling beneath
the skin, they all need iron, and our ancient predecessors fought
them for it. Viewed in this way it makes perfect sense that we
didn't develop a mechanism to get rid of excess iron, because
we didn't need to; our parasitic "friends" did it for us. What we
needed was the ability to tenaciously hang on to every molecule
of iron we could get—and the ability to hide it from invaders
when necessary.

It's interesting to note that when anthropologists study the
remains of ancient populations, they find that prehistoric hunters
had almost no evidence of iron deficiency, whereas it was widespread in their agricultural descendants.[5] If you think about it, it's
easy to see why. The hunters lived in small bands and were usually
on the move in search of game. When they found it, they got a lot
of iron. Agriculturists, on the other hand, didn't move around
because they were tied to their land, and, sanitation being what it
must have been in those times, they were more prone to be heavily infested with parasites and other microorganisms looking for
iron. To compound their problem, they ate a grain-based diet that
was loaded with phytates and oxalates that prevented maximal
absorption of iron. So they had the triple whammy of not as much
iron intake as the hunters, more parasites, and food filled with
substances that inhibited the absorption of what little iron they
ate. It's no wonder they were all iron deficient and sickly.

As hunters we lived in a sort of symbiosis—a semipeaceful
coexistence—with parasites; as agriculturists we fought mostly a
losing battle. But in either case we didn't have to worry about
storing too much iron, at least not until John Snow came along.
John Snow was a society physician in London in the mid 1800s

5. Iron-deficiency anemia produces changes in the bones, notably a moth-eaten
appearance on the top of the skull called porotic hyperostosis and the same changes in
the upper part of the eye socket called cribra orbitalia. When anthropologists find skeletal remains of ancient populations with these signs, which are common in the skulls of
agriculturalists and almost nonexistent in those of hunters, they know these peoples
were iron deficient.

who, among his other accomplishments, attended the births of Queen Victoria's daughters and founded a new medical discipline. When a deadly outbreak of cholera that had swept through Europe killing thousands hit London in 1845, Snow, like the rest of London's physicians, treated his share of cholera patients. During this outbreak he got the notion that since cholera was a disease of horrendous diarrhea, it might be transmitted from infected sewage—which, it turns out, is correct. What made his thinking astounding is that it took place years before the great German scientist Robert Koch proved that microbes cause disease. Snow tracked down a large number of households that were stricken with cholera and found that the vast majority of them got their water from one of the two water companies servicing the residents of London. He then checked out a number of families who were getting their water from the other company and discovered that almost none of them had been infected. When he tracked down the sources of the water from both companies he found that although both got their water from the river Thames, the one providing service to the families infected with cholera got its water just downstream from the main sewage dump, whereas the other drew its water upstream. Snow published his findings in 1855 and launched the science of epidemiology, the study of disease patterns. Thanks to the work of John Snow and others who followed, we now enjoy clean drinking water and relatively germ-free food in most of the Western world. We only hear about cholera, dysentery, and a host of other awful diseases in news stories about Third World countries, where poor sanitation and crowded living conditions are the norm, or when natural disasters disrupt our sanitation systems. Aside from the pinworms we may have had as kids, most of us have probably never had a serious parasitic infection. But, alas, it seems that all medical triumphs come at a cost, and the eradication of parasites was no exception. Our bodies, molded by millennia of fighting for iron, conserve iron and hang on to it through thick and thin, and never give a thought to getting rid of it. We now find ourselves with no indwelling parasites and more iron than we know what to do with.

Is Anemia Then Only a Disease of Ancient Farmers?

Does this mean that we can never become anemic because we have no way of getting rid of excess iron? No, not at all. It just means that anemia is much less common than previously thought. And we do have a way of getting rid of excess iron. Its called bleeding. You probably think of bleeding as in a cut or other trauma, which certainly can cause a loss of iron, but for most of us, trauma is an infrequent occurrence in our modern world. Premenopausal women lose blood every month during their menstrual periods and are the group most likely to experience iron-deficiency anemia. But because the body clings to iron so tenaciously, true iron-deficiency anemia occurs relatively infrequently even in menstruating women. Menstrual blood loss accounts for only about 0.6 mg of iron loss per day,[6] which taken together with the normal 1 mg or so of usual daily loss, is still an amount easily replenished by the normal daily iron intake. And even if a particular woman's iron intake falls below this amount, her body will compensate by absorbing a greater percentage of the dietary iron traveling through. So if a woman consumes a normal diet, typical menstrual blood losses generally don't lead to anemia. Some women—especially teenage girls, many of whom may follow a near vegetarian diet—can develop iron-deficiency anemia if they don't eat enough iron-containing foods and have unusually heavy menstrual bleeding.

Bleeding from the digestive tract also commonly causes anemia. A number of diseases, such as esophagitis, gastritis, ulcers, stomach cancer, colon cancer, and a few others, cause bleeding into the digestive tract that passes out with the stool. Depending upon the severity and location of the bleeding, patients may or may not see this blood. Although it may be bright red and visible, often the bleeding is slow and occurring in such tiny amounts that

---

6. Averaged over a thirty-day month. The actual loss per day varies with the length of the cycle.

it can be identified only with a chemical test. This is the type of bleeding doctors look for when you provide a stool sample for a colon cancer test. Other times, mainly when the bleeding comes from the stomach, the stool appears black and sticky, like tar. In any case, bleeding in the digestive tract over a long period of time can deplete the body of iron and lead to anemia. In those who don't get their recommended annual checks for colon cancer, sometimes the first sign of this disease is anemia. This happened to one of our physician friends. He had an incredibly busy practice, and one day after a particularly exhausting procedure, he collapsed. His coworkers rushed him to the emergency room, where he was found to have severe iron-deficiency anemia. When a male has iron-deficiency anemia, the first thing you think of is gastrointestinal bleeding, which turned out to be the case with our friend. His bleeding, unfortunately, was caused by late-stage colon cancer, and he died a few months later in his mid fifties of a death that could have been prevented had he taken the same advice he gave to hundreds of his patients and gotten an annual test for blood in the stool. His sad story, which we will revisit later, will prove to be a cautionary tale about the perils of iron overload.

Once testing identifies the underlying cause of anemia, treatment should start to eradicate the cause. The anemia itself responds to the administration of iron, whether by pill, injection, or by increasing the intake of easily absorbable iron-rich foods such as red meat. The key point to remember is this: you should not take supplemental iron unless you are sure you are actually anemic and that your anemia stems from an iron deficiency. Most physicians use the measurement of the hemoglobin and the size of the red blood cells to determine anemia, an inaccurate method at best; a few look at the serum iron along with the hemoglobin, which is a little more accurate but not much. The only way to truly diagnose iron-deficiency anemia is to test the blood for levels of ferritin, the molecule that stores excess iron. Later in this chapter we will show you what to look for in your laboratory results to evaluate whether you have too little or too much iron. You're now familiar with the relatively uncommon problem of too little iron, so let's consider what happens when we get too much.

The Iron Man (or Woman) Rusteth

Despite the fact that we need it to live, iron is an incredibly dangerous substance that the body handles with kid gloves. Iron is a potent pro-oxidant. Pro-oxidants are the opposite of antioxidants. They are stimulators of free-radical formation. Iron is one of the most hazardous free-radical promoters we harbor in our bodies, and it is responsible for most of the tissue damage that occurs in heart attacks and stroke.

From the moment iron starts its trek through the gut, the body handles it delicately and with utmost respect for its fearsome potential for free-radical formation and tissue damage. Before enterocytes pull the iron in, they first wrap it in a protective cloak (a molecule called integrin), and then transfer the cloaked iron to a transport molecule (called mobilferrin). Flavonoids (antioxidants) shepherd the entire process to make sure the iron stays contained within its cloak and doesn't pop off a free radical or two on the way in. If the body needs iron, the mobilferrin then carries it through the interior of the intestinal cell and, via a process that is still poorly understood, hands it over to transferrin, the major iron-transport protein inside the body. This process accelerates if the body needs more iron, increasing the absorption and increasing the amount of iron delivered to the tissues. If the body has plenty of iron, the mobilferrin transfers most of its iron to a molecule inside the enterocyte called ferritin, the specialized storage protein evolved over the millennia of our development to tuck iron safely away within our cells and tissues. The enormous ferritin molecule, somewhat resembling a geodesic dome, usually holds about two thousand iron atoms in a nontoxic form similar to rust and keeps them from damaging the surrounding tissue. As part of their normal turnover these iron-rich enterocytes slough into the interior of the bowel, become part of the stool, and so leave the body.

The body quickly surrounds the iron from food that does get through the lining of the bowel into the circulation along with the iron from the breakdown of red blood cells, binding it tightly to transferrin, which serves to transport it safely along in the bloodstream, like a dangerous prisoner, keeping it from harming the tissues. Transferrin takes its captive iron to the bone marrow, where the body can use it to manufacture new red blood cells. Whatever it can't transfer to the forming red blood cells, it transports for storage in the spleen and/or liver, the bone marrow's partners in blood cell production. But the transferrin also carries excess iron to other tissues, especially glandular tissues such as the pancreas, thyroid, and gonads.

These iron-filled ferritin molecules can behave like little time bombs distributed throughout the body; as more of them accumulate they become collectively more and more dangerous. Nature designed the ferritin molecules to keep iron locked away like nuclear waste (which in a way it is, because free iron in the body initiates the production of free radicals in the same way that nuclear radiation does), letting it out only when necessary and then only with rigorous care. When the body needs iron, ferritin releases it through tiny openings in its structure, placing it directly into the custody of transferrin to be taken where it is needed. As long as ferritin does its job of sequestering the iron, everything is okay, but just as with nuclear power plants, accidents happen. And just as with nuclear power plants, when accidents happen they can be disastrous.

Iron on the Loose

What kind of accidents are we talking about? Well, let's look at a heart attack for example. Without iron in the picture, most heart attacks would resolve pretty quickly without much damage. But since we do have stored iron and sometimes a lot of it—heart tissue, in fact, has a greater affinity for iron than many other tissues do—that isn't the case. When a clot lodges in a coronary artery or a piece of plaque breaks off and travels downstream to a narrower part of the artery, it lodges and either stops or decreases blood flow to points beyond. All the tissues that get their blood from that artery are suddenly deprived of the oxygen the blood carries. Deprived of oxygen, some cells in the downstream tissue start to die and break apart, damaging, among other things, ferritin molecules, which release their load of stored iron into the tissues, setting the stage for trouble. Indeed, it is when fresh new blood finally forces its way past the blockage and into the tissues that have been without oxygen that the real disaster occurs. When the oxygen-rich blood hits the free iron, an enormous free-radical explosion occurs, severely damaging the surrounding tissue, sometimes irreversibly. So, ironically, it's not really the lack of oxygen while the artery is blocked that causes the majority of the damage; it's the explosive iron-oxygen reaction that occurs in its wake. Physicians refer to this phenomenon as a reperfusion injury.

Stroke is another example of a reperfusion injury. The same thing happens in the brain that happens in the heart. In fact, some physicians refer to strokes as brain attacks. A clot lodges in a small artery in the brain, depriving the brain tissue downstream of oxygen. The lack of oxygen causes the ferritin to break down and release its iron, priming the tissues for a catastrophe. When the oxygenated blood pushes through the blockage and hits the tissues loaded with free iron, the resultant free-radical reaction devastates the brain tissue and causes all the symptoms that accompany a stroke.

We suspect that there are many other situations in which reperfusion injuries can occur that don't have the obvious immediate disastrous effects of a heart attack or a stroke. Let's say you are sitting on a hard chair waiting your turn at the department of motor vehicles. If your state is like ours, you could wait for a very long time. As you sit, the tissues in your rear end are under pressure and the arteries are squeezed, reducing blood flow to the area. Over time the reduced supply of oxygen to the area could cause the breakdown of ferritin molecules and the release of free iron into the tissues. When your name is finally called, you jump up, and fresh, oxygenated blood flows into the tissues of your derrière, and a reperfusion injury occurs. Now, granted, not a lot of iron is stored in your skeletal muscles and fat tissues compared to your heart muscle, so in all likelihood the damage is slight. But if you go throughout the day accumulating the free radicals from these many slight reperfusion injuries, you could consume a great deal of your antioxidant capacity in neutralizing them.

The line from the old Roger Miller song "Well, they tell me you're runnin' free . . ." is not something you want to hear about your iron. Iron running free in the tissues is disastrous because when combined with oxygen it can, and typically does, precipitate an enormous free-radical cascade that can brutally and permanently damage the surrounding tissue. Free iron can promote the formation of the hydroxyl radical, the most dangerous free radical of all because it can directly attack DNA, causing mutations and possibly the initiation of cancer. And, the more free iron loose in the tissues, the greater the potential for harm.

An Iron Sword Has Two Edges

Although the ability to hoard iron served our ancestors well, it has turned out to be a mixed blessing to us. We live in a time of iron plenty, and instead of worrying about not getting enough iron or having to fight parasites for it, many of us are now at the other extreme of the Goldilocks story: we have too much iron, in some cases, *way* too much. What we want is just the right amount.

Most Americans consume a diet that has plenty of iron in it, and, unfortunately, many of us eat foods that override the body's only mechanism to prevent excess iron accumulation: controlled absorption. Look at a typical fast-food meal and you'll see what we mean. If we analyze a meal consisting of a burger, fries, and a soft drink, we find that there are about 2.5 mg of iron in the beef patty along with 1.5 mg in the bun and almost 1 mg in the fries. Of the 2.5 mg in the beef patty only about 40 percent, or 1 mg, is heme iron; the remaining 1.5 mg is nonheme. All the iron in the "enriched" bun is nonheme, and an extremely easily absorbable nonheme at that. So we have 4 mg of nonheme iron, the least absorbable of the two types under normal circumstances, but here we're not under normal circumstances. The burger is consumed with a soft drink that nowadays is sweetened with high-fructose corn syrup, and fructose is one of those compounds that increases the rate of nonheme-iron absorption tremendously. The iron in the bun gets in easily on its own while the fructose in the soft drink enhances the absorption of the nonheme iron in the beef patty and the fries. So, instead of the normal 10 to 20 percent absorption of 0.5 to 1 mg of iron, we could get double that—1 to 2 mg, an amount equal to or exceeding our daily losses—in just this one meal. If we add a typical breakfast into the mix, we heap on even more iron. Let's say we have a bowl of Cheerios; that's another 4.5 mg of iron.[7] If we add a couple of pieces of toast or a bagel, we add an additional 1.5 mg. So with just a typical breakfast and lunch we take in 11 mg of nonheme iron of the easily absorbable variety and 1 mg of heme iron. Even with just 10 percent absorption, that gives us 1.1 mg, an amount that in most cases exceeds our daily losses. If, in addition to these meals, we take a basic, run-of-the-mill multivitamin supplement such as Centrum,[8] we get an additional 18 mg of easily absorbable iron along with whatever vitamin C the supplement contains, which makes the iron even more absorbable. Any other iron absorbed throughout the day is in excess and is packed away in ferritin.

A few extra milligrams here and there doesn't seem like a lot, but over a lifetime a few milligrams of excess iron per day begins to add up. The more iron we have stored, the greater potential we have for damage if that iron gets loose in the tissues. And indeed that's the case. A number of studies have shown that people with excess stored iron have more heart disease and stroke and greater rates of cancer. They also have a higher incidence of such glandular disorders as diabetes and hypothyroidism (sluggish thyroid).

Does Iron Loss Prevent Disease?

Males are the group at greatest risk for excess iron storage because they have no way to get rid of iron. Women, conversely, get rid of up to 18 mg of iron with each menstrual cycle and up to 500 mg with each childbirth. If you look at figure 8.1, a graph of the amount of iron stored over time, you can see that women accumulate very little until they reach menopause, at which point they rapidly catch up to men. The interesting point about this diagram is that it reflects not only iron storage but also the differ-

---

7. A bowl of Cheerios contains a typical amount of iron for a fortified breakfast cereal. If we choose a bowl of General Mills' Total or a bowl of Kellogg's Product 19, we get 18 mg of iron.

8. Centrum has one of the lowest iron contents among supplements. Some supplements contain up to 50 mg of iron; a prescription iron supplement could provide as much as 150 mg.

FIGURE 8.1

Age-Related Storage of Iron

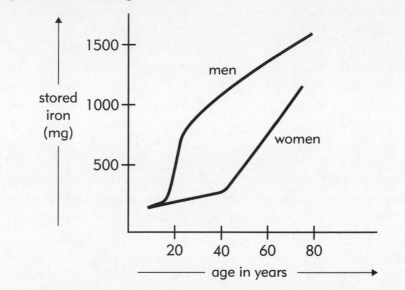

Adapted from J. D. Cook, C. A. Finch, and N. J. Smith, *Blood* 48 (1976): 449–455.

ence in heart disease between the two groups. It is well known that women don't have much heart disease to speak of until they are beyond menopause, whereas men begin to have heart attacks as early as their late twenties in some cases. As women go beyond menopause, however, they rapidly find themselves on the same mortality tables with males. Why?

Many people, most physicians included, believe the estrogen theory explains the gender disparity in the incidence of heart disease. This theory holds that since women produce large amounts of estrogen before menopause and very little after, estrogen somehow protects against heart disease. Based on this theory, researchers gave estrogen to men who were at risk for heart disease only to discover to their surprise that these men developed even more heart attacks: clearly estrogen did not protect *them*. Investigators in a twenty-four year study of 2,873 women found that, as expected, they developed an increased risk for heart disease within just a couple of years of menopause. Was estrogen their protector during the premenopausal years? Probably not. When the researchers compared the rates of heart disease of women who had undergone hysterectomies that removed only the uterus to the rates of women who had had their estrogen-producing ovaries removed along with their uterus, the results told the tale. If estrogen were truly protective, those women who lost only their uterus would have been protected while those women who lost their ovaries (and the presumptive protection of estrogen) would have begun to develop heart disease. What the researchers found, however, was that both groups began to develop heart disease at greater rates than premenopausal women. These findings imply that it is the loss of the uterus that increases the risk for heart disease, not the loss of the ovaries. Since the ovaries produce estrogen and the uterus loses blood, it appears that blood loss is more important than the output of estrogen, at least as far as heart disease is concerned.

Another finding that casts doubt on the estrogen theory is that women who have taken oral contraceptives (birth control pills) have a three-to-four-times higher risk for developing heart disease than those who haven't. Why? No one knows for sure, but studies have shown that women who use these medications have shorter menstrual periods with lighter blood flow, leading to decreased iron loss and the increased potential for iron storage.

The idea of premenopausal blood loss protecting against heart disease is just one of many observations that begin to make sense when viewed from the perspective of iron storage. For example, it's long been known that native populations living in Africa have almost no heart disease. Denis Burkett, who lived with and studied these peoples for many years, attributed their resistance to heart disease to their intake of large amounts of fiber. In fact, Burkett's writings almost single-handedly launched the fiber craze that was prevalent a few years ago and that still persists. All the studies that have been done to date show at most a slight protective effect of fiber but nothing that would come even close to conferring the degree of protection that these African people have. If it has to be something other than fiber, then how about iron? As we discussed earlier, most of these people have parasitic infections, and if they eat primarily grain-based diets, we can expect much of their dietary iron to be bound up with the phytates in grain, making it difficult to absorb. We believe their low levels of iron, not their fiber intake, protect them, although, admittedly, the grain does inhibit the absorption, so it is secondarily responsible—but not for the reasons everyone has suspected.

Take aspirin, we're told, to prevent heart disease. Research theorizes that aspirin inhibits platelet aggregation and blood clot formation thought to initiate a heart attack. Could be, but aspirin also causes a low level of gastrointestinal bleeding that, over time, can approximate the loss of blood from normal menstruation. Perhaps the real protective effect of aspirin is in the iron loss it causes, not the clot formation it inhibits. More likely, it is a combination of the two.

Research has also shown that the regular consumption of fish oil loaded with omega-3 fatty acids protects against heart disease. Once again, the mechanism for this protection hasn't been fully explained. There is no doubt that fish oil acts as an antiarrhythmic agent, stabilizing the heart tissue against erratic beating. And there is no doubt that fish oil, like aspirin, inhibits platelet aggregation. And there is likewise no doubt that fish oil, again like aspirin, causes blood thinning, which is frequently accompanied by slight gastrointestinal bleeding. The bleeding may be too slight to even be noticed, but it's there nevertheless. Could a part of fish oil's protective benefit be that it, too, causes those who consume it regularly to lose iron?

Iron and Cancer

Scientists have long known that iron in the presence of oxygen behaves as a carcinogen, a cancer-causing substance. What makes the iron-oxygen combination so deadly is that it creates the incredibly dangerous hydroxyl free radical. (See also chapter 5, "Antioxidant Use and Abuse.") The hydroxyl radical attacks the DNA molecule, causing genetic mutations that can lead to the formation of cancerous cells. But iron doesn't stop there. Iron itself becomes a food for the cancer. In order for cancer cells to divide rapidly they need to manufacture DNA for the new cells, a process that involves a key iron-containing enzyme. If the body has a lot of iron available, the tumor can grow rapidly. Remember, one of our body's defenses against rapidly multiplying cells is to withhold iron—that's why most people diagnosed with cancer will be found to have low blood iron levels. If we have Goldilocks's "just right" amount of iron, we can lock most of it away in ferritin to deprive the growing cancer of the iron it desperately needs and perhaps slow it down enough for our immune system to destroy it.

Have studies shown that people with elevated iron storage (high ferritin levels) develop more cancer? Indeed they have. One large study published in the *New England Journal of Medicine*[9] showed that men with higher ferritin levels developed lung, colon, bladder, and esophageal cancers at an increased rate compared to those with lower ferritin levels. The relationship between iron storage and cancer in women was inconclusive in this study, but the authors pointed out that the women with the highest levels of stored iron appeared to have the most cancer. There is no question that excess iron stored in the liver leads to a much greater incidence of cancer in that organ. Some studies have shown that people with hereditary hemochromatosis, a genetic disease of greatly increased iron storage, have liver cancer at over two hundred times the rate of the normal population. Why liver cancer specifically? Because when we store too much iron, a substantial portion of it gets tucked away into the liver; development of any other type of liver disorder, such as hepatitis or cirrhosis, can then damage the ferritin storage molecules, break them down, and release their stored iron. Once released into the liver tissue, the free iron generates the hydroxyl radical that can cause mutations and cancer formation. While we were writing this chapter a lead article appeared in the *New England Journal of Medicine* documenting that the incidence of liver cancer in the United States has *risen by 70 percent* over the past twenty years. Maybe the government-mandated-iron-fortification-of-bread-and-cereals chicken has come home to roost as a contributing factor in this dramatic rise.

You'll likely have read or heard that eating red meat (the best source of heme iron) causes colon cancer. So does it? It's a ques-

---

9. R. G. Stevens et al., "Body Iron Stores and the Risk of Cancer," *New England Journal of Medicine* 319, no. 16 (1988): 1047–1052.

tion we routinely get from audiences when we speak. Although the connection has been suggested by some epidemiological studies (the kind not worth much, remember; see page xxiv), there's never been hard clinical evidence proving that this is the case. In fact, the associations with colon cancer are much stronger for lack of natural vitamin D (see chapter 10, "Sunshine Superman") and as a component of the insulin-resistance metabolic syndrome than for meat-eating. Red meat is the best dietary source of zinc, a mineral critical for immune health; coenzyme Q10, a potent antioxidant to defend against the "rusting" effects of free iron; and sulfur-containing amino acids necessary for the body's own powerful free-radical scavenger, glutathione peroxidase, important protection against DNA damage by the hydroxyl radical. From that standpoint, meat serves as the *protector* against colon cancer, not the promoter, as research published in the *British Medical Journal* (August 1999) clearly seems to prove.

And while we're on that subject, let's look at one other advantage of not having a large amount of stored iron. Remember our physician friend who died from advanced colon cancer? He found out that he had this cancer when he became so anemic from blood loss from the tumor that he passed out. Since he was a middle-aged male, we can safely assume that he had plenty of stored iron when his cancer started growing, so it took a long time for the cancer to deplete him of his iron stores to the point that he became seriously anemic. Let's suppose that he hadn't had a ton of excess iron stored; let's assume that he had had just the right amount in storage. On a simple blood test, he would have been found to be anemic much earlier in the course of his disease and would probably have been diagnosed long before his cancer had reached an advanced and untreatable stage. He might still be alive today, because colon cancer is curable if detected early enough.

How Do I Know If I've Got Too Much Iron?

If you have any of the disorders of the Metabolic Insulin-Resistance Syndrome, you should ask your physician to order a test to detect excess stored iron. The best laboratory test you can get to determine your stored iron levels is a serum ferritin test.

It's a simple blood test that measures the amount of empty ferritin "storage containers" that seep into the blood. Researchers have been able to correlate the amount of this empty ferritin in the blood with the actual amount of iron stored in the tissues of the body; the ratio is 1:10. To determine your total stored iron in milligrams all you need to do is to multiply the units of ferritin on your lab report by ten. (Serum ferritin is measured in a couple of different ways depending upon the lab involved: as units of nanograms per milliliter or as micrograms per liter of serum, which are different ways of saying the same thing.) So, for example, if your ferritin level is 100, then that 100 units times 10 means that you have 1,000 mg (or 1 gram) of iron stashed away.

How much iron should you have in storage? Probably around 500 mg or a little less, which corresponds to a serum ferritin of 50 or lower. For safety (in case you should suffer a major trauma with significant blood loss, for instance), you want to have at least 150 mg of stored iron (a ferritin of 15), and should have no less than 100 mg (a ferritin of 10). A ferritin of 10 or lower is an indication of true iron-deficiency anemia and should be treated by a physician.

Getting Rid of Your Iron

If your ferritin level is 100 or over, you probably have much more iron than you need, and you should consider getting rid of some. How do you do that? It's easy. In fact, of all the medical treatments or therapies you could possibly undergo, the treatment for excess iron is the least demanding and the least expensive. How do you get rid of your excess iron? The simplest way is to bleed, and the easiest and most charitable way to do that is to call the Red Cross, set up an appointment, and donate. They'll be happy to relieve you of some of your iron. What's excess to you could save a life.

Unless you have hereditary hemochromatosis (which we will address later), each time you give a unit of blood you should, *in theory,* reduce your iron stores by about 200 to 250 mg (women are at the lower end of the scale; men at the higher), or your ferritin levels by 20 to 25 units based on the amount of iron a unit of blood contains. At one donation every two months (the Red Cross requires a minimum two-month wait between blood donations), it would take you a little over two years to get rid of your excess iron. We say in theory, however, because in reality you'll probably get rid of your excess iron much more quickly.

A unit of blood contains roughly 250 mg of iron, representing a ferritin of 25. In theory, each unit of blood you give should reduce your ferritin by around 25 units, but in the excess iron storage associated with the Metabolic Syndrome, it usually reduces it by much more. As part of the standard evaluation in our clinic, we check ferritin levels on each of our patients. Since most of our patients are middle aged and have had plenty of time to store a fair amount of iron, it's not unusual for us to discover ferritin levels in the 300 to 500 range and sometimes even higher. We counsel these patients to give blood. When we see them again and recheck their ferritin levels, we usually find that if they have given blood just once, they have reduced their ferritin by anywhere from 100 to 200 units, not the 25 units that we would expect. As ferritin levels drop closer to the 40 to 50 level that is our goal, we find that each donation comes closer to bringing about the expected 25-unit decrease. In a person with a ferritin of 400, we would typically see the level drop to around 250 after the first donation, then to 125 after the second. The third donation would bring it down to the 75 level, and the fourth down to the ideal level of 50 units. So, instead of taking fourteen donations spread out over more than two years, it takes only four donations over eight months to bring iron stores to a safe level (see table 8.1). Why is this? We don't know for sure. Our guess is that the ferritin measurement is much more accurate in the lower ranges, at least in patients without the genetic form of excess iron storage, hereditary hemochromatosis. In patients with hemochromatosis, the ferritin falls at the 25-units-per-donation rate no matter what the starting ferritin. The iron storage in this serious hereditary disorder differs from the accumulation seen in most people. Let's see how.

Hereditary Hemochromatosis

Hereditary hemochromatosis is an inherited disorder of iron absorption that is one of the most common genetic diseases found

TABLE 8.1

Approximate Donations Needed to Reduce Stored Iron

FERRITIN LEVEL	NUMBER OF DONATIONS
75 to 100	1
<200	2
<300	3
<400	4
<500	5
<600	6

After each donation, wait at least two months, then recheck ferritin level. Sometimes the levels will drop even faster and fewer donations will be needed. Continue to donate until your level is near 50.

in our population. Researchers estimate that as many as one in ten to twenty people carries the gene for hemochromatosis, and that one in four hundred has both genes, the condition necessary for the full-blown syndrome. Victims of hemochromatosis don't have the ability to regulate the absorption of iron in the intestine, and, consequently, they absorb large amounts of iron throughout their lives. Despite their propensity to absorb iron easily they, like people without the disease, have no built-in way to get rid of their stored iron. As these people reach middle age they have accumulated an enormous amount of iron, sometimes as much as 30 to 40 grams (and sometimes even higher!), which translates into a ferritin level of 3,000 to 4,000.

The tremendous amounts of iron these individuals store gets packed away in their livers, hearts, joints, gonads, pancreases, adrenals, thyroid glands, and skin, putting them at risk for a whole host of diseases. Many of these people develop cirrhosis of the liver and have an almost two-hundred-fold increased risk of developing liver cancer; they develop a multitude of glandular disorders such as diabetes, hypothyroidism (sluggish thyroid), and hypogonadism (loss of libido and other sexual dysfunctions). Since the iron accumulates in the heart, these people are at risk for certain types of heart disease called restrictive or congestive cardiomyopathies, which, if untreated, can lead to heart failure.

The most common symptoms of hemochromatosis, found in

almost 90 percent of the cases when first presenting for treatment, are weakness and fatigue. Unfortunately, iron-deficiency anemia causes these same symptoms, and the medical literature is filled with cases in which hapless hemochromatosis patients were actually treated with iron supplements. In fact, it is estimated that hemochromatosis victims typically consult more than five physicians over a period of around five years before they finally get a correct diagnosis and can begin treatment.[10] Other less common symptoms include abdominal pain, joint pain, loss of libido, impotence, menstrual irregularities, and some vague neurological symptoms—not one of which points specifically to hemochromatosis.

Individuals with hemochromatosis who are undiagnosed and untreated have markedly shortened life spans. But the good news is that with early diagnosis and treatment, victims of hemochromatosis can live a normal life free of the many pathological developments they would otherwise suffer. How is hemochromatosis treated? By giving blood, and lots of it. People newly diagnosed with hemochromatosis typically give blood weekly until their ferritin levels begin to fall. As they get rid of their excess iron, their blood-letting frequency lessens, but they have to make regular blood donation a part of their lives. And as long as they do, they remain free of the iron-related disorders they would otherwise develop.

An exceptionally high ferritin reading suggests the possibility of hereditary hemochromatosis, and the testing physician needs to perform several additional measurements to differentiate simple metabolic iron storage (more about which shortly) from the hereditary form.

It's vital for you to know if you have hemochromatosis so that you can begin giving blood immediately, and, since hemochromatosis is an inherited disorder, so that you can make sure that all your relatives are evaluated and the ones affected can also begin taking steps to remove their iron. You should avoid alcoholic beverages and never take vitamin C supplements, as both

---

10. Part of the reason for this is that most medical schools emphasize the treatment of anemia while relegating hemochromatosis to the status of a rare disease.

will markedly increase your absorption of iron. And you ought to avoid cooking in iron pots because the iron can leach into the food, especially if it is acidic, and then this iron can leach into you. If you take these few precautions, monitor your blood iron levels regularly, and give blood as often as needed to keep your ferritin levels down, you will have the same life expectancy as someone without hemochromatosis.

While relatively rare, hemochromatosis still affects a large number of people, but the iron storage associated with the Metabolic Insulin-Resistance Syndrome affects a vastly larger number of people, potentially as many as 75 percent of adults in this country.

Iron and the Metabolic Syndrome

In our clinical practice we have noticed that most of our patients with insulin resistance have elevated ferritin levels in varying degrees. A number of medical researchers throughout the world have observed the same phenomenon and published papers linking excess iron storage to the Metabolic Syndrome. A group of French researchers studied this issue in depth and published their findings in the British medical journal *The Lancet* a couple of years ago.[11] They compared a group of patients who had greatly elevated ferritin levels (an average of 566 micrograms/liter) and many of the symptoms of the Metabolic Syndrome (hypertension, obesity, diabetes, and so on) but no indication of hereditary hemochromatosis to a group of patients with similar ferritin readings who did have hemochromatosis. They treated both groups of patients by phlebotomy (blood letting) and discovered the same thing we have seen repeatedly in our clinic: patients with iron overload associated with the Metabolic Syndrome reduce their ferritin levels much more quickly than those with hemochromatosis.

At this point no one knows for sure why people with the Metabolic Syndrome tend to accumulate iron more readily than people

---

11. R. Moirand et al., "A New Syndrome of Liver Iron Overload with Normal Transferrin Saturation," *Lancet* 349, no. 9045 (1997): 95–97.

without it. We have our own theory, which is that people with insulin resistance and hyperinsulinemia consume a lot of carbohydrates. The primary high-carbohydrate foods that people eat are breads and cereals, both of which are heavily fortified with iron. Couple this diet high in easily absorbable iron with the main sweetener in use today—high-fructose corn syrup, an enhancer of iron absorption—and you've got a surefire way to raise ferritin levels.

Breaking Out of the Iron Cage

While the change to a *Protein Power LifePlan* diet will confer enormous health benefits and help to slow the further accumulation of iron, if you have an elevated ferritin level, you need to give blood to get it down. By doing so, you'll go a long way toward reducing your risk for some pretty sinister diseases—and you will achieve some immediate benefits as well. Let us show you what we mean.

Free iron in the tissues stimulates the production of free radicals; enough stored iron in the glandular tissues often prevents the glandular cells from performing their functions efficiently. For example, if the body packs away a lot of iron in the thyroid gland, often the thyroid cells won't be able to function as they should. In most cases the thyroid will continue to do its job, but just not quite as efficiently as it used to. People with this problem may feel a little sluggish, have skin that is a little drier than they would like, note some roughness to the elbows and knees, and be a little cold intolerant, but they won't develop an overt case of hypothyroidism. In fact, their thyroid tests are probably pretty normal. As we've seen more times than we can count, whenever these patients give blood, they feel better almost immediately, and more often than not, these symptoms of a marginally functional thyroid clear up.

The body often uses the pancreas as a storage bin for excess iron. The pancreas contains the beta cells that make insulin, and often these cells don't function properly in the face of excess iron in the pancreas. In fact, in patients with hemochromatosis, the huge amount of iron in their pancreas often damages their beta cells to the extent that many of these patients quit producing insulin and develop insulin-dependent diabetes. We usually find an improvement in the glucose tolerance of our patients after they have reduced their iron levels. It's difficult to tell how much of their improvement comes from changing their diet and how much comes from reducing their iron, because they do both things simultaneously. A few studies, however, have shown that reducing stored iron does bring about improvement in glucose tolerance and insulin sensitivity.

Since the body often stores iron in the gonads and in the pituitary gland, patients with iron overload frequently have diminished sexual function. Both men and women lose their libido, and men sometimes become impotent and even develop breast enlargement and loss of body hair. In addition to a diminished libido, women can have menstrual problems of varying kinds: some may experience heavy bleeding, in others the bleeding may be scanty and unpredictable, and in both cases, the cycles may be irregular with missed periods; and, not uncommonly, these women may have difficulty becoming pregnant. All of these problems are routine in people with untreated hereditary hemochromatosis, but they are also common to a lesser extent in the iron overload associated with the Metabolic Insulin-Resistance Syndrome. In both cases blood donation solves the problem as long as patients begin treatment before the problems become irreversible. (And there's no sure measure of how long-standing the condition must be before permanent damage to the glands can occur.)

Some researchers and authors have developed programs to reduce iron that involve meticulously avoiding foods with significant iron content. We have found this to be a slow and ineffective way of reducing blood iron levels. A little back-of-the-envelope analysis shows how absurd this idea is. If you cut your iron intake to 5 mg per day, and if—and it's a big if—your body doesn't respond by increasing its rate of absorption, you will end up taking in about .5 mg of iron. If you're a male you need about 1 mg per day to replace your iron losses, so by taking in only half that you create a deficit of about .5 mg. If your excess iron stores were in the range of 2,000 mg, represented by a ferritin level of 220

(200 of the 220 represents the excess; the remaining 20 you need), you would have to follow this diet for two thousand days or *almost five and a half years* to get your stored iron levels into the ideal range. And not only that, you would have to avoid much meat and other iron-rich foods that provide many other nutrients essential to good health. Remember, early man didn't keep his iron levels low by watching what he ate; his parasitic companions did it for him. If you don't wish to become a scientist in New Guinea and contract a nice parasitic infection, you can simply let the Red Cross play the role of blood letter, and help your fellow man to boot. We have included table 8.2 to help you find where you are in the spectrum of iron overload. This table is not meant to take the place of your doctor, but it will help you get a better handle on your iron situation.

When you take the simple step of donating blood you reduce your risk of cancer, heart disease, and multiple endocrine abnormalities. You can also reduce your risk for infection because low iron stores don't provide much sustenance for invading microbes. It would seem, then, that compared to nondonors, blood donors should be an all-around healthier bunch. And, indeed, a number of studies have shown that blood donors live longer and experience better health than nondonors (but these are epidemiological studies, so don't put too much stock in them). Given what you now know about iron, it makes sense that people who routinely

TABLE 8.2

Determining Your Iron Status

IRON STATUS	SERUM IRON	FERRITIN	HEMOGLOBIN
Optimal	50 to 100	<50 to >10	Male 13 to 18 Female 12 to 16
Iron overload	Normal to high	>100	Normal
Hemochromatosis	Elevated	>100*	Elevated
Infection	Low	>100	Normal to low

*Usually much higher, along with an elevated serum transferrin saturation level.

get rid of their excess iron, albeit in a different manner than their prehistoric ancestors did, would reap the benefits. It's simple, and, best of all, it's free. Who knows . . . maybe if our friend had given blood a few times (he was and is a nondonor) he wouldn't have fallen prey to the pig virus, and maybe he would be happily married to the "pig woman" today.

BOTTOM LINE

I ron is absolutely essential for life. We must have it to build red blood cells to carry oxygen in the blood; to make new proteins to repair wear and tear of our tissues; to make new enzymes that run the millions of chemical reactions going on inside us at all times; to keep our hormones working properly; and to produce the substances needed to efficiently burn fat for energy. Humans must have iron to live, but so must other living creatures, including microbes.

Early humans lived in a natural world, with no means of decontaminating the foods they ate or the water they drank. As a consequence, they were riddled with parasites, bacteria, viruses, and fungi, all of which need iron to thrive. With no antibiotics available, the human body learned to defend itself from attack by hiding its iron from the microbes when needed—in effect, starving them of iron. Parasites regularly robbed our ancestors of much of their iron (through low-level, constant intestinal bleeding), and in order to survive, the human body developed many methods to increase absorption of iron and store it away with virtually no means of getting rid of any excess. Nowadays, without the constant assault of parasites and a hostile environment, we tend to accumulate iron.

But iron is a two-edged sword: although it's necessary, it's also quite dangerous. Iron behaves as an oxidant, powerful enough to turn the steel body of a truck into a rusty heap. This same oxidant power can damage us, too. For instance, the most severe damage from a heart attack comes not from the blockage preventing blood flow but from the explosive reaction that occurs between stored iron released during the attack and the oxygen-rich blood returning to the heart muscle after the obstruction has been relieved. And so the body handles iron carefully, wrapping it for storage in packets called ferritin to prevent its getting loose and "rusting" us.

Accumulation of iron in the tissues—the heart, the liver, the thyroid gland, the pancreas, and others—can not only prove dangerous as an oxidant but can hamper the function of the organ in question. And people with the Metabolic Syndrome, for reasons that remain unclear, tend to accumulate iron readily. All people with insulin-resistance disorders should ask their physician to evaluate them (by a simple blood test called a serum ferritin) for iron-storage disorder. A reading under 50 mg/dl is a healthy ideal; in people who have substantially higher readings, we recommend donating blood to the Red Cross. If you believe you may have excess iron storage, please refer to the sections "How Do I Know If I've Got Too Much Iron?" and "Getting Rid of Your Iron" for further details.

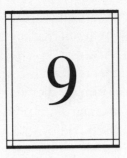

THE MAGNESIUM MIRACLE

A reckoning up of the cause often solves the malady.
—CELSUS, 25 B.C.–A.D. 50

M odern humans have departed from the diet the forces of nature designed for our well-being in a variety of ways— our reliance on cereal grains, our higher intake of sodium, our low intake of good-quality essential fats, to name a few—but we've made no more critical step off the Paleolithic path than the startling decrease in our intake of the mineral magnesium, along with an equally dramatic increase in our intake of its "opposing partner" mineral, calcium. And this imbalance has brought with it a plethora of modern ills. Let's first examine what *was* through the lens of history, with a look at what the diet of our ancient ancestors provided, and see how we measure up.

Paleolithic nutrition researchers Loren Cordain and Boyd Eaton have devoted innumerable hours of thought, study, and analysis to the reconstruction of a modern model of the diet our ancestors thrived on. By their estimates, the magnesium intake of early man appears to have been as much as 800 to 1,500 mg per day. Interestingly, this amount of magnesium approximately equals what Dr. Cordain estimates the daily calcium intake to have been at that time, giving early humans a calcium-to-magnesium ratio of about 1:1. Look at how things have changed; contrast those Paleolithic figures with the intake of Americans today. We now on average consume a diet that provides only an estimated 200 to 300 mg of magnesium and 1,200 to 1,500 mg of calcium, making our modern ratio not the 1:1 of old but 5:1 or even as high as 15:1 by some estimates. Nowadays we're taking in five to fifteen times more calcium than magnesium much to the detriment of our health.

Consider this list of the *known* conditions that research has correlated with deficiency of magnesium: heart disease and sudden death, diabetes, high blood pressure, asthma and chronic bronchitis, chronic fatigue syndrome, migraine headaches, muscle cramps, premenstrual syndrome, depression and other psychiatric disorders, and susceptibility to the brain-damaging effects of food additives such as aspartame and monosodium glutamate (MSG). Quite an impressive list, and that's not even the half of it.

Our readers and patients in our clinic often ask us, "If you could take or prescribe only one supplement, what would it be?" And the answer is simple: magnesium. It's already been identified as a required cofactor for more than three hundred enzymatic reactions in the body—and who knows how many more have yet to be uncovered? Although we wrote of it in *Protein Power,* based on what we now know and the new research that's accumulating, we feel that we didn't stress its importance sufficiently. In fact, we feel that magnesium is so important to your health that we've devoted an entire chapter of this book to it. If it's so important, you may be thinking, why don't you hear more about it? Again, the answer is pretty simple: magnesium has no commercial lobby to tout its benefits on the airwaves. Calcium has the dairy lobby, fiber gets its media boost from the grain producers and cereal manufacturers, vitamin C has the citrus growers trumpeting its many benefits, but poor old magnesium is a media orphan. However, waves of interest have begun to form, and some private citizens' groups have begun to act on magnesium's behalf. What's all the hullabaloo about?

Too Good to Be True?

How can one simple element have such diverse and potent physiological actions? One important way that magnesium works its miracles is through its influence on and regulation of calcium, a mineral that's gotten more than its share of media play in recent years. You'd have to have been locked in a cave on the most remote corner of Bora-Bora not to have heard the hype—particularly aimed at women over forty—about taking more calcium to prevent deficiency and keep bones strong. And so now we have the entire nation chomping calcium antacids by the handful, drinking calcium-fortified orange juice, downing calcium supplements of all kinds in an effort to raise their intake of calcium. But guess what the calcium hype fails to point out? It takes both calcium and magnesium (along with vitamin D; see chapter 10, "Sunshine Superman") as well as an entire intricate symphony of bit players (molybdenum, boron, phosphorous, adequate protein, and bone-building hormones) to properly build and maintain bone. In fact, high levels of calcium in the blood can actually *weaken* bone and make it more brittle. And to make matters worse, taking excessive amounts of calcium without magnesium will promote magnesium deficiency, leading to the development of any of the host of diseases we mentioned above. While it's true that our bones need plenty of calcium to make them strong, if it reaches excessive levels *within other cells,* it's quite harmful—a situation that can easily arise in the face of an unbalanced intake of calcium and magnesium. Let's see how this works.

Beyond its role in making bones hard, calcium serves as a critical stimulating component in the generation of electrical impulses in many tissues throughout the body—notably, the heart, the muscles, and the brain and nerves. Calcium resides in the tissues in the fluid that bathes the outside of the cells—and that's where the cells want calcium to stay until it's called for. When it's needed for the generation of an electrical impulse, the cells open tiny channels in their membranes—called, appropriately enough, the calcium channels—to admit a controlled number of calcium ions. The inrush of these calcium ions alters the electrical charge within the cells and creates the spark for transmission of an electrical impulse. As soon as it has done its job, however, the cell hustles the calcium back out. In fact, calcium inside the cell is so toxic that the cells expend an enormous amount of energy keeping it in its proper place—on the outside. When too much gets in and remains inside the cell, bad things happen.

Many disease processes occur because the tight regulation of the calcium channel fails, permitting calcium ions to flow into the cells unabated. Rising calcium levels within a cell activate its energy-production systems, setting into motion a variety of effects depending on the tissue in question. For example, calcium flowing unrestrained into the smooth muscle cells in the coronary arteries of the heart can bring on arterial spasm and the chest pain called angina. Calcium overstimulation of the cells in the muscular layer of the temporal arteries (or others supplying blood to the brain) can cause migraine headaches. Excess calcium entering the cells of the smooth muscle surrounding the small airways in the lung causes constriction—called bronchospasm—and the resultant wheezing of asthma and other restrictive lung disorders. If too much calcium flows into the delicate cells of the brain, the repeated discharge of energy that follows may deplete their energy stores, killing the cells!

Pharmaceutical companies have developed an entire family of drugs to prevent this excess flow of calcium into the interior of the cells. These drugs, called calcium channel blockers, are among the most versatile drugs on the market, currently approved for a wide range of medical indications. This single class of drugs can reduce or eliminate the chest pain from heart disease by preventing coronary arterial spasm, alleviate the blinding pain of migraine headaches and prevent their onset, treat high blood pressure, reduce asthmatic attacks, and even relieve vasomotor rhinitis, the drippy nose often associated with severe allergies. All these disparate diseases respond to a single action: preventing excess calcium from entering the cell by blocking the calcium channel. Ah, the miracles of modern medical technology! But here the story gets even more interesting, and it's one reason we titled this chapter "The Magnesium Miracle."

Magnesium is nature's calcium channel blocker, acting as a natural retardant to the flow of calcium ions into the cells. Adequate magnesium levels on the inside of the cell prevent calcium's entry from without, and all is well within the cell. If the interior of the cell becomes magnesium deficient, however, watch out! Calcium can then enter at will. Medical researchers have repeatedly demonstrated a low level of magnesium inside the cells in virtually every disorder treated by calcium channel blocking drugs. So why don't doctors treat these patients with magnesium instead of the terribly expensive prescription medications? For one thing, because drug companies can't patent natural substances, there's no army of pharmaceutical representatives knocking on the doctors' doors, crowing about the advantages of simple, cheap magnesium in treating these disorders. But the information does slowly trickle down, and the good news is, many physicians are beginning to use more magnesium in the treatment of disease.

In the emergency room, physicians now routinely give magnesium directly into the vein to relieve severe chest pain, stabilize the heart rhythm, and reduce or prevent the death of heart muscle cells during a heart attack. And more and more in the ER, astute physicians, recognizing the power of magnesium to relax the spastic respiratory muscles and open the airways, have begun to give it by the IV route to break asthmatic attacks. (Several research studies have demonstrated that magnesium deficiency occurs nearly uniformly among asthma suffers and that replacing it will reduce the number of attacks.) Obstetricians have been on the magnesium bandwagon since long before we did our medical training, routinely giving intravenous injections of magnesium sulfate to treat toxemia of pregnancy, rapidly reducing the malignant high blood pressure sometimes associated with labor and delivery. And since the discovery that virtually every patient admitted to the medical intensive care unit is deficient in magnesium, its intravenous (IV) supplementation in these critically ill people has become commonplace. Unfortunately, most physicians don't yet use magnesium to prevent these disorders, mainly relying on it to treat diseases after they're present. As is too often the case with modern medicine, we close the barn door after the horse has gotten away. But that approach, we hope, is changing.

We routinely use magnesium—both as an oral supplement and intravenously—in our office to treat these conditions in our patients, and we recommend it to them before they develop problems. Sometimes we even use it before patients become patients. A few months back, a new patient came to our office for preliminary blood work prior to an evaluation by our partner, Dr. Rosedale, who happened to driving in from the airport after speaking at a medical conference. In the course of his evaluation, the nurse had taken the patient's blood pressure and discovered it was extremely elevated. Since many patients come to us for treatment of hypertension, the finding of an elevated blood pressure wouldn't normally have inspired much excitement in our nursing staff, but this patient's reading was through the roof! Our nurse came flying through the door to our office with his eyes the size of saucers, reporting what he'd found, and seeking our immediate intervention. We, of course, went straightaway to evaluate the situation, rechecking the pressure ourselves (always the first order of business anytime a dramatic reading shows up) to be sure there was no mistake. And indeed, there was not; we, too, got dangerously high numbers—of a magnitude that would send this patient to the hospital if we were unable to reduce the pressure fast. And the fastest way possible? Some fancy high-dollar drug with an unpronounceable name? Nope. We had the nurse quickly insert an intravenous butterfly catheter and we administered—you guessed it—plain old magnesium in as rapid a drip as we deemed safe. And as usual, it worked its miracle magic and quickly brought his pressure down to a manageable level. Blood drawn from his arm prior to putting the magnesium into his vein indeed showed his blood (serum) magnesium to be on the low side of normal—not unusual, since like potassium magnesium lives inside the cells. The body uses this giant reservoir of intracellular magnesium to keep the levels in the blood within a normal range, leaching a little out as needed to maintain an adequate amount in the blood. Once the blood levels of magnesium fall below normal, you've got bodywide intracellular depletion—true deficiency that can take months of oral supplementation to restore adequately. A check of his intracellular magnesium level—a more accurate measure of what's inside the cells, determined at a few labs around the country from a sampling of the cells on the inside of the cheek— revealed that he was indeed low on magnesium where it counts most, inside the cells. And this deficiency, most likely, lay at the root of his dramatically elevated blood pressure, perhaps not the only player in the game, but a ring leader, nonetheless. But blood pressure isn't the only disorder that magnesium deficiency appears to figure into; the list is already long and growing. Let's take a closer look at some others.

Magnesium plays major roles in the whole Hyperinsulinemia/Insulin-Resistance cluster. In patients with every disorder so far associated with hyperinsulinemia—diabetes, high blood pressure, heart disease, elevated cholesterol, low HDL cholesterol, elevated triglycerides, and obesity—lab studies have demonstrated decreased magnesium levels. Because of this broad connection, an alternative school of thought—called the Ionic Hypothesis of Syndrome X—has begun to develop, attributing the entire syndrome to low magnesium instead of chronically elevated insulin levels. Other researchers believe that low magnesium may cause the insulin resistance in the first place—in effect, magnesium deficiency may trigger the disease cluster—based on research showing that experimental animals deprived of dietary magnesium develop insulin resistance. We believe that the lowered magnesium common to sufferers of hyperinsulinemia comes from a combination of dietary inadequacy and the well-documented loss of magnesium in urine that elevated insulin causes; that is, it's the hyperinsulinemia that causes the low magnesium and the beginning of a vicious cycle of insulin resistance and further magnesium loss. (It's sort of a chicken-or-the-egg dilemma that has not yet been completely sorted out by research but surely will be in time.) Once the levels of magnesium inside the cells fall there's no question that all the diseases of the Hyperinsulinemia/Insulin-Resistance Syndrome worsen. But equally true is the reverse scenario, that restoring magnesium to normal levels greatly improves them. Let's look at some specific disorders and see how magnesium deficiency may be involved.

Not Enough of a Good Thing

Perhaps you've known someone who has developed high blood pressure (a parent, grandparent, friend, perhaps even yourself); it's such a common disease, you'd be hard-pressed not to have. If so, do you recall the first treatment prescribed for them when their physician diagnosed their high blood pressure? In most cases "water pills," diuretic medications designed to make the kidneys throw off excess sodium and with it excess water to lower the pressure. And certainly, at least for a time, diuretics probably did lower their blood pressure. But here's the catch: the same mechanism that causes the diuretic drug to deplete the body of sodium and excess water depletes it of potassium and magnesium. Every person on diuretic drugs becomes magnesium deficient, but virtually none of them receive instructions to supplement magnesium. All physicians supplement their patients on diuretics with potassium, but in the face of low magnesium, it's tough to keep potassium levels in the proper range, since one of magnesium's three hundred–plus jobs is to help regulate potassium levels. And while lowered potassium levels can cause the rapid development of dramatic symptoms (such as abnormal heart rhythms, muscle cramping, and profound fatigue), the effects of magnesium deficiency, while more subtle, can actually cause more harm in the long run. However, few people on diuretics take magnesium supplements. Isn't it ironic that most patients take diuretic drugs for an elevated blood pressure resulting from a magnesium deficiency, and in the process they make their deficiency worse?

A whole host of disparate diseases have been laid at the door of magnesium deficiency. In asthma, for example, research has shown that even a slight increase in magnesium intake can improve the movement of air—a great benefit for people gasping for an easy breath. It does this not only by relaxing the muscular wall of the airways and opening the passages wider but also by reducing the inflammation and swelling of the airway walls and increasing the release of the powerful dilator nitric oxide. (You may be familiar with this substance in the wake of the Viagra revolution; increasing the release of nitric oxide is how the drug works its magic to improve sexual potency.)

And here's another example of magnesium's far-reaching effects. You've no doubt heard of chronic fatigue syndrome, a modern epidemic of uncertain origins that afflicts hundreds of thousands of people. Although theories abound as to its cause, no one has yet come up with the definitive theory of what brings it about, and, consequently, the pharmaceutical wizards have not yet been able to offer any specific medication to treat it. But, interestingly, researchers have recently discovered that sufferers of chronic fatigue syndrome almost without fail have low levels of magnesium inside their cells and, even more important, that replenishing the deficiency with a particular form of magnesium (magnesium malate, available at most health food stores) brings relief in 40 to 50 percent of cases, making supplemental magnesium the most potent "drug" discovered to date for treatment of this frustrating disorder.

And the list goes on: the sudden death of young athletes, premenstrual syndrome, allergic reactions, sudden cardiac death, abnormal blood fats, many diseases of aging (transient ischemic attacks, the so-called mini-strokes, Alzheimer's disease, and senility), seizures, sudden infant death syndrome (SIDS), susceptibility to the development of toxic shock syndrome in young women, anxiety and panic reactions, schizophrenia, and a host of others may all be—at least in part—the unhappy consequence of low intracellular magnesium. If the idea that a single nutrient could be behind such a vast and variable number of disorders stretches your credulity, remember that magnesium's critical involvement in more than three hundred important enzymatic processes influences actions all over the body. And the modern pervasiveness of these disparate disorders of magnesium deficiency, if indeed we might lump them together as such, becomes easier to comprehend when you realize that despite living in a nation that enjoys unparalleled peace, plenty, and downright excess, the vast majority of Americans don't consume enough magnesium.

A 1995 Gallup survey (as well as a number of studies) showed that as much as 72 percent of the population of the United States may not get the recommended amount of magnesium each day. And that number becomes even more startling when you realize that these surveys measured the deficiency not according to some elevated standard set by a company selling vitamins but according to the ridiculously low standards of the recommended daily allowances (RDA), which most researchers and nutritionally aware physicians find woefully inadequate in all categories. Bear in mind that the RDAs set by the National Research Council represent the minimum amounts of the various nutrients required to prevent observable nutritional-deficiency diseases, such as scurvy, pellagra, and beriberi, not the amounts required to promote optimal health. (Our colleague, nutritionist Robert Crayhon, terms the RDA minimum-wage nutrition. How true!) With the limits set so low, most people eating even a halfway adequate diet can get considerably more than 100 percent of the pitifully inadequate RDA for virtually every nutrient category listed. Except for magnesium. Over half of our population consumes a meager 75 percent of the RDA for magnesium, and, astoundingly, one-third of us get less than 50 percent of the requirement! If nearly three-quarters of the population don't meet even the minuscule RDA levels for magnesium, is it any wonder we're awash in a flood of magnesium-deficiency disorders or that calcium channel blockers are among the most widely prescribed drugs in the cardiology clinics across the land?

Why Don't Americans Get Enough Magnesium?

We've spent a considerable amount of time pondering this issue, trying to make sense of what seems hardly possible in a time of such tremendous food availability, and we have a number of theories about the possible causes, among them poor absorption from food, depletion of magnesium from farming soils, loss in modern food-processing techniques, the vilification of dietary fat, and the softening of our water supply. Let's look at each of these in turn.

Poor Absorption from Food. Even when we're young and the "new" hasn't yet worn off our intestinal tract's nutrient-absorbing machinery, we have a hard time absorbing magnesium from food; kids absorb only about 25 to 35 percent of the dietary magnesium they take in. And as we age, our ability to absorb magnesium falls to under 15 percent. So even if we're eating what ought to be enough—which, as you've seen, the vast majority of people don't do—the magnesium may not make it in through the intestinal tract very well. We have to work to take in enough—or, better said, more than enough—if we're to overcome the difficulty we have in absorbing it. (We'll give you some guidelines about how much that should be in a bit.)

Depleted Farming Soils. As they grow, plants take their minerals from the soil, naturally filling their leaves, stems, flowers, and fruit with such important nutrients as magnesium, selenium, nitrogen, phosphorous, potassium, and whatever else the plant needs that the soil may contain. By taking up these mineral nutrients, however, growing plants deplete them from the soils in which they grow. Cycle after cycle of crop growth without rest and replenishment can potentially leave the soil deficient in some minerals. To replace the loss, commercial farming methods typically use potash to fertilize the soil, replenishing the phosphorous, nitrogen, and potassium but not necessarily the magnesium or other essential minerals. In theory it's certainly conceivable that crops grown in mineral-depleted soil might not contain as much of some of these minerals as they once did or that the published agriculture literature would suggest, although, to be fair, there continues to be some debate about whether soil depletion does in fact cause the production of relatively mineral-deficient foods.

A plant uses magnesium as the core around which it builds the green pigment, chlorophyll, in much the same way that we humans use the iron molecule to build the heme of hemoglobin, the pigment that imparts the red color to our blood. For plants to build chlorophyll, which they must do to convert sunlight to energy for their growth, they must have magnesium. Dark green, leafy vegetables, therefore, should normally be good sources of magnesium, since by their color we can tell that they have plenty of green chlorophyll, and that's probably why these vegetables give you the best cluck for your buck when looking for food sources of magnesium. But just as is the case with our blood, which can sometimes be iron-poor and still bright red, plants can become relatively deficient in magnesium. Nuts and seeds, normally good sources, may not prove on actual analysis to be as rich as you'd expect since these structures don't contain much chlorophyll; in a relatively magnesium-deficient state, the plant concentrates it in the leaves and stems, not necessarily in the seeds or fruit. And however much modern nuts and seeds contain, it's very likely not as much as the ones gathered from the trees and bushes grown in the mineral-rich soils of the Paleolithic garden by your ancient ancestors. Still, they're among the better food sources for this mineral available today.

Food-Processing Techniques. While most people have become aware that food-processing techniques raise the sodium content of canned, frozen, and packaged foods (the higher sodium intake today being another of the important departures from our Paleolithic nutritional past), few realize that commercial processing almost entirely depletes the food of magnesium. Flash-freezing techniques cause less loss, and foods prepared in this fashion still contain amounts of many nutrients relatively comparable to fresh produce.

Avoidance of Dietary Fat. In an effort—albeit a sadly misguided one—to purge fat from their diets, many people have eliminated or reduced their intake of dairy products, seeds, and fatty nuts, some of the best food sources of magnesium. A cup of almonds, for example, all by itself, contains over 400 mg of magnesium, almost an entire day's requirement for the mineral; that 1-cup serving also contains 167 grams of fat, an amount that would make any dyed-in-the-wool low-fat dieter blanch. So nuts and seeds have been verboten during the low-fat reign. (Fortunately, blind avoidance of higher-fat foods isn't going to be a cause of magnesium deficiency for you if you follow the *Protein Power LifePlan.*)

When the low-fatters eliminate nuts and seeds, that leaves only fat-free dairy products to take up the slack. But remember, just taking in more magnesium isn't the whole story; we eat far too much calcium relative to our deficient intake of magnesium. And even though milk, yogurt, and cheeses provide a fair amount of magnesium, these and other dairy products (which, of course our ancient ancestors didn't eat) contain about ten times more calcium, further upsetting the balance. Now that's not to say that we discourage your eating good-quality dairy products as a part of your diet; just be aware that dairy products contain too much calcium for you to rely solely on them as your magnesium source. When you choose to eat cheeses, yogurt, milk, and cream, you'll need to increase your intake of magnesium from other sources to close the gap between magnesium and calcium that dairy products widen.

The Softening of Our Water Supply. The most crucial magnesium loss in our modern diet has come not from our food, but from our water. Certainly for early humans and throughout most of human history, the single most available source of magnesium has been drinking water. As the glaciers of the Ice Age formed, scraping up into their vast bulk the mineral deposits of the land over which they crawled, then receded, and melted, they filled the rivers and streams with mineral-rich water—hard water, we term it today. This hard mineral water, available to our ancient ancestors, provided a wealth of trace minerals, including an abundance of magnesium. But unfortunately that's changing. Not that people are drinking any less water (although that may also be true), but they're quite certainly drinking more bottled water and commercially softened water and less of the mineral-rich variety. While a few bottled "mineral" waters have a low but measurable mineral content, few have much magnesium, because, in general, the higher the mineral content, the more pronounced the distinctive hard-water taste. (We've provided a list of several waters and their magnesium content in table 9.1.)

Unlike some people who object to the mineral taste of hard water, we love it ourselves, preferring it over the chemical-antiseptic-chlorine taste of the product turned out by many municipal water systems; it calls up pleasant memories of cool well water in the hot summers of our respective southern childhoods. But nowadays hard water has fallen out of vogue—no one wants it. It causes a buildup of mineral scale that clogs modern plumbing and appliances; soap doesn't form suds well in it; and it tastes . . . well . . . like minerals. So municipalities, towns, and cities throughout the country go to great lengths to treat their water supply with softening agents—in other words, to remove most of the minerals (and add back in chlorine and fluoride). And in doing so they rob us all of our best and historically most important source of magnesium.

The Basic Diet You Eat. And of course diet plays a role. The basic composition of the diet you eat makes a difference in your body's ability to absorb and use magnesium. A number of studies

TABLE 9.1

Magnesium Content of Bottled Waters

We've included in this list those products from around the world that contain the most magnesium per liter, but we have also given you their calcium to magnesium ratio—remember that we're striving for equal amounts in the overall diet, so that selecting one with a ratio of 2.0 or less (the lower the better) will be of great benefit. We've tagged these choices with an asterisk (*). We've also included some popular brands that don't measure up, so that you can see what you're really getting. There are many more waters available, some with good ratios, but as the list shows, some with magnesium content so low that you'd have to drink 20 liters a day to get enough to matter. Still, if the ratios are good, at least they won't make calcium-to-magnesium matters worse!

BRAND	AMOUNT OF MAGNESIUM (MG) PER LITER	CALCIUM TO MAGNESIUM RATIO
Mendocine	130	2.4
Rosbacher	128	2.0*
St. Gero	121	3.4
Vittel Hepar	118	4.9
Gerolsteiner Sprudel	113	3.2
Vichy Novelle	110	0.6*
Vichy Original	110	0.9*
Apollinaris	104	0.9*
Badoit	100	2.0*
Noah's Spring Water	96	almost zero*
Sao Lourenco Fonte Oriente	65	1.0*
San Pelligrino	57	3.6
Abbey Well	36	1.5*
Golden Eagle	37	0.6*
Evian	24	3.3
La Croix	22	1.7*
Bru	23	1.0*
Naya	20	1.9*
Mountain Valley	8	8.5
Diamond Pure	1	7.0
Crystal Geyser, Alpine Spring	6	0.0*
Volvic	6	1.6*
Panna	5	2.8
Perrier	4	41.4
Poland Spring	2	0.0*
Ozarka	1	18.4
Calistoga	1	7.0
Quibell	0	—(virtually mineral free)

Sources: Arthur von Weisenberger, *H₂O: The Guide to Quality Bottled Water* (Woodbridge, 1989) and Maureen Green and Timothy Green, *The Good Water Guide* (Rosendale Press, 1994).

have demonstrated that in the face of an elevated insulin—which, remember, 75 percent of Americans may have to one degree or another—the kidneys waste magnesium, leading to an increased loss of magnesium in the urine of more than 30 percent. So America's decade-plus love affair with the high–complex carbohydrate, low-fat diet (a surefire way to keep insulin levels high) has also played its part in depleting the population of magnesium. On the other hand, a diet designed to reduce insulin levels maximizes your body's ability to hang on to magnesium, allowing you to more quickly and effectively restore deficient levels to normal. Taking large doses of magnesium without the added symbiosis of the proper diet might ultimately correct the deficit—and would no doubt be a step in the right direction—but combining it with the nutritional strategy we offer in the *Protein Power LifePlan* produces a truly powerful rejuvenating force.

Determining Your Need

So how do you know where you stand in the magnesium department? For starters, consider where you are in the insulin-resistance spectrum. If you currently have diabetes, obesity, high blood pressure, elevated triglycerides, low HDL "good" cholesterol, or suffer from asthma, migraine headaches, or chronic fatigue syndrome, the chances are pretty good that you've got a low level of magnesium inside your cells. In fact, it's so likely that you might as well assume you're deficient in magnesium.

To test the assumption—or to find out where you stand even if you've not yet developed any of these problems—you can check the level in your blood with a simple blood test, which is cheap but fraught with error. If the level in your blood turns out to be low, you know you're deficient bodywide, but here's the clinker: if your blood level falls within the normal range, you still don't know where you stand. Remember that magnesium lies mainly inside the cells, leaching out to keep the blood level in a stable, "normal" range. That means that you could be getting quite low on magnesium inside the cells, where it counts, and still have a "normal" level in your blood. To get a more accurate reflection of whole-body magnesium stores once meant undergoing an elaborate test that required collecting all the urine passed in a twenty-four-hour period, measuring the amount of magnesium in it, injecting the patient with a quite painful shot of a known amount of magnesium, re-collecting all the urine for twenty-four hours, and assessing how much of the injected dose of the mineral the body kept versus what it threw off in the urine. Quite a miserable and lengthy (not to mention painful) undertaking for all concerned. But again, twenty-first-century technology has come to the rescue with a noninvasive testing procedure that gives an even more specific measurement of what's going on inside the cells. Although it's a more expensive test than a simple blood measurement, it's head and shoulders above the old cumbersome inject-and-measure method. For these reasons, we rely on this newer method of measurement of intracellular magnesium levels as an accurate reflection of magnesium status when symptoms or history suggest it may be low but blood levels remain in the "normal" range. Only a very few specialty labs around the country can reliably make such a determination from a specimen of cells obtained by swabbing the inside of the cheek; we've included information in the Resources section of the appendix on how to contact the group we use if your physician wishes to undertake this evaluation for you.

Mineral Reconstructionism: Restoring Your Magnesium Levels

So how do you get your level of magnesium back up into the normal range if it's low? Simple: take in more magnesium. Okay, that's the short answer, but how? Actually there are several paths that will lead to that end. But first we need to offer a word of medical caution: although almost everyone needs some extra magnesium, and for the vast majority of people supplementation brings only health benefits without any risk, two groups of people—*those with kidney failure and those with high-degree AV (heart) block*—*should not take magnesium supplements except with the express permission of their doctors, specifically, their kidney or heart specialists.* In these conditions, the body doesn't eliminate magnesium rapidly, and with supplementation the levels of magnesium can become dangerously high; as is the case with so many bodily processes, too much is as bad as too little. But for the vast bulk of the rest of us, let's take a look at the ways to increase magnesium intake.

One easy way, of course, is to increase the magnesium content of your drinking water—that is, remineralize it—by adding a few drops of any of a number of concentrated mineral solutions you can find at most health food stores. This option offers the advantage of being the least expensive, but you'll need to be mindful of the quality of water you're remineralizing. If you depend on a well for your water (as we do when we're in Colorado), be certain to periodically have a local water-testing authority examine it for mineral content and impurities; afterward, get the printed results, so you, too, will know what's in the water you drink. We always filter our water at home to remove impurities, chlorine, bacteria, etc., and we encourage you to do the same. Even if it's "city" water, you'd be amazed at the impurities and chemicals it may contain! If you choose to remineralize your water, look for a brand of mineral solution that doesn't contain measurable amounts of heavy-metal toxins, such as aluminum, iron, and mercury, because you certainly don't need to pile more of those into your body.

Another option is to drink more of the few bottled waters that *do* contain some magnesium (see table 9.1) or eat more of the higher-magnesium foods, such as nuts, seeds, dairy products (unless you're adopting the Purist approach), and dark green, leafy vegetables. But by far the easiest and surest way to take in an adequate amount of magnesium is to use one of the many supplements currently on the market. There are dozens, so you'll need to know which one and how much to take. If you're like many of our patients, one trip down the aisles of your neighborhood health food store or vitamin shop will convince you that magnesium supplementation is a bit more complicated than just grabbing the first bottle that says magnesium on the label and throwing back a few tablets. A bewildering array of products lines the shelves, all claiming to provide magnesium in large and absorbable doses—and since our ability to absorb magnesium isn't so hot to begin with and declines with age, ease of absorption matters. The labeling of magnesium supplements can confuse even the most conscientious label reader, but never fear: we'll guide you through the magnesium maze—it's really easier than it looks.

For example, you could take tablets or capsules of plain old elemental magnesium. It's the least expensive form but not necessarily the best, and here's why. The body absorbs elemental minerals—ions—through tiny channels called single-ion channels in the intestinal cell membranes; the name itself describes the problem with taking minerals in this form. The bottleneck of the single-ion channel limits the amount of mineral ions that can pass into the cell, setting the stage for competition between ions for admittance. (Recall that we mentioned that chomping calcium tablets not balanced with magnesium can lead to magnesium deficiency? If there's a lot more calcium around in the stomach and intestine than there is magnesium, more of the calcium will make it through the channels.) The upside of taking elemental minerals is, of course, they're cheap; the downside is they're the least absorbable form. Granted, they will work if you take a bigger dose to make up for the low-absorption factor, but with magnesium, taking the higher dose needed to overcome this factor commonly causes diarrhea (the Milk of Magnesia effect that those of you who grew up like us in the 1950s will surely remember!). And if you've got to take more of a cheaper form to get the desired effect, it may not be as cost effective as it looks at first blush. If you choose to take elemental magnesium, such as magnesium oxide, you'll want one that provides a dose of 300 to 400 mg of elemental magnesium in a reasonable number of capsules. The labels of elemental magnesium are pretty straightforwrad—that is, if it says a dose provides 400 mg of elemental magnesium, that's what's in it.

Chelated magnesium products offer another option. They're a little more expensive but much more absorbable and a bit less likely to stimulate diarrhea, so you may actually get to keep more of what you pay for. With our patients in the clinic we've had better luck using these forms of magnesium for supplementation—at least our patients seem to tolerate them better. What are they? The term *chelate* derives from the Greek word meaning "claw." In the process of chelation, amino acids, the subunits of protein, grab—in clawlike fashion—onto mineral ions, joining their structures together to form a cage around the mineral. Wrapped in this protein cage, the mineral ion can bypass the ion channel by masquerading as protein and be absorbed by the intestine as such. Once inside, the body disassembles the cage of amino acids, liberating the mineral. The danger of using a chelate, however, lies in the fact that all chelating agents don't work equally well with every mineral. While some of them work like a charm, others can fall apart too soon or resist disassembly at the appropriate time to ensure adequate absorption. When you purchase a magnesium chelate, look for the words *citrate, malate,* or *aspartate,* all of which we've found work well with magnesium. It's really here that the labels can become confusing, because some manufacturers state on the label that the product contains 1,000 mg or more of, for instance, magnesium malate. When you pick that bottle up, you think, Wow! 1,000 mg! Why, I'd only have to take half a tablet or capsule to get 500 mg! But that's not usually the case. Quite often, the product label lists the total weight of the mineral *plus the chelating agent,* of which there is substantially more. And it's the magnesium you're after, not the malate. But usually somewhere on the label, often on the back or side, you'll find a section of text that will say something on the order of "This product provides 75 percent (or 90 percent or 130 percent or some percentage) of the RDI for magnesium." And it's that portion of the label that actually tells you how much magnesium is there. Since the RDI for magnesium is 360 mg, if a product provides 100 percent of the RDI, it provides 360 mg of magnesium. If, on the other hand, it provides only 50 percent of the RDI per capsule, then each dose contains only 180 mg of actual magnesium, regardless of what the milligrams on the front of the package say.

We recommend that our patients take at least 300 to 400 mg of extra actual magnesium (usually as the citrate, malate, or aspartate chelate) each evening if they're in apparent good health, with adequate or lowish but normal intracellular levels. In those people who have already developed any of the problems related to insulin resistance, we bump the daily dose up to 400 to 600 mg (if the patient can tolerate the dose without developing diarrhea and if they have no medical reason that would prevent their safely taking the mineral). In these people, if we've uncovered low intracellular levels of magnesium, we begin whenever possible to replenish the deficiencies by the intravenous route first and then follow with supplementation in capsule form as testing shows the levels rising. In cases where the oral route is our only ongoing means of supplementation, we keep tabs on our progress by rechecking the intracellular magnesium levels (by the cheek-scraping method) in about twelve to sixteen weeks.

Magnesium supplementation (by mouth) takes time to show benefit, but sometimes the results can be dramatic and sometimes in a matter of just a few weeks. Patients who have suffered for years with chronic headaches describe welcome relief; at long last intractably elevated blood pressures being to decline; fluid retention lessens; tight breathing eases; sleep improves; constipation resolves. So much benefit from one simple mineral. No wonder we—and our patients—call magnesium a miracle nutrient. Restoring your levels to that of your Paleolithic ancestors will also take you a step closer to the ancient diet you were designed to eat and the wellness you were born to enjoy.

BOTTOM LINE

Modern humans have departed from the diet designed by millennia of human development in many ways, such as reliance on cereal grains, a much higher intake of sodium, and not eating enough good-quality essential fats and too many poor-quality ones. But the most striking departure of all is that we consume far too little of the mineral magnesium (and relatively too much of its partner, calcium). The ancient diet contained approximately equal amounts of these two minerals, while in our modern one we consume five to fifteen times more calcium than magnesium—to the detriment of our health.

Consider this list of the known conditions that research has correlated with deficiency of magnesium: heart disease and sudden death, cholesterol and triglyceride abnormalities, diabetes, high blood pressure, toxemia of pregnancy, asthma and chronic bronchitis, chronic fatigue syndrome, migraine headaches, muscle cramps, premenstrual syndrome, anxiety, depression, and other psychiatric disorders, susceptibility to the brain-damaging effects of food additives such as aspartame and monosodium glutamate (MSG), and susceptibility to toxic shock syndrome. Quite an impressive list, and that's not even the half of it.

How can one mineral play a part in such widely diverse diseases? For starters, it's involved in more than three hundred biological reactions throughout the body, giving it broad influence. One important action involves its regulation of calcium. While it's true that our bones need plenty of calcium to make them strong, if it reaches excessive levels within other cells, it's quite harmful—a situation that can easily arise in the face of an unbalanced intake of calcium and magnesium. Too much calcium inside the cells can cause spasm of the arteries of the heart, leading to heart attack; spasm of arteries of the brain, causing migraine headache; spasm of the breathing passages of the lung, causing asthmatic wheezing; and the effects go on and on. To combat these disorders, physicians often prescribe drugs called calcium channel blockers, designed to prevent too much calcium from entering the cells. Magnesium is nature's calcium channel blocker. If there's enough inside, calcium can't enter to cause problems.

More than 75 percent of Americans fail to get even the pitifully low RDI for magnesium, and that, in large part, explains the epidemic of the magnesium-deficiency disorders we currently see in this country and around the world. We fail to get enough for several reasons: we absorb it poorly from food; food-manufacturing processes (canning, freezing, and so on) destroy most of what the food contains; crops may contain less of it from depletion of the farming soils without adequate replacement; softening of our water supply, which once provided over 25 percent of our intake, removes most of it from the water we drink. Our modern reliance on bottled waters has also had an impact, since many of these "mineral" waters have little magnesium (see table 9.1).

We recommend that you eat more foods that contain magnesium—dark green, leafy vegetables, nuts, seeds, and some dairy products—and that you drink water with a higher content of magnesium if possible. To ensure you get enough of this crucial mineral—and to help you reclaim the good health you were born to enjoy—we also encourage you to increase your intake with a magnesium supplement (using a good chelated form of the mineral, such as magnesium malate, magnesium citrate, or magnesium aspartate) in a dose of 300 to 600 mg each evening.

10

SUNSHINE SUPERMAN

*Organisms become adapted to the environment through
natural selection in their search for a better world . . .
[one example being] the discovery that sunlight can be
eaten. . . . This inexhaustible food supply . . . created
the kingdom of plants; and the discovery that plants can
be eaten created the animal kingdom.*
—KARL POPPER

There is little doubt that early humans lived in a warm symbiosis with the sun, like all free-living creatures that by natural inclination will seek out even the tiniest patch of sunlight to bask in. There's no reason to assume that our early ancestors—free-living natural creatures themselves—would have done otherwise. And they did so without benefit of broad-brimmed hats, long-sleeved clothing, zinc oxide ointment, or an SPF 45 sunblock. But there is likewise little doubt that in this day and age the incidence of skin cancer, especially malignant melanoma, the deadliest of all skin cancers, is sharply on the increase, a specter that, justifiably, frightens the modern descendants of these early sun-loving people. Because in the minds of many, the sun is the chief culprit behind the rising rates of skin cancer—a premise that is not entirely correct—the once warm symbiosis we had with the sun has devolved into cool suspicion. We're cautioned by current medical wisdom, warned by the media, and bombarded with advertise-

227

ments, all telling us to cover up and protect ourselves from exposure to the sun as though it were merely some cancer-causing
toxin and not also an essential human nutrient beneficial to our
health. So what's a modern human to do? Slather with sunblock?
Hide indoors? Avoid the sun? Our position is absolutely not! In
this chapter, we'll take a look at the medical and scientific evidence; the findings may surprise you.

Based on our study and wide reading of the recent—and not
so recent—medical and scientific literature on this topic, we've
concluded that the benefits of sunlight clearly outweigh the risks.
And speaking from that position, we'll make some recommendations concerning what we feel is the role of sunlight in a healthy
lifestyle.

What Is This Thing Called Sunlight?

Let's first look a little more deeply into what sunlight actually
is. It's energy—electromagnetic energy that radiates from the sun
in waves not unlike those on the ocean, with regularly occurring
peaks and valleys. The length of the various types of waves—that
is, the distance from one peak to the next, as shown schematically
in figure 10.1—ranges from very long (over three thousand miles)
to minuscule (less than one-billionth of a millimeter). Only a portion of the total electromagnetic spectrum of waves radiating from
the sun reaches the surface of the earth. The remainder is hin-
dered by the atmospheric layers that surround our planet (figure
10.2). Some of what does reach us our eyes can see; this is called
the visible spectrum of light, with wavelengths ranging from 380
to 760 nanometers. Contained within it are all the colors of the
rainbow, from longest to shortest: red, pink, orange, yellow, green
blue, and violet. Although the human eye cannot perceive the
longer (infrared) and shorter (ultraviolet) waves also present in
the sunlight reaching us, their impact on life and health is profound. The infrared spectrum provides us with warmth, and the
ultraviolet with a nutrient crucial to life: vitamin D.

The ultraviolet light, which we refer to in shorthand as UV
light, can be further subdivided into waves of differing lengths,
designated UVA, UVB, and UVC. It's important to note that 90

FIGURE 10.1

Wavelengths of Sunlight

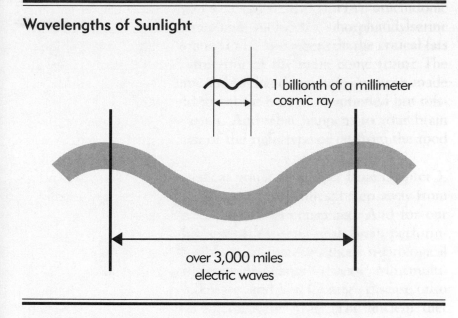

1 billionth of a millimeter
cosmic ray

over 3,000 miles
electric waves

to 95 percent of the ultraviolet light in sunlight falls into the UVA group, with UVB making up most of the remainder. It is within this ultraviolet spectrum that we find most of the beneficial effects of sunlight. But like mentioning the thorns that come with the roses, we'd be remiss not to note that it is also the UV range of sunlight that ages and damages our skin and that has the potential to cause certain skin cancers, topics we'll delve more deeply into later in the chapter.

The Sunshine Vitamin

Probably the most widely known benefit of sunlight is its essential role in production and regulation of vitamin D—a role that earned this vitamin the name *sunshine vitamin*—and thereby in the maintenance of strong, healthy bones. Lack of vitamin D brings about one of the classic vitamin-deficiency diseases: rickets. In this disorder, which, although rare in the United States and western Europe, still ravages children in certain areas of the world, the bones fail to mineralize—that is, to take up the cal-

FIGURE 10.2

Types of Rays from the Sun

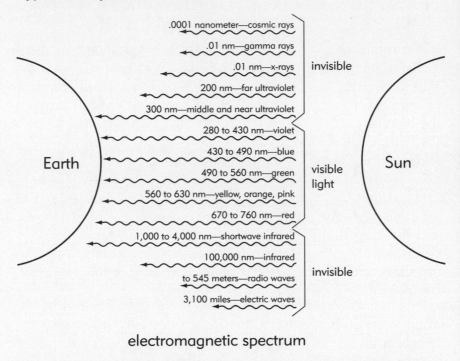

electromagnetic spectrum

cium, phosphorous, and other minerals that make them hard and strong. As a result, the bones bend and deform; in extreme cases, children with rickets cannot support their own weight, cannot walk, cannot breathe easily from deformities of their rib cages, cannot absorb calcium, and ultimately can die from lack of vitamin D. Yet childhood rickets can be both prevented and cured by a few minutes a day of strong sunlight.

And while adults deprived of sufficient vitamin D don't develop rickets (since their bones have already formed), they do suffer loss of bone mineral and weakening of their bones, a disorder termed osteomalacia. And again, exposure to sunlight—our chief and best source of vitamin D—will solve the problem. How does sunlight work its magic to provide us with a steady and correct supply of vitamin D? It's a matter of simple chemistry. (Fear not, those of you who do not view chemistry as simple in any circumstance, we're not going to go into the heavy details.)

EATING THE SUN: THE MIRACLE OF VITAMIN D PRODUCTION

In a nutshell, the chemistry of vitamin D production is this: When sunlight strikes exposed skin, the UVB portion of it causes a chemical change in a special type of cholesterol present in the skin, converting it to an inactive precursor (forerunner) form of vitamin D. From the skin, this inactive vitamin D travels through the bloodstream to the liver, where it is again chemically altered (by hydroxylation, the addition of a hydrogen-oxygen complex) and finally to the kidney for its final alteration (another hydroxylation) to a substance called in scientific parlance 1,25-dihydroxy-cholecalciferol or, more simply, active vitamin D—and that's what we'll call it from here on. Three organ systems (the skin, the liver, and the kidneys) work in concert to provide our bodies with a steady, sufficient, and controlled amount of vitamin D, but the first and essential step, without which vitamin D cannot be made, is exposure of our skin to natural sunlight.

THE CONSEQUENCES OF BLOCKING THE SUN

What happens when we slather on the sunblock? Many of the sunblocking agents currently on the market block the UVB portion of sunlight but offer little to no protection against the full complement of UVA wavelengths, which make up 90 to 95 percent of the UV light. And as you'll soon see, this spells trouble by lulling users into a false sense of security about their true safe duration of exposure to the sun.

It may surprise you to learn that the SPF (sun protection factor) numbers on the labels refer only to UVB screening. An SPF of 8, for example, means that the average individual using that strength of block can stay in the sun eight times longer than without it before burning, because the blocking agent screens out the "harmful burning UVB rays." An SPF of 15 permits fifteen times the duration before burning. An SPF of 45? Forty-five times longer protection against burning the skin, but also forty-five times longer "protection" against the production of natural vitamin D—and, most important, forty-five times the unprotected exposure to UVA, the wavelengths of UV light that appear to promote the development of the deadliest skin cancer, malignant melanoma. (More on that topic shortly.) Research has shown that a single application of sunblock with an SPF of only 8 can effectively prevent the conversion of cholesterol in the skin to vitamin D, robbing the body of one of its most valuable bone-building and cancer-fighting nutrients.

What then will protect our skin against UVA radiation? Nature has endowed humans with built-in sun protection: the ability of the skin to tan. With gradual "unblocked" exposure of skin to sunlight, the UV waves (both UVA and UVB) stimulate pigment-producing cells within the skin (called melanocytes) to produce and rearrange little packets of a pigment called melanin—our naturally produced sunscreen. The body can regulate the amount of pigment produced to handle the amount of daily sun exposure, naturally protecting the deeper layers of skin from the damaging and potentially cancerous effects of UVA and controlling the product of natural vitamin D (in the upper layers). But recognize that the buildup of pigment within the skin—especially in fair-skinned people, who tan with difficulty and burn with ease—develops slowly, requiring short, frequent exposure to sunlight to achieve protection without injury. You'll find the how-tos of safe sun exposure later in this chapter.

About now, you may be thinking that the pharmaceutical and cosmetic industry is bound to come up with a full-UV sunblock. Why don't we just slather that on and protect ourselves that way? Granted, a few UVA-blocking agents have come on the market in recent years—titanium oxide and others—but at best they fully screen only about half of the UVA wavelengths. And that still leaves the other half of the UVA spectrum to worry about. How can you tell if a sunscreen blocks UVA?[1] Some manufacturers in addition to providing the traditional SPF rating are now using a star system to denote the amount of UVA protection provided by their block, with one star (*) offering the lowest degree of protection and four stars (****) the most. But so far, all the products

1. Even the U.S. government gives sunblock a C to D rating (on an A = excellent scale) because the purported benefit (preventing skin cancer) is only presumed and has never been scientifically substantiated.

that block up to half of the UVA also block virtually all of the UVB, with the same unhealthy consequence of robbing the body of natural vitamin D production and preventing the skin from protecting itself with pigment. But aside from the issue of blocking vitamin D production, the sunscreening agents themselves may not be without risks. Some research has suggested that PABA (para-aminobenzoic acid, a common UVB sunblock agent) can be altered chemically by solar radiation to produce a potential cancer-causing compound. Talk about your Catch-22: you cover yourself in PABA to prevent skin cancer, go into the sun, and turn the sunblock into a carcinogenic chemical! As a consequence, many manufacturers have removed PABA from their products— and usually proudly announce it on the label. But the problem is this: What about other blocking agents? Could they, too, undergo transformation to a malignant substance when exposed to the sun's energy? The scenario is possible, although at this point research hasn't answered that question definitively.

You may be thinking, But wait. If I don't put on a sunblock when I go to the beach, I'll surely burn! And indeed you will if you overexpose your unprotected skin. Reddening of the skin from UVB exposure is a built-in warning that you've stayed in the sun too long. To silence that warning signal with a UVB blocking agent and far exceed your safe exposure time for UVA is a fool's bargain. Your best strategy is to cover up at the first sign that your skin is beginning to slightly redden (get into the shade, put on a hat, a shirt, long pants), rest your skin, and slowly build up your pigment protection day by day. Doesn't it make more sense to simply let the skin do its job providing us with vitamin D and a natural sunscreen at the same time? We think clearly so, and to that end we've included detailed recommendations on how to safely build up your natural pigment block later in the chapter.

But Couldn't I Just Take Vitamin D Pills?

Vitamin D is not abundantly found in the foods we eat. Fish-liver oils provide the richest amounts, with a little found in meat and eggs and vitamin D–fortified dairy products. Consequently, our bodies depend upon regular exposure of our uncovered skin to sunlight as the primary source. Granted, you could supplement vitamin D in the diet in pill form, but that choice is fraught with some risk, since in excess, dietary vitamin D is quite toxic, as the British discovered in the 1950s when they sought to ensure adequate levels of it by adding it to much of their food supply. Instead of making a healthier population, they ended up creating an epidemic of vitamin D–toxicity syndrome, the cardinal symptoms of which are weakness, excess calcium in the blood, calcification of tissues in the body, development of atherosclerosis and kidney stones, and elevated cholesterol.

While the body has a number of checks and balances to regulate the activation of the forerunner of vitamin D found in our skin, it has no means to control absorption of preformed dietary vitamin D and will continue to absorb it even when there's already too much. Vitamin D is a fat-soluble vitamin, which means that it can and will be stored in the liver to exceedingly high, toxic, and potentially fatal levels. Again, wouldn't it be a better idea simply to allow skin to do the job?

Human skin (along with its production partners, the liver and kidneys) is uniquely adapted to perform the task of supplying our bodies with natural vitamin D safely and efficiently—but only when we need it. When the body has sufficient levels of it, the conversion to the active form slows down or stops entirely, so there's no risk of reaching toxic levels of natural vitamin D, no matter how much sun exposure we receive.

Research has shown that 1 square centimeter of lightly pigmented skin can manufacture 18 IU (international units) of vitamin D in three hours of sunlight exposure even in northern latitudes. To produce the minimum daily requirement of 400 IU would demand a mere 20 centimeters of exposed skin, or about the size of the cheeks of a toddler, even bundled up on a cold winter's day. With slightly more exposure, say, the average adult's forearm (a body part often open to the sun), sufficient vitamin D can come from just 5 to 10 minutes of strong summer sunlight. The greater the amount of pigment in the skin, however, the slower the rate of conversion, since the pigment itself acts as a natural sunscreen and is, in fact, one means the body has developed to regulate vitamin D production in regions close to the equator. For this reason, dark-skinned people are far more susceptible to vitamin D deficiency and the development of rickets in children and osteomalacia in the elderly. The risk heightens in areas where sunshine isn't plentiful, such as in northern climates (in the Northern Hemisphere above 36° latitude) in winter or in urban areas with high levels of atmospheric pollution that may block the UVB portion of winter sunlight. Other groups at obvious risk of sun deprivation and the diseases it causes include underground workers (miners and others), shut-ins, bedridden hospital patients or nursing home residents, and Muslim and some Hindu women and children who subscribe to the custom of purdah and by design live their lives secluded indoors. Rates of rickets in children and osteomalacia in adults run high among these groups. Without sunlight to initiate the production of vitamin D, bones suffer. Think of what just a short bit of daily sunlight therapy would do to reduce physical disability among the elderly—in just fewer hip fractures alone!

You may be thinking, Yes, but that doesn't describe me. Think then of the many people who spend their lives indoors as a matter of routine, from their early-morning commute shelter in their cars to their fluorescent-lit offices, back to their cars, and by dusk or full dark into their houses again. Their entire day spent indoors, their only sunlight coming through window glass that provides an effective screen against much of the UV light. All told, they may spend only a few minutes outdoors, and that in the early morning or late evening, when the sun lies low on the horizon and its rays are their weakest. Research has shown that during the winter months, particularly in northern climates, vitamin D levels fall in these people, too, sometimes even to the point of clinical deficiency. And again, bones suffer.

How Sunshine Builds Strong Bones

Once manufactured in the skin and modified by the liver and the kidneys, the active vitamin D becomes the body's chief director of bone health in several ways. First, it acts as an incredibly potent stimulator of dietary calcium and phosphorous absorption from the intestine. In fact, even in the face of an adequate dietary calcium intake, without enough active vitamin D, the body will not absorb calcium properly. That's bad news for the millions of menopausal and premenopausal women trying to fend off osteoporosis by gobbling calcium tablets by the handful while at the same time doing all in their power to avoid exposing their "unblocked" skin to the rays of the sun.

In the face of vitamin D deficiency and the consequently poor absorption of dietary calcium and phosphorous that it brings, the levels of these two bone minerals in the blood begin to fall. As a result, mineralization of new bone becomes defective, and the bones themselves become mechanically weak and at higher risk for fracture. It's important to understand that even though our bones stop growing longer and thicker once we've reached maturity, they continually renew and remodel themselves throughout our lives, so we're all constantly making new bone tissue. It is here, in the remodeling and renewal of our bones, that active vitamin D exerts a direct influence through a hormonelike action that stimulates the bones to lay down minerals and to remove old bone and replace it with new healthy tissue. This role for vitamin D should come as no surprise if we take a moment to think about its chemical structure; active vitamin D closely resembles the male and female reproductive hormones and the "mother hormone" DHEA, all of which the body also manufactures using cholesterol as the beginning framework and all of which play important roles in bone building and maintenance. In fact, vitamin D *is* a hormone in its own right—a hormonal gift from the sun.

Taking hormones to ensure bone strength isn't a new concept. Women the world over have come to accept the effectiveness of taking estrogen after menopause to prevent osteoporosis, recognizing the power of that hormone to curb bone loss—although not without its own price in terms of increased cancer risk. Indeed, the risks of estrogen involve cancers more serious by far than the skin cancers the sun is typically thought to contribute to. What may surprise you is that while estrogen works pretty well to curb further bone loss, it isn't a particularly strong bone-*building* hormone. Natural active vitamin D is. Perhaps a better approach might be to use the power of sunlight and the "sunshine hormone," along with proper nutrition, to build and maintain bones throughout life.

Sunlight and Skin Damage

There's no real debate about the fact that solar radiation, particularly of the UV type, can age the skin. The damage occurs both by UV light's direct assault on the DNA (the genetic material within the cells responsible for directing all the cells' functions—in effect, the "brains" of the cell) and by the production of free radicals within the skin (see chapter 5, "Antioxidant Use and Abuse"), which once formed, may initiate a chain reaction and, in the onslaught, damage the tissues involved.

Unfortunately, the portion of sunlight that instigates the formation of free radicals—the UV portion—is the very portion necessary to begin the activation of vitamin D. So how do we reconcile this dilemma? Why would nature have given our ancient forebears—and us, by virtue of our inheritance of their biological makeup passed down through the millennia—this two-edged sword? Why create a system that requires exposure of our skin to the sun to obtain a crucial nutrient (vitamin D) if by that very exposure we risk skin damage and even skin cancer formation? How can we make sense of this contradiction?

Simply. Nature also provided our skin with protection against such damage in the form of antioxidants. Within the skin—as throughout the body—such substances as vitamin C, vitamin E, beta carotine, alpha-lipoic acid, glutathione, and coenzyme Q10 act as powerful scavengers of the free radicals generated by sun exposure and other toxins in our environment. Research has shown that exposure to UV light depletes the levels of these antioxidants in the skin, lending credence to their protective role against the damaging effects of sunlight. Replenishing the levels of these antioxidants in skin, therefore, would be a critical step in maintaining our natural protection against sun damage. For a modern human, that task is quite simple—we can trot down to the local health food store and pick up some selenium (needed to make glutathione), vitamin E, alpha-lipoic acid, and coenzyme Q10. But what of our ancient ancestors? Where did early humans get the antioxidants to replace what the sun baked away? From food!

Nature's vitamin shop provided all the critical nutrients necessary for early humans, just as it can for us today on the *Protein Power Lifeplan,* the difference being that modern nutritional technology allows us the luxury of supplementing nature with know-how. By maintaining sufficient antioxidant levels in our skin—through the foods we choose to eat and the antioxidant supplements we take—we can retard aging of the skin and still receive the sun's many other benefits. But age spots and wrinkles aside, let's tackle head-on the biggest fear concerning sun exposure: skin cancer.

Exactly what is the connection between sunlight and cancer? While there's little doubt that inappropriate or prolonged overexposure to the sun can burn and damage the skin and lead to the development of superficial skin cancers (called squamous cell carcinomas of the skin), it may surprise you to learn that sunlight can actually *prevent* the development of some much deadlier cancers. Let's see how.

The Sun and Skin Cancers

The American actor George Hamilton, renowned for his year-round, deep golden tan, when asked whether he feared he was increasing his risk for skin cancer by tanning, is said to have once quipped, "The best protection against skin cancer is a good tan!" The audience laughed at his glib response, and syndicated cartoonists lampooned his naïveté. But the joke's on them; as it turns out, Mr. Hamilton is probably right. Gradually and safely building up a protective layer of natural sunscreening skin pigment designed by nature to fend off the penetration of the UVA rays may indeed be the best way to protect against the development of skin cancers, including the deadliest form, malignant melanoma. While we hasten to add that we're not advocating a return to endless baking in the sun, we want to dispel the notion that exposing yourself to it can only do you ill. The sun, like all powerful forces, is best used wisely; recognize its great potential both to help and to harm and *never, never let your skin burn!* With that in mind, let's examine some of the evidence about the development of skin cancers and what seems to prevent them.

Skin cancers arise of three main cell types: *Squamous cell* cancers form in the most superficial, "flaky" layers of the skin; *basal cell* cancers are found in the bottom-most or base layer of epidermal (skin) cells; and *melanomas* form deeper within the skin in the pigment-producing cells, the melanocytes. The incidence of these cancers has risen dramatically in the last two or three decades—during which time, we should add, the use of potent UVB-blocking sunscreens has also skyrocketed. The most recent estimates from the American Cancer Society tell us that 1 million Americans will develop squamous and basal cell cancers each year, and 41,600 Americans were diagnosed with malignant melanoma in 1998. While the first two types of skin cancer grow slowly, rarely spread widely to distant sites within the body, and tend to be cured by early removal, such is not always the case for malignant melanoma. This type of skin cancer is the second-leading cause of death for young white men between the ages of fifteen and thirty-five. It tends to be aggressive, to spread quickly (often before it looks ominous to the untrained eye), and to be exceedingly difficult to treat once it does spread. If detected early, melanoma is highly curable, with ninety-five out of one hundred people alive and well five years after their diagnosis. However, if melanoma spreads to distant sites within the body, the five-year survival rate falls precipitously to sixteen out of one hundred. What causes these cancers to develop? Is it sun exposure?

For many years, UV light has been implicated as the primary cause of skin cancers, including malignant melanoma. And while there's less controversy—based on studies of both animals and humans—about its role in the development of squamous cell cancers and basal cell cancers, the case for sunlight as the cause of melanomas isn't as clear-cut.

Research has shown that exposing laboratory mice to a combination of the UVA and UVB wavelengths found in sunlight resulted in the development of skin cancers similar to squamous cell cancer in 80 percent of the animals, while exposure to UVB wavelengths alone caused such cancers to develop in only 17 percent of animals. Clearly, the impact of UVA light far exceeded that of UVB in promoting squamous cell skin cancers. However, with regard to melanomas, while exposure to UVA light easily promotes their growth in lab mice, even doses of UVB radiation sufficient to severely redden and damage the skin will not.

Can we conclude then that the cancer risk from sunlight rests primarily with the UVA portion of the spectrum and that as far as significant cancer risk goes UVB is safe? Probably so, although the relationship of sunlight and melanoma is a complex one, and while UVA seems to be the more likely culprit, it alone may not be solely responsible. In some studies exposure to UVA—even with a partial UVA-blocking screen—still promoted the development of melanoma in lab mice, leading the researchers to speculate that since they'd blocked the UVA light with the screen, other triggering factors must have been at work. (This connection of UVA and melanoma should be cause for concern for the millions of people who bake to a golden brown in tanning beds equipped with "safe tanning" UVA lights or who spend endless hours in sun worship, under the "protective" security blanket of a UVB-blocking sunscreen, even if it contains a partial UVA blocker.)

What's unclear from these studies is whether the researchers took into account the sunscreen-turned-carcinogen factor. That is, did the UVA radiation convert the benzophenone-3 and PABA (used as UV screening agents in the experiment) into cancer-causing compounds and by that means increase the occurrence of skin cancer in the mice? Or is there some other as yet unidentified cancer-causing agent triggered by UVA exposure? The issue isn't settled, but one fact is clear: in people, the development of a layer of natural sunscreening skin pigment brought about by gradual, regular, year-round exposure to sunlight offers the melanocytes lying deep in the skin as good or better protection from the harmful effects of UVA light than any currently available chemical sunscreens—without the added risk of conversion of the screen into a carcinogen. Again, it's simply better to let the skin do the job that eons of human development and refinement designed it to do. But the skin does more to protect us from skin cancers than just producing pigment to screen out harmful UV rays. And once again, the production of natural active vitamin D plays a central role.

Sunlight and Cancer Prevention

Numerous research papers have shown that metabolites (breakdown products or derivatives) of active vitamin D can actually suppress the growth and spread of malignant melanoma cells. Your eyes aren't playing tricks on you. We indeed just said that active vitamin D can retard the development and spread of melanoma. It is a tumor-inhibiting hormone. And what's more, its effects reach much farther than the skin; research has shown that active vitamin D can also impede the growth and development of breast cancer, colon cancer, and cancer of the prostate. And where do we get active vitamin D? From the sun—from the interaction of the UVB portion of sunlight with the special cholesterol in our unblocked skin. If adequate sunshine and vitamin D production can impede the development of these malignancies, then it stands to reason that inadequate amounts may promote them. And indeed that appears to be the case. Some researchers have even speculated that the inadequate vitamin D production that occurs in people with heavily pigmented skin living in geographic locations with limited sunlight, such as in northern latitudes and in the winter, might in part explain why these cancers behave so much more aggressively in black Americans (who, because of heavier pigment, may require more sunlight for adequate vitamin D production) than in white ones. (The same might be true for the millions of people who would never dream of going outside without covering every exposed inch of skin with a strong sunblock to "protect them.")

Indeed, even international cancer statistics bear out the cancer-preventive effect of sunshine. The incidences of breast, colon, and prostate cancer are lowest in the sun-drenched countries near the equator and increase as you move toward the polar regions of the globe. Not surprisingly, their occurrence also increases in areas of high air pollution, which blocks a significant portion of UVB from reaching us at the surface. And, as you have seen, without sufficient UVB exposure, the production of active vitamin D falls, robbing the sun-deprived populous of a potent anti-cancer weapon.

Researcher H. Gordon Ainsleigh in work published in the February 1993 issue of *Preventive Medicine* hit the nail on the head with this statement: "Frequent regular sun exposure acts to cause cancers [that result] in 2,000 U.S. fatalities per year, [but also] acts to prevent cancers that [result in] 138,000 U.S. fatalities per year." And since 1993, when that article appeared, the rates of these "preventable" cancers have continued to climb. Dr. Ainsleigh went even further, stating that "there is support in the medical literature to suggest that the 17% increase in breast cancer incidence during 1991–1992 may be the result of the past decade of pervasive anti-sun advisories from respected authorities, coinciding with effective sunscreen availability." And finally he went so far as to speculate that "trends in the epidemiological literature suggest that approximately 30,000 U.S. cancer deaths yearly would be averted by the widespread public adoption of regular, moderate sunning." From where we sit, that looks like a pretty decent bargain: risking a slight increase in the chance of superficial (and treatable) skin cancer for a substantial decrease in risk for cancers of the colon, breast, and prostate, as well as malignant melanoma.

Add to moderate sun exposure the *Protein Power Lifeplan* diet, containing, as it does, plenty of complete protein, good-quality fats, and antioxidants, and you've got a recipe not only to reduce the risk of colon, breast, and prostate cancers and malignant melanoma but even to lessen the risk of superficial cancers and retard skin aging. On the subject of dietary fat (a topic covered in detail in chapter 3, "The Fat of the Land"), an additional word about its relationship to cancer seems in order, because the fat you eat has clear implications in your risk of developing cancer. But not in the way you may think.

As you'll remember, the fats that you eat wind up in the walls of the cells throughout the body—including the skin—and influence both the critical functioning of the cell membrane and the production of the microhormone messengers (called prostaglandins or eicosanoids) that regulate many cell functions, including, perhaps, susceptibility or resistance to cancers. Research has shown that lab mice fed diets rich in Menhaden oil (a source of the omega-3 fat EPA, which is found in cold-water fish) resist the development of skin tumors, whereas those fed corn oil (a source of linoleic acid, a common omega-6 polyunsaturated fat) develop them more readily. Some cancer researchers believe that eating corn oil and other vegetable oils may be a necessary ingredient for the development of breast cancer—at least in lab mice. Other studies suggest that this connection may translate to the human plane as well.

In a study of people who developed malignant melanoma, all of those afflicted stated that they had eaten less saturated fat and more polyunsaturated fat in the ten months prior to their diagnosis. And this dietary modification was borne out in samples of the fat tissue taken from under the skin of patients with melanoma. Their fat tissues contained greater amounts of the polyunsaturated linoleic acid than those of people without the cancer.

Why would polyunsaturated fats in the walls of our skin cells heighten the risk for cancer development? Because of their inherent instability. You may recall that unstable oils under the influence of heat or oxygen will form damaging and potentially cancer-causing compounds called lipid peroxides. This transformation also takes place under the influence of the sun's heat and UV energy in the unstable fats (read: polyunsaturated fats) that find their way into the walls of our cells in the skin and throughout the body. (And the same transformation can occur in the oily bases of commercial sunblocks you apply to your skin.) So eating a diet high in corn and vegetable oils, in effect, sows the seeds of cancer throughout the walls of every cell in the skin, where they lay dormant waiting for the sun to help them grow. In a country where a misguided "cholesterol phobia" has spurred an increased consumption of these cheap oils, and the use of high-strength UVB-blocking sunscreens has become pervasive, is it any wonder we're facing an explosion of skin (and other) cancers? We interfere with the natural relationship our bodies have developed with sun and food through the millennia to our peril.

Sunlight and Other Health Issues

When we adopt modern living habits that disrupt our connection to the sun, bones weaken, cancers arise, and we fall heir, not to the wellness that is our natural birthright, but to a host of problems ranging from mood disorders (sunlight alleviates depressive symptoms) to multiple sclerosis and psoriasis (where the added vitamin D may offer hope for remission). Let's explore some of these now.

SKIN DEEP IS DEEP ENOUGH

Although the effects of intense light therapy go deeper than the skin, the surface benefits, too. People suffering from the persistent and difficult-to-treat skin disorder psoriasis understand the healing power of sunlight and know that their symptoms will generally improve in the sunny summer months and worsen in the gray of winter. This correlation led to the development of therapies using artificial UV light alone or in combination with sun-sensitizing chemicals called psoralens. The combined therapy (abbreviated PUVA, standing for psoralen + UVA light) has proven somewhat helpful in the treatment of this disorder; however, the risk of skin cancers from repeated UVA exposures limits its use. For most people UVB has proven to be a better and more efficacious therapy choice. In one clinical trial, the majority (86 percent) of psoriasis patients responded with clearing of their skin rashes and improvement of the joint pains that often accompany the disorder by exposure to artificial UVB light treatments administered three to five times a week for a total of thirty-five treatments. Interestingly, however, in this same trial, treatment with natural sunlight (instead of artificial UVB) resulted in clearing of symptoms in 94 percent of patients; in other words, they both work, but the plain old sun works better. What is it that the sun (or the UVB light) is doing to treat this disorder? To answer that question, we need to back up a bit and give a little background on psoriasis itself.

In psoriasis, the body produces an overabundance of the flaky cells of the upper most skin layer, resulting in inflamed, red, scaly patches on the skin. (The inflammation is thought to be a consequence of the body's own immune-defense system "turning on" itself both in the skin plaques and in the joints.) In some areas, these excess flakes build up, forming a thick, silvery, scaly plaque, especially prominent over the elbows and knees. Research has shown that vitamin D decreases the rapid production of these skin cells and normalizes their development. Clinical trials have shown that taking a form of vitamin D by mouth or rubbing it on as a cream results in improvement of the scaly patches of psoriasis. Although this therapy has proven effective, some clinicians and researchers have had reservations about its long-term safety, since, as you've already learned, taking vitamin D by mouth (or even absorbing it as a cream) can lead to the buildup of toxic levels in the body. Creams and pills are a nice idea to be sure, but the perfect vitamin D delivery system already exists: the UVB portion of sunlight striking skin. It produces the proper amount of natural active vitamin D, without fear of toxic side effects and without cost. How do you improve on the perfection honed by millennia? To our way of thinking, you don't even try, and we encourage those people plagued by psoriasis to view a daily sunbath in the same way as they would a daily dose of curative medication.

GOOD NEWS FOR SUN LOVERS WITH LOVE HANDLES

Way back there in 1939, a researcher named Ellinger published findings in the journal *Radiology* that exposure to UV light influenced body weight. The research had shown that laboratory animals receiving sunlight treatments lost weight on a given diet, while those not exposed to sunlight did not.

Apparently there is something in sunlight that boosts metabolism. In fact, it turns out that there are many "somethings" that it boosts. For example, it's been shown that exposure to sunlight stimulate the thyroid gland to produce thyroid hormone; it increases the production of testosterone, growth hormone, epinephrine (adrenaline) and norepinephrine (noradrenaline), all of which are intimately involved in the regulation of the metabolic rate and body weight. The metabolic rate climbs and remains elevated following a sunbath just sufficiently long to cause a slight "blushing" of the skin. Upon further study of these metabolic effects of sunlight, it appears, once again, that they involve the actions of vitamin D. In fact, active vitamin D and its derivatives have direct effects in more than thirty different tissues in the body, many of which relate to the metabolism. To our way of thinking, the most important connection thus far has been demonstrated in work published in 1997 by K.C.R. Baynes and colleagues, who showed that depletion of vitamin D results in poor glucose tolerance, hyperinsulinemia, and insulin resistance.[2]

And that means that in those people seeking to boost metabolic rate, burn calories more efficiently, build lean body mass, and trim down the love handles, a daily sunbath may help. For others, sunlight may actually be life saving. Let's see how.

CAN SUNLIGHT STOP MS?

Multiple sclerosis, the crippling disease of nerve and muscle that strikes eight thousand adults each year in the United States, has frustrated patients and medical practitioners alike, both because of its variable and unpredictable course and because of the difficultly in formulating effective treatments to deal with it. There's little doubt of a strong genetic pattern in the disorder— that is, people inherit a susceptibility to develop it—but genes don't explain everything in MS. Some predisposed individuals will develop it while others will not, leading researchers to search for an environmental trigger.

Interestingly, the disease shows a striking geographic pattern, with virtually no cases of MS found in regions near the equator and the incidence climbing sharply as you move toward either pole—a clear solar relationship. Even within countries, there is a geographic pattern; in Switzerland, for example, MS occurs with greater frequency in low altitudes, where less sunlight makes it to the surface, and less often at higher altitudes, where the thinner atmosphere admits a greater percentage of the sun's UV rays. This geographic-solar distribution has led researchers to speculate about a possible protective role of the sunshine vitamin in preventing MS.

And indeed, research published in 1997 by C. E. Hayes and colleagues at the University of Wisconsin seems to verify the con-

2. K.C.R. Baynes et al., "Vitamin D, Glucose Tolerance and Insulin Resistance in Elderly Men," *Diabetalogia* 40 (1997): 344–347.

nection. The research team demonstrated that by giving active vitamin D to laboratory mice, they could completely prevent their developing the mouse equivalent of MS. The work, as yet, can't be looked upon as conclusive, but just the glimmer of hope of preventing it in susceptible people or lessening its impact once present with something as innocuous as a daily dose of sunshine is cause for celebration.

DOES A SUNBATH A DAY KEEP THE DOCTOR AWAY?

If you're one of the millions of people who suffer from periodic recurrences of painful herpes simplex virus sores on your lips every time you get a cold, a fever, or spend too long in the sun, you'd probably answer no to that question. For some people, exposure to sunlight clearly causes eruptions of these sores. In fact, there's little doubt that anything that causes a dip in the vigilance of the immune-defense system can bring on a crop of those ugly blisters, no matter what caused the dip. So to be fair, we'd be remiss if we didn't include the UV portion of sunlight right along with a cold, fever, trauma, and stress as a cause of these troublesome outbreaks. But does that mean that sunlight exposure causes a dip in our immune function? And if so, does that mean we'll be at greater risk for infections or cancer formation from a daily sunbath? We think not, but let's look at what the research has to say.

Before we delve into this area, we want to point out that the lion's share of the research on this topic has been done on laboratory mice and not on humans, and there seems to be a big black hole in current scientific understanding of whether or not the findings can apply to us as well.

There have been numerous experiments in which researchers exposed laboratory mice to various wavelengths of UV light and then studied various measures of immune-defense system "health." Pretty much across the board, exposure to UV light, particularly UVB and UVC (which we don't get much of naturally on earth), caused a drop in what's termed cell-mediated immunity. This type of defense is what we rely on to help us recognize viruses, fungi, and precancerous or cancerous cells and to attack and eliminate them. It's also what goes awry when we develop skin allergies or sensitivities. Cell-mediated immunity causes us to react to such environmental miseries as poison ivy or gives us hives. And while having your skin not itch and blister on exposure to poison ivy sounds appealing, having your immune defenses fall asleep at the wheel when a virus or cancer cell lurks nearby doesn't.

On the other hand, a number of early scientific studies done in the United States, Europe, and Russia showed that exposure of both children and adults to UV light, especially in winter, reduced the rate of upper respiratory infections. It seems the literature is of two minds here. Does sunlight help or hurt the immune-defense system?

We felt we needed some resolution to this dilemma before we could recommend daily sunbathing as a clear benefit. And so, as we often do when things just don't add up, we looked at the problem through the Paleolithic lens, and when we did, we couldn't see why nature would have provided us so many benefits from sunlight—stronger bones, better mood, sounder sleep, a metabolic boost, and improved insulin sensitivity—if it also crippled the immune system. Remember that in the days of our early human ancestors, an infectious disease was quite literally a mortal enemy. And a solar-crippled immune system would certainly not have been conducive to survival of our species. So we delved deeper still into the research literature. And a solution appeared.

Virtually all the mouse studies, and most of the few human studies, have been done with short exposures of artificial UV light insufficient to give the skin time to adapt. We felt that we were on to something with this line of reasoning and finally we found the missing link: you have to continue the experiment to see the effect of *frequent, regular sunning.* Even though the immune defenses go into a slight slump with short amounts of exposure, Kripke and colleagues in 1977 found that after two to three months of chronic UV irradiation, the mice regained their normal degree of immune function.[3] The immune dip appears to be tem-

3. M. L. Kripke et al., "In Vivo Immune Response of Mice during Carcinogenesis by Ultraviolet Irradiation," *Journal of the National Cancer Institute* 59, no. 4 (1977): 1227–1230.

porary. And that makes sense, because how could something (UVB to be precise) that appears to prevent a number of cancers cripple the immune system? The answer is, in the long run it doesn't.

So yes, if you have led a "sheltered" life devoid of the sun, your sun blisters will blossom when you go out and get too much sun at one time. And that's why we encourage frequent, gradual exposure to the sun. And yes, if you turn your untanned, unadapted skin lobster red at the beach, you might get "sun sick" from the release of immune-suppressing substances from your burned skin. And that's another reason we say *never, never allow yourself to burn!*

But when all the facts are in, we believe that if you use the sun safely in conjunction with proper nutrition, your daily sunbath can indeed keep the doctor away.

THE SUNBATH

Safe sunbathing takes some explanation, though, because what is a "safe" amount of time for a given person depends on a wide variety of factors, including skin coloring, geographical location, time of year, time of day, setting, and the use of medications, soaps, and cosmetics that could make the skin burn more easily. We'll take these factors one at a time and then try to give you some basic rules of the sunbathing game so that you can come up with a sensible regimen that will work for you.

Skin Coloring. An almost limitless variety of skin tones exist within every ethnic group, so you should think of skin color as referring not to ethnicity but to amount of pigment. Those with more of it can spend more time in the sun before burning than those with less since, as you've learned, the skin's natural melanin pigment serves as an effective UV sunscreen. But except for the few people whom we can classify as true genetic albinos (those very rare individuals who can produce no pigment whatsoever), all of us have some pigment and all of us—even very fair-skinned people—can "train" our skin to protect us from the sun.

For example, if you're a person with little native pigment (in other words, if you're likely to say of yourself, "I don't ever tan, I just burn!"), you will need to take it very slowly to encourage pigment production. In direct summer sun, you may need to begin with exposures as brief as two to three minutes per side per day. And although with your fair natural coloring you're not likely to ever develop a deep golden "George Hamilton" tan, you'll produce enough pigment and thickening of the superficial layers to protect you from burning so readily and to produce plenty of natural vitamin D for health.

Safe sun-exposure limits loosen up somewhat as skin pigment increases. If you're one of those people whose skin tans a little but with some difficulty, a starting point of five minutes of summer sun per side per day would be prudent. Those who tan with relative ease could begin at the "winter white" stage with ten or even fifteen minutes or more per side per day, and those with heavily pigmented skin may begin at thirty or more minutes per side per day. Specific times will of course vary depending on the season of the year and the latitude at which you're sunning. Think of the numbers given here as good general ballpark figures, but use your common sense and your skin's built-in timer—the development of the first slight pink blush—to determine when you've had enough sun. In bright sun, it can be hard to detect the slight blush. You may need to go inside and check your skin color once your eyes have adjusted to the indoor light. (If you've got very darkly pigmented skin, of course, it won't develop a pink blush and you'll have to go more by feel, stopping when the skin feels warmed and tingling.) Whatever you do, no matter what your level of natural skin pigment, *don't let yourself burn!* When you first begin to feel or see a blush, you're through for the day—no matter what the clock says. Go inside, get into the shade, or cover up and sunbathe again tomorrow.

Geographic Location. The sun's rays must pass through the earth's atmosphere before making it to the surface, and this means that the amount of sunlight you receive depends on where in the world you are. Locations near the equator receive the most direct rays of sunlight (see figure 10.3); safe sun-exposure time there will be less than anywhere else on earth. As you move farther from the equator toward the poles, the spherical shape and tilt of the earth on its axis causes the rays of sunlight to strike at a steeper angle, forcing them to traverse the atmosphere for a much longer distance before making it to you on the surface. This

FIGURE 10.3

Atmosphere for Ultraviolet Rays to Pass Through by Season

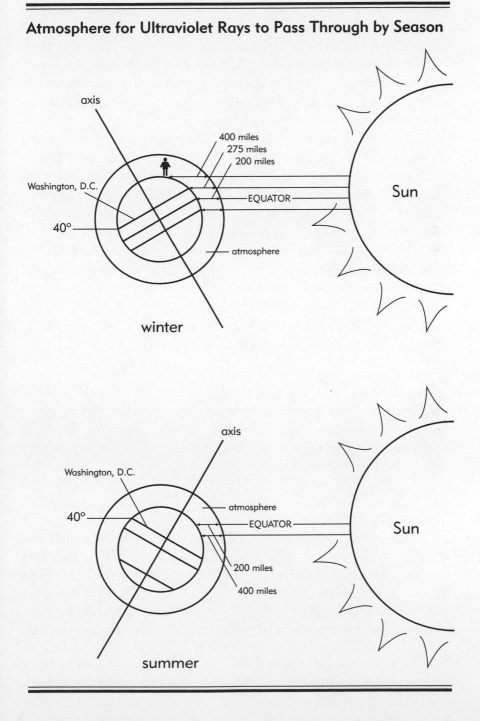

lengthier traverse diminishes some of the power of the rays, particularly in the UVB spectrum. This means that, in general, you can't safely spend as much time in the tropical sun as you can in the Alaskan sun.

Time of Year/Time of Day. Time of year or day doesn't matter much near the equator, where there's not a lot of difference in day length and sun strength between the seasons; cautious, gradual exposure should be the byword for the tropical sun in all people with untanned skin at any time of the year. But if you live or sunbathe outside the tropics, time of year alters the length of time you can safely sunbathe without risking a burn.

We encourage you to sunbathe year-round for maximum health benefit. The concept of winter sunbathing may not seem like a feasible notion at first, but in most locations, you'll find that the sun's rays will keep you warm and toasty if you block the wind. We'll sunbathe on sunny days in January in Colorado with a foot of snow on the deck and be comfortable.

During the winter months, in the Northern Hemisphere at least, the sun rides low on the horizon, with its slanting rays losing power as they pass through the long distances of atmosphere. The farther north you go, the weaker the winter rays become, so that even at high noon the sun still rides so low in the sky in the northern United States and Canada that almost no duration of exposure would cause burning. In these northern locales, winter sunbathing in the early morning or late afternoon won't be very effective in providing you with UVB and vitamin D. Consequently, during the period from November through February, the best times to sunbathe will be near noon (between 10 A.M. and 2 P.M.), when the sun is at its highest point. At this time of year, untanned, fair-skinned people in much of the United States can probably tolerate as much as thirty minutes to an hour per side without burning. (Exceptions are Hawaii, the coastal South, desert Southwest, southern West Coast, and high-altitude mountainous regions, where winter sun is still pretty strong and duration of safe sunning considerably less.)

During the sunnier months of the year (March through October) in areas from the middle of the United States to points north, it may take as little as fifteen to thirty minutes of exposure between the hours of 8 A.M. and 4 P.M. to slightly redden untanned light skin. In more southerly locations, only a few minutes may be enough. But we urge you once again to let your skin itself guide the duration. Whatever the season or time of day, consider your sunbath over when your skin first begins to blush, whether you've been at it five minutes or fifty-five. We've summarized the sunbath duration by season and location in table 10.1.

Setting. The effectiveness of the sun's rays also depends on the setting for your sunbath. Reflective surfaces will, as the word implies, reflect the incoming sunlight, enhancing its effect. That's one of the reasons you will burn more easily while snow skiing or on a white-sand beach. Snow provides the strongest influence, reflecting 85 percent of the UV rays, almost doubling your exposure; a white-sand beach returns about 17 percent of the incoming UV rays; and grass and water reflect only about 3 percent. (Contrary to what you may have thought, water isn't an especially good reflector of the sun's rays.) So in estimating your safe sun-exposure time, you must consider what kind of surface you'll be on. If you're on snow (especially) or sand, your safe sun-exposure time drops considerably, and you should take that into account.

TABLE 10.1

Average Time to Redness

MONTHS	TIME OF DAY	LATITUDE OF LOCATION	AVERAGE TIME OF EXPOSURE*
Year-round	8 A.M. to 4 P.M.	3 to 40°	15 minutes
Mar. to Oct.	8 A.M. to 4 P.M.	40°	30 minutes
Nov. to Feb.	10 A.M. to 2 P.M.	40°	60 minutes
Apr. to Sep.	8 A.M. to 4 P.M.	60°	30 minutes
Oct. to Mar.	anytime	60°	limitless

*This is the approximate time required to produce redness in unblocked, untanned white skin.

(And that brings up another point: What do you do if you're not fully tolerant of the sun and intend to enjoy a sun-filled vacation? If you're snow skiing or at the beach, for example, you've probably come for the day or for the week, and it's not practical to limit your ski or beach time to the amount of sun exposure your exposed skin—often just your cheeks, forehead, ears, and neck in skiing—can tolerate without burning. In these instances, it's probably most prudent to harvest your vitamin D with the amount of sun you can tolerate on your unblocked skin and then apply an oil-free full-spectrum sunblock to prevent your burning during the remainder of the day. It's not a perfect option but a compromise to permit your enjoyment of skiing or playing at the beach without risk of burning your skin. Recognize, however, that a potential risk of prolonged sun exposure in skin unadapted to sunlight is the development of skin cancers—even with the use of sunblocking agents. The better option, of course, would be to pre-adapt to the sun gradually throughout the months prior to your trip.)

Medications, Soaps, and Cosmetics. We've already mentioned that ingredients in these kinds of products can sensitize the skin to the sun, making it burn or develop a rash more easily. Once you adopt the practice of frequent sunbathing, you should check with your physician or pharmacist anytime you must take medications of any sort to be certain there's no known sun-sensitizing effect. (See table 10.2.) If there is, you should plan to reduce your exposure time accordingly until the medication is no longer necessary. For example, once you begin a new medication, cautiously check your sensitivity by dropping back to a two-minute-per-side maximum and working gradually up until your exposure causes no more than a slight blush. Do not exceed this new limit while on the medication.

With regard to lotions, soaps, perfumes, and cosmetics, they should not be on your skin when you sunbathe. We recommend that you shower using a natural soap that does not contain perfumes or antibacterial agents such as chlorine or fluoride derivatives, and then thoroughly rinse your body under the running stream of water prior to your daily sunbath. (It's also probably a good idea to check the chlorine and fluoride content of your home's water, too, since most communities add these chemicals

TABLE 10.2

Sun-Sensitizing Medications

The following chemicals can exaggerate or potentiate sunburn or stimulate the development of skin rashes with sun exposure. It is a partial list, with new members added frequently. It's a good idea to check with your pharmacist to discover if any medication you take has been shown to cause sun sensitivity.

Antibiotics (*Tetracycline and Sulfa families*)
Anti-fungal medications (*Griseofulvin*)
Anti-nausea medications (*Phenergan*)
Antiseptic agents containing halogens (*chlorine, fluoride*)
Diabetic medications (*Sulfonylurea family*)
Diuretics (*Thiazide family*)
Heart rhythm medications (*Quinidine*)
Sunscreen (*PABA*)
Tranquilizers (*Thorazine family*)

to city water. Several companies now make showerheads that will remove these potentially sun-sensitizing chemicals from your bathing water.) Do not apply perfumes, talcum powders, lotions, sunscreens (obviously), tanning boosters, moisturizers, or makeup to your skin prior to your sunbath, since ingredients in them might promote burning. Additionally, the oils in some of these products may not be stable when exposed to UV light and could form lipid peroxides—meaning that you would have spent time carefully applying a coating of carcinogens to your skin. After your sunbath, when you're no longer actively exposing your skin to UV light, if your skin feels dry, you can use a moisturizer. Prudence dictates that for chronically sun-exposed areas, such as the face and hands, you choose an oil-free moisturizer with antioxidants or simply use a little pure vitamin E oil.

The Basic Rules of the Sunbathing Game

1. Sunbathe year-round.

2. Build up sun time slowly, beginning with just a few minutes per side per day, never exceeding the point of a faint blush of the skin. *Never, never let your skin burn.*

3. Sunbathe with clean skin, free of lotions, soaps, perfumes, or cosmetics.

4. Do not use sunblock: the production of both vitamin D and melanin pigment are UVB dependent.

5. Reduce sun exposure time on snow or white sand or in tropical or high-altitude locations.

6. Do not exceed safe daily limits! When you've reached your limit, get out of the sun, put on a broad-brimmed hat and light clothing, or carry a "sunbrella."

7. Enjoy the sun!

We think that after taking a look at the wealth of scientific information that explains all of the good that you'll receive from natural sunlight, you'll come to revere the life-giving power of the sun, just as your ancient ancestors did for millions of years before you. So we encourage you to make the sun a part of your life, and in doing so, take one more step closer to the natural lifestyle we all once knew and to the birthright of wellness that is rightfully ours.

BOTTOM LINE

From our humblest human beginnings millions of years ago, we co-existed happily with the sun, seeking its life-giving power and warmth. Far from fearing the sun, early man reveled in it and even worshiped it—without the benefit of high-powered sunscreens. In modern times, however, our belief in the sun's power to cause wrinkles, age spots, and skin cancer has made us slather ourselves with sunscreen to "protect ourselves" from it. If you're worried about age spots and wrinkles from sun exposure, fear not. Antioxidants present in your skin and body tissues will protect you from damage caused by the sun, but you have to replace them regularly in your diet. Be certain it includes plenty of beta carotene, vitamin E, selenium, good-quality fats, animal protein (vegetarians must supplement their diet with sulfur-containing amino acids), and magnesium so that your body can replenish its antioxidant stores.

The rise in use of sunscreens has mirrored a rise in many cancers, including cancers of the breast, colon, prostate, and the deadliest form of skin cancer, malignant melanoma. It seems that far from protecting us, the use of powerful sunscreens has made things worse. We discourage the use of sunscreens, since they simply encourage you to bypass your natural warning signal of too much sun exposure (the sunburn) and create a false sense of security. Unfortunately, most commercially available sunscreens do not block the full spectrum of harmful ultraviolet (UV) rays, allowing through wavelengths of sunlight that could cause damage to the deeper layers of skin and increase the risk of malignant melanoma. They do, however, effectively block out the beneficial UV rays in sunlight and rob the body of an essential health-promoting nutrient.

This theft of nutrition—along with the fact that some sunscreens may be transformed into cancer-causing compounds by exposure to sunlight—may in part explain the rise in rates of cancer. Although it may sound strange, we humans "eat" the sun as a nutrient. Just as plants use sunlight to produce energy, the action of sunlight on our skin produces the "sunshine vitamin," natural vitamin D. The health benefits of this miraculous vitamin are legion, including building and strengthening bones, regulating calcium metabolism, influencing our mood, alleviating depression, boosting metabolism, and, amazingly enough, preventing the growth of cancers of the breast, colon, and prostate and even malignant melanoma.

Because only a few foods contain vitamin D (fish-liver oils, sardines, fortified dairy products, with just a bit in eggs and meat), we depend on sun exposure for vitamin D production. Granted, you can supplement vitamin D artificially in pills or add it to foods, but unlike the vitamin D that we make in our skin, the body has no means of regulating vitamin D that you take by mouth. Even when the body has taken in plenty, you'll continue to absorb dietary or supplemental vitamin D, allowing dangerous and even toxic levels to build up. A daily sunbath, however, can provide you with plenty of vitamin D to protect you from weak bones, sad moods, a slow metabolism, and cancers, all without the expense or risk of a toxic vitamin D overdose.

We recommend regular sunbathing as a necessary step back to the natural lifestyle we were born to live. By building up "sun time" slowly, you'll encourage the skin to increase its production of nature's best sunscreen—skin pigment. This process will happen even in fair-skinned people, but naturally, they must take it very slowly and cautiously.

The amount of time you can safely spend in a regular sunbath depends upon a number of factors: skin pigment, geographic location, time of year, time of day, and the setting of your sunbath. For complete details, see pages 249 to 256. For safety, begin sunbathing two to three minutes per side per day, assess your response, and work up in one-minute increments from there. Those people with greater levels of skin pigment can begin at five to fifteen minutes per side per day and work up, and those with heavily pigmented skin may begin at thirty minutes per side per day. Consider your sunbath ended at the first sign of a pink blush, regardless of what the clock says. Enjoy your new relationship with the sun, but remember its power and *never, never allow yourself to burn!*

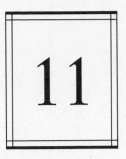

CALISTHENICS FOR THE BRAIN

All that we are is the result of what we have thought.
The mind is everything. What we think, we become.
—BUDDHA

A lifestyle program that maximizes physical health but ignores mental, spiritual, and emotional health is half a program. If we truly are born to be well, that must mean well in all senses—physically, mentally, and spiritually well. Just as sloth, gluttony, and abuse can destroy the physical wellness that is our genetic birthright, so, too, can nutritional abuse, mental laziness, and taking the path of least resistance dull and age our minds.

The human brain is a wondrous organ, designed to think, to problem-solve, to synthesize new and challenging information. When, through laziness, we fail to ask it to do this kind of work for us, its circuits rust, its myriad interconnections become weak and slow. The brain, like a racing thoroughbred, demands a regimen of constant exercise to stay in peak form. It wants to run, to test its limits; it will atrophy and age if left unattended in the stall or merely asked to plod along a well-known course.

When we are young, our brains must naturally confront new challenges regularly, and young brains, like young bodies, are supple, agile, and quick. As we age and the routine of adult life settles around us, most of us devote our mental energies less and less to the new and unfamiliar and more to the work we engage in day to day (which, no matter what the endeavor, with time becomes monotonous and unchallenging). While we may become more and more proficient in our chosen field, with age, thinking outside our "area" becomes increasingly more difficult. Sloth then comes into play, as we unconsciously opt not to put forth the effort that such thinking now requires.

As a part of your strategy to reclaim the whole-body wellness you were born to enjoy, we're going to prescribe a regimen of brain calisthenics along with brain nutrients to keep your mind as active and sharp as your body. Your job will be to find the areas that interest you and dive in. What sounds good to you? Learning a new language, reading philosophy or the classics, taking up golf, solving brain-teaser puzzles, rekindling an acquaintance with mathematics, learning to play an instrument, listening to classical music, learning to fly or scuba dive, taking up painting, working with clay, or beginning yoga, dance, or tai chi? All these and many more are possibilities, and you'll find that you can undertake many of these new activities without ever leaving home. In the Resources section of the appendix, we've included a number of at-home audio, video, music, and book suggestions for your learning pleasure. In addition, we've sought out adult summer vacation programs at college and university campuses, where you may further your enlightenment if you choose. The world of mind expansion is open to you; you have but to reach out to it from wherever you live to reap the rewards. Let's take a look at the scientific evidence validating the importance of brain exercise and proper nutrition.

You're a Fathead

Insulting as the phrase may be, it's absolutely true. The brain—yours, ours, everyone's—is indeed made mostly of fat. In fact, more than 60 percent of the complex structure of the brain is composed of fats of one kind or another, including a large percentage of the much-maligned cholesterol. But along with cholesterol, there's also a wide array of lesser-known but crucially important fats, such as docosahexanoic acid (DHA), arachidonic acid (AA), and two fat-containing molecules, phosphatidylserine (PS) and phosphatidylcholine (PC). And where do the critical fats needed to maintain the structure of the brain come from? The diet. And how can we hope to build and maintain an organ made of fat if we're made afraid to eat fat by well-intentioned but misguided media hype? We can't. And what happens to your brain when you don't get enough of the right type of fat from the food you eat? Disaster.

In the area of dietary fat (as you'll remember from chapter 3, "The Fat of the Land") we've taken a significant step away from the kinds of fats our ancient ancestors consumed. And for our trouble we've reaped a harvest of less-than-peak brain performance, depression, and possibly even more insidious neurological disorders, such as schizophrenia, Alzheimer's disease, MS (multiple sclerosis), Parkinson's disease, and Lou Gehrig's disease (also called amyotrophic lateral sclerosis, or ALS). The ancient diet contained a fair amount of cholesterol and some arachidonic acid, both of which we can easily obtain in eggs, dairy products, or red meat. But nowadays, something critical is missing. Recall that early humans also consumed a diet rich in DHA (an omega-3 fat absolutely crucial for brain development and health), provided by the meat and the brains of the game animals on which they feasted and in some areas by fish.[1] It's here in the DHA department that too many of us fall far short. Unlike meat from wild game, meat from lot-fed or grain-fed beef or chicken contains almost no DHA. For optimum brain health, good sources of DHA should become a regular part of your diet; we encourage you to eat sardines and fatty fish (or their oils) as often as possible, aiming for at least three or four times a week. (See chapter 3 for more details.)

---

1. With the advent of Mad Cow disease, dishes containing animal brains, once considered a delicacy, no longer find their way onto America's tables. And although in many instances eating brains may be safe, the specter of this devastating disease militates against this practice today. We therefore do not encourage the eating of animal brains as a source of DHA—even though it would be an excellent one. Instead we recommend increasing seafood, especially sardines, as a safe and excellent source. Vegetarians may instead wish to use the commercially available DHA "farmed" from algae.

Pass the Eggs, I'm Feeling Blue

For the last several decades, the cholesterol-is-deadly hypothesis has held sway in this country. We live in the grip of a national anti-cholesterol hysteria, with virtually every respected authority trumpeting the supposed dangers: Reduce cholesterol! Cut out eggs! Don't eat red meat! Keep cholesterol down or it will clog your arteries and you'll have a heart attack! And so the race to a zero-cholesterol diet has been going on apace. Fast-food establishments no longer cook their fries in cholesterol-laden lard; instead "healthy vegetable oils that contain no cholesterol" now boil and bubble in their deep fryers. (And you now know what happens to polyunsaturated vegetable oils after a few hours in the tank: they become truly deadly lipid peroxides!) And legions of adolescents, teens, and adults belly up to the counter to super-duper-size their orders of potato starch soaked in trans fats, unaware or unconcerned that the bad fat they're eating will wind up in cell membranes everywhere—including their brains. But we digress; we'll explore the subject of trans fats and your brain in greater detail shortly. Let's look first at what happens when the brain doesn't get enough of what it does need. One of those things is dietary cholesterol, and avoiding it can bring on the low-cholesterol blues.

In studies of both primates and humans, researchers discovered that depriving their subjects of dietary fat—and in particular dietary cholesterol—resulted in changes of mood and disposition that included depression, social withdrawal, and aggressive behavior. Furthermore, providing an adequate amount of fat but devoid of sufficient cholesterol resulted in the same depressive and/or aggressive symptoms. A brief examination of the biochemistry of cholesterol makes at least one reason for these findings clear: cholesterol acts in the brain to block the reuptake of the mood-enhancing brain chemical serotonin. This is precisely the action of the burgeoning class of anti-depressants typified by the drug Prozac. So it appears that a stable sense of well-being and contentment depends on getting enough of nature's serotonin reuptake inhibitor, cholesterol, from the diet. And certainly, examination of the diet of our ancient ancestors bears out their having eaten a fair amount more of it than modern-day nutritional recommendations deem "healthy."

Other research has shown that apart from the amount of cholesterol a person (or chimp) eats, the level of cholesterol in the blood may also correlate with mood and behavior—and in particular with violence. In one study, subjects with low blood cholesterol levels were found six times more likely to die violently from causes including suicide, auto accidents (which may often be disguised suicide), and homicide. Yes, homicide. The research doesn't make the cause clear, but perhaps having too low a cholesterol reading can make your disposition unpleasant enough to move even *other* people to violence!

This information is not based on the cherry-picking of a few studies in osbcure journals. In fact, a review of the medical literature done by Beatrice A. Golomb, M.D., uncovered no fewer than 163 studies linking low cholesterol to violence.[2] How low is too low? Through analysis of a number of these studies, statisticians have pegged a low limit for cholesterol levels, at least in the males of our species. Men whose cholesterol readings run below 160 mg/dl have 50 percent more violent deaths than men with higher readings. The connections held true both in people who had lowered their cholesterol readings too far with a low-fat diet (although that's tough to do unless you're eating both a very low-fat and low-carb diet) and in people who used any of the dozen or so currently available cholesterol-lowering medications to reduce their cholesterol to these low levels.

But other blood fats have an impact on the brain's normal functioning and play a part in depression as well. Research has also demonstrated that depression occurs quite commonly in people with elevated triglycerides (which you now know are a major marker of the insulin-resistance syndrome and are related to carbohydrate intake and not to eating fat). Reducing triglyceride levels—and there's simply no more powerful tool to do so than *Protein Power LifePlan* nutrition—brings about a lifting of the depressed mood.

2. Beatrice A. Golomb, "Cholesterol and Violence: Is There a Connection?," *Annals of Internal Medicine* 128 (1998): 478–487.

By following the nutritional recommendations of the *Protein Power LifePlan,* you, too, should benefit from a more stable mood by keeping your triglycerides and cholesterol within a healthy range and providing your brain with enough dietary cholesterol to keep it happy—by eating eggs, enjoying red meats, shellfish, and seafood, and indulging in butter. So if you're feeling blue, instead of popping Prozac, we advise you to eat your eggs and feel better naturally.[3]

But important as it is, cholesterol is only half the story on fat intake and depression. Once again, the essential fat DHA comes into the picture. Studies have also documented that depletion of DHA may occur following pregnancy in women who do not sufficiently replace it in their diets. This finding has led to speculation that this deficiency may underlie the sometimes severe depression that can occasionally follow pregnancy. If indeed deficiency of DHA in the diet can bring about depression, then it should follow that depression should be rare in societies that consume plenty of it. And indeed, such is the case. Examination of the inhabitants of Japanese fishing villages (chosen because fish-dependent diets are usually high in DHA) by trained psychological interviewers found only about 1 percent of the population to be depressed. Moreover, the rates of depression in North America and much of Europe are as much as ten times higher than in societies around the world that rely heavily on fish (particularly those that eat more fatty cold-water fish, such as sardines, mackerel, salmon, and herring—all rich sources of DHA).

Fat Deficiency and Faulty Insulation

The brain is only part of the nervous system, and essential dietary fats play crucial roles in other areas as well. Most important, fat makes up more than three-quarters of the insulating tissue—called the myelin sheath—that covers and protects all nerve fibers. Patches of loss of this sheath—bare areas, if you will—are

---

3. We do not intend that readers misinterpret this advice as a message to discontinue current medications for depression except under the direct supervision of their prescribing physicians.

the hallmark of multiple sclerosis (MS). Studies of people suffering from MS document an increased rate of depression, hardly a surprising correlation given the frustrating nature of their disorder. But what's more to the point, from a fat perspective many of them have low levels of DHA in their tissues, which, as you've already seen, also appears to correlate with depression. So perhaps the two disorders are linked, both being manifestations of a DHA (and possibly cholesterol) deficiency.

In the development of MS, an oversimplified explanatory scenario could go something like this: low levels of these essential fats in the tissues (perhaps from birth) lead to less raw material for nerve-sheath maintenance, which leads to potholes in the nerve's insulation, which leads to short-circuitry of nerve function. The circumstantial evidence connecting MS and essential-fat deficiency is pretty strong. For example, there's evidence to suggest that MS arises more often in adults who were fed with DHA-deficient cow's milk or formula instead of breast milk. Also, the disease occurs less commonly in geographic locations where fish comprise a substantial part of the diet. Furthermore, there's a fair amount of empiric clinical data to support the use of supplemental essential fats in the treatment of MS. Do we believe that eating a diet higher in essential fats will cure MS? That this devastating disorder is merely a fat-deficiency disease? No, it's probably not that simple, and certainly the data thus far aren't totally convincing, but the intake of good amounts of essential fats is important for so many aspects of health, that we think everyone should make a conscious effort to increase dietary sources. And people suffering from MS might be doubly advised to learn to love sardines.

Invasion of the Frankenstein Fats

As we detailed in chapter 3, another major departure of our modern diet from that of our ancient forebears occurred with the introduction of partially hydrogenated vegetable oil (trans fats) after the Second World War, following which their consumption skyrocketed. Chips—a staple of children, teens, and many adults throughout the country—may contain as much as 47 percent of these fats; french fries, deep-fried fish and chicken, and dough-nuts contain even more. Many Americans, and especially kids, may subsist almost solely on a diet of these kinds of foods. A number of researchers now feel that the explosion of ADHD (attention deficity hyperactivity disorder), learning disabilities, behavior problems, and possibly even increasing teen depression, apathy, and suicide can, at least in part, be laid at the door of diets containing poor-quality fats, little good-quality cholesterol, far too much sugar and starch, and an abundance of altered fats. The impact on our national health is frightening, but more frightening yet is research showing that these altered fats readily cross the womb from a mother to her unborn child and also appear in her breast milk.

Remember, the fats you eat find their way into the cell membranes of every tissue and organ in the body, including the brain and nerves; this holds true whether they're "good" fats or "bad" ones. Each of the good-quality essential brain fats—cholesterol, DHA, AA, PS, and PC—has a specific role in maintaining the shape, structure, fluidity, and function of the cell membranes. But nowhere in our Fred Flintstone physiology do trans fats fit in. Since Fred didn't have access to them through his couple of million years of refinement, he developed no means of dealing with their structure. And consequently, as heirs to his physiology, we have no use for them either. Because of their abnormal shape, when they're taken up as raw material for the cell membranes, they simply don't fit properly. They stack too neatly, pack too tightly, and make the cell membrane less malleable. When this happens, receptors fail to function properly, brain-signaling chemicals can't transmit their messages normally, the insulating properties of the nerves break down, and the brain fails to perform optimally. And we may fall prey to depression, mood disorders, fuzzy thinking, sleep disturbances, and the whole host of brain and nervous system diseases that we mentioned earlier. Eating trans fats is like eating brain poison. We urge you to avoid them wherever you can. We feel strongly enough about the dangers of trans fats to your brain and to your general health to make this trans fat avoidance recommendation across the board—regardless of which level of commitment you've selected for your rehabilitation.

It will take a while—sometimes only weeks but often six months or longer—for your dietary changes to make a noticeable impact on your brain and nerve tissues. It takes time to replace the poor-quality fats that may now be lurking in your tissues with good-quality ones. But one of the great things about the design of the human body is that it constantly renews, and because of this miracle, with good nutrition you can in time rebuild a healthier body and brain.

The Windows of the Brain

While ancient philosophers could endlessly debate the question of whether the eyes are the windows of the soul, we believe that your eyes are at least the windows of your brain. They are an elegantly sophisticated pair of sensory-collection devices that transform light energy into chemical and electrical impulses that the brain then interprets in pictures. The business of image collection occurs on the retina, a highly specialized type of nervelike membrane located at the back of the eyeball. Each day, the retina sheds some of its image-processing, or photoreceptor, cells, necessitating replacement with new cells, which, of course, requires adequate amounts of the correct raw materials. Like all nerve tissues, the composition of the retina relies heavily on fat-based molecules—particularly our old friend DHA; in fact, concentrations of DHA are higher in the retina than in any other tissue in the body. This essential fat must be present in sufficient amounts during pregnancy for normal development of eye structures to occur and after birth for continued development and sharpening of vision. Because of the regular shedding of retinal cells, we can assume that maintaining good vision requires the regular intake of DHA (or sources for its production) throughout life.

Chronic exposure to the light—an obvious requirement for seeing—makes the eyes vulnerable to accelerated aging from the potentially damaging effects of ultraviolet radiation. As occurs with the skin and other sun-exposed tissues, ultraviolet light rays cause the production of free radicals (see chapter 5, "Antioxidant

Use and Abuse," for more details) that can damage the delicate eye structures, leading to the formation of cataracts in the lens or degeneration of the most highly sensitive portion of the retina, the macula densa. Since the job of the eyes is to see, we can hardly escape the necessity of allowing light into them. But if with light comes damage, what can we do to prevent the damage?

At first blush, it may seem that the best defense for your eyes would be to always wear dark sunglasses that block the UV rays. However, while there may be some protective benefit there (and we ourselves wear them when the occasion demands), sunglasses may not necessarily be your best option. Hiding behind tinted glass may be giving you a false sense of security. Not all sunglasses provide protection from 100 percent of all potentially damaging UV rays, and if they do not, the tinting allows your pupils to widen comfortably, admitting more UV light and raising the possibility of surreptitious damage from the sun. Beyond that, by always wearing dark UV-filtering glasses, you'll rob yourself of the mood-elevating properties of natural sunlight. A broad-brimmed hat can cut the percentage of sunlight entering the eye by as much as half without completely altering the spectrum of waves that enter the eye and stimulate the brain. Certainly in some situations—snow skiing comes immediately to mind—wearing a broad-brimmed hat simply won't work, but you will burn your eyes without some form of protection. In such instances, sunglasses make infinitely more sense and we certainly recommend their use, but you should try to select a pair that will offer 100 percent UV light protection.

However, the protective screen you put above or in front of your eyes may not be as important as the invisible screen of anti-oxidant nutrients you put into your tissues. Research has shown that a variety of foods, if eaten regularly, can help to retard aging not only of the eyes but also of the brain and nervous system. In studies animals have demonstrated improved brain function (at least when it comes to the learning abilities of middle-aged rats) on diets enriched by such foods as spinach, kale, blueberries, strawberries, raspberries, broccoli, and tomatoes—all foods high in natural antioxidant and free-radical-scavenging compounds. And since they're all foods prominent in your *Protein Power LifePlan* regimen, meeting that goal will be a snap.

As you now know, we don't recommend the wholesale gobbling of individual antioxidants for good health. It's not always
helpful and sometimes downright harmful (as in the case of the
CARET beta carotene smoking study; see chapter 5). Apart from
a bit of extra vitamin E, alpha-lipoic acid, and coenzyme Q10,
and on occasion some extra vitamin C, we recommend that you
increase your antioxidant intake with whole foods. Certainly what
you eat (the raw materials you take in) matters most in developing, rehabilitating, and preserving the structure and functioning
of your brain and nervous system (including your eyes). Enhancing their performance and keeping them agile require that you do
brain work. Let's explore this area in greater detail.

Brain Aerobics: Pumping Your Noggin

Imagine yourself in a gym, curling a dumbbell with your biceps. As you work the muscle, your body sends extra blood to it
to nourish it during its exertion. The biceps puffs up slightly after
the workout because it is filled with blood—at the gym, they call
it "being pumped." If you keep doing those curls regularly, the
biceps muscle will actually become larger by building more muscle
tissue, losing fat, and gaining definition (your buddies at the gym
would smile approvingly and dub your biceps buff or ripped!).
Well, the same thing happens to your brain when you work it
regularly: your brain becomes buff, at least in theory.

To investigate this hypothesis, researchers at Washington University studied blood flow to the brain using a special type of brain
scan (called positron-emission tomography, or PET scan) while
their subjects took tests involving language, practiced the piano,
or played a sport. Their results documented an increase in blood
flow to the area of the brain involved in that particular type of
learning or concentration. But what's even more interesting is that
these researchers were able to map increased blood flow to different areas of the brain, depending on whether the activity being
done was a new and unfamiliar one or one that had already been
learned. And this is why we encourage you to regularly undertake
the study of subjects or activities that are new and unfamiliar to
you. Based on this research, "new" learning should open up more

blood flow along new circuits and pathways within the brain, while repeating familiar tasks will keep blood flowing along the same circuits. Both endeavors have their place.

Recall that we mentioned not just opening new circuitry but the possibility of exercising your way to a buff, ripped, expanded brain. What about that? In *Brain Workout* (St. Martin's, 1997), a fascinating book by Arthur Winter, M.D., and Ruth Winter, M.S., the authors describe some intriguing primate research on the part of R. J. Nelson and colleagues that indicates that beyond the forging of new connections, *repeated* use of pathways—for example, regular practice of an instrument, study of a new language, or developing skills in a new sport—may actually increase the size of the brain in the areas controlling those activities. At least it appears so for apes and chimps. But what about humans?

M IS FOR MUSIC, M IS FOR MOZART

Utter the words *genius* and *music* in the same sentence, and if you're at all a fan of classical music, try to suppress a mental image of Mozart. It's almost not possible to do. Nowhere in all of human history can we find a better example of inherent talent landing in the right place at the right time. In the instance of Mozart, the potential for specific genius, the desire to develop it, and the nurturing environment needed to do so converged, and the world will be forever enriched. To those people with the desire or ability to learn to play the piano we heartily recommend learning selections of Mozart—or his classical contemporaries Beethoven and Haydn—as an exercise in brain building.

And it's a good thing that miraculous convergence occurred also for those people who love music but whose musical talent extends mainly to playing the stereo. If that describes you, don't despair. You can still use the music of Mozart to brush the cobwebs from your brain. While compelling research shows the potent benefits of actually attempting to learn to play an instrument (doing so may facilitate learning in many areas, including improvement of verbal skills), a wealth of research has also shown that simply listening to the beautiful melodies that Mozart and the other classical masters left us can improve concentration and learning, unlock creative channels, relieve chronic pain, and fine-tune the brain for almost any task. We recommend that our patients—especially expectant mothers, infants, and all people under stress—listen to the music of Mozart. Research has shown a high likelihood that even babies in the womb appreciate the tonal and rhythmic perfection of this music. Developing infants respond with less kicking, as though the music relaxes them and they settle in to enjoy the concert. The complex construction of Mozart's music also seems to improve babies' ability to learn after they make their arrival into the world. Continuing to play the music softly in their rooms calms them and increases the likelihood of their developing musical facility later. (See the Resources section of the appendix for recordings of Mozart's music suitable for expectant mothers, infants, and children.)

PARLEZ-VOUS FRANÇAIS? SPRECHEN SIE DEUTSCH? PARLA LEI ITALIANO?

Among the activities that can strengthen the adult brain, one of the best—and one with practical ramifications if you're like us and love to travel abroad—is learning a new language. The complex skill of communication involves many areas of the brain, and working those connections conditions and strengthens them. Interestingly, in exercises involving repetition of words, PET scans show increases in blood flow to different areas of the brain, depending upon whether a given word comes from the subject's first language or a second language being learned. For most adults, learning a new language is difficult, but it's work worth doing because it exercises wide areas of your brain, forces you to use your memory, often calls upon you to control different kinds of facial, mouth, and tongue musculature to make a variety of new sounds, and in general improves your cognitive skills across the board.

If this appeals to you, we recommend that you purchase a set of audio- or videotapes to guide you, and dive in. Just a few minutes a day spent making this effort will be a boon to your brain; you'll begin lighting up whole new areas! We've included a variety of sources to help you in your language quest—tape series, software, and books—in the Resources section in the appendix.

ROSES ARE RED, VIOLETS ARE BLUE . . .

And while we're on the subjects of language and music, we'd be remiss not to mention the study of musical language—poetry. Whether writing your own poetry or reading out loud the great poetry of others, the metered discipline of poetic verse improves not only thinking skills and verbal skills but spatial skills and memory skills as well. To exercise your memory in this way, take a flashback trip to your grammar school days and set yourself the task of memorizing lines of poetry or entire poems that appeal to you. Daily practice and recall exercise yet another area of your brain—and besides, once you've built your repertoire and have lots of lines of poetry at the ready, you'll be the hit of the party when you can call up an appropriate snippet of verse for just the right toast.

But any new learning—on subjects outside your comfort zone or chosen field—can be of benefit in brain building. Although it may be too late to go back to college (or perhaps it's not, as the burgeoning number of older adults at colleges and universities will attest), you can still expose yourself to the thoughts of great thinkers and the words of great teachers through any of a number of series of video- or audiotaped or in-residence programs on a wide variety of subjects ranging from classical literature to philosophy to political thought to religion to history and more. Peruse the Resources section of the appendix for suggestions.

Each of us possesses latent talents that we can uncover only by daring to venture into new areas of learning. Perhaps you have an unmined gift for writing or poetry, for playing the flute or guitar, for sculpting or painting. You'll never know, unless you work the connections in those brain areas by trying your hand at a wide variety of new tasks. Remember, Grandma Moses, the famous painter of folk art, didn't begin exploiting her gifts until very late in life. And even if you discover that your abilities in art, music, or poetry aren't sufficient to make you give up your day job, we still encourage you to try any new activity that seems appealing; like performing aerobics with your brain, the effort will improve circulation, increase oxygenation, and keep the circuitry polished and in good repair.

LEARNING BY DOING: REFURBISHING A RUSTY CEREBELLUM

Brain-building exercise doesn't have to mean book-learning, however. New physical activities can also reopen and hone the circuitry. In fact, as we age, continuing to engage in physical activities that require balance skills may have health implications more far-reaching than just improving brain function, such as by reducing the chance of falls and hip fractures in the elderly. For a moment, we ask you to engage in a simple exercise: Imagine yourself at the age of ten. You're in a park, surrounded by flowers, shady trees, and a carpet of verdant grass. A parking barrier made of upright 2-foot-high railroad tie timbers edges the grassy expanse. The twenty timbers are set about 3 feet apart; yellow daffodils and clover have sprung up around their bases. The sun warms the breeze, as puffy, white clouds dot a clear blue sky. Take a minute with your eyes closed and really envision this scene. Feel the sun on your face. Smell the scent of the daffodils on the breeze. Really try to be a kid again, there in this place. What does the ten-year-old in you immediately do?

Chances are you hop up on the first timber and thoughtlessly and effortlessly leap from one to the next—all twenty in a row and back without a slip. No work involved; no fear of falling. Now return to the present; become the adult you. Would you even consider (except perhaps in an inebriated condition) engaging in this game? Probably not, and that's a shame. One of the consequences of age is that we opt out of activities that keep the balance and agility centers of the brain oiled and running smoothly. We walk around barriers rather than hopping over them. But let us pose a question: Do our circuits become rusty with age because we opt out of these activities, or do we opt out of them because we're getting old and rusty? Although the research doesn't yet clearly establish the answer to this question, we believe it to be the former: we first rust because of disuse and then the fact of our rustiness makes the use difficult. And if that is the case, dusting off those circuits can only help.

Balance is a complex skill, requiring your brain to make myriad minuscule adjustments in a milli-instant. While we're not going to recommend that you rush out and begin to leap parking barriers from pole to pole—if you really haven't done that since you were ten, you might end up with your nose bandaged and your arm in a sling—we do encourage you to begin once again to engage in activities that improve your balance, such as dancing, yoga, tai chi, or any of your own invention, or even just standing on one leg.

SWING YOUR PARTNER

If you're the gregarious sort or would like to couple calorie-burning exercise with balance improvement, you might enjoy taking up some sort of dance; whether your inclination runs to ballroom or swing dancing, country-western line dancing, square dancing, tap dance, modern or jazz dance, or classical ballet, any form of dance will improve your balance and agility. You should be able to find classes in some or all of these dance forms through dance studios or private dance instructors listed in your newspaper or telephone book. And in many communities local colleges, universities, athletic clubs, churches, or the Y offer dance classes. By becoming involved in these areas, you may not only improve your balance and agility but expand your circle of friends as well.

But perhaps you'd prefer a more ancient form of balance improvement, such as the oriental arts of tai chi and yoga. These most controlled disciplines, properly performed, can offer a lifelong venue for learning, demanding patience, balance, strength, and flexibility—and calling upon memory skills to boot! Although we think personal instruction by a qualified teacher is the best way to learn yoga or the martial arts, including tai chi, there may not be an instructor in your community, and if not, you can try one of the video instruction programs available at many bookstores.

A LITTLE LEARNING IS A DANGEROUS THING . . .

A scholar and terrific teacher of high school English (MDE's mother) began each new school year by inscribing the following quote and her addendum to it on the classroom chalkboard:

"A little learning is a dangerous thing."
Live dangerously, learn a little!

That's one of the important take-home messages from this chapter. We urge you, for the sake of your brain, to feed it properly and to continue learning throughout your life. Try anything that intrigues you, and let your imagination soar: try your hand at painting, take a class in pottery making, sign up for a course in canoeing, learn to play an instrument (it doesn't matter if it's the harp or the harmonica; the benefit is in the effort). Learning keeps the channels open, so we challenge you to live really dangerously and learn a lot!!

BOTTOM LINE

The human brain was designed to think, problem-solve, and synthesize new and challenging information. When, through laziness, we fail to ask it to do this kind of work for us, its circuits rust and it becomes weak and slow. As we age and the routine of life settles around us, most of us devote our mental energies less and less to the new and unfamiliar and more to the work we engage in every day. To keep the brain sharp, we prescribe a regimen of brain calisthenics by encouraging you to continually attempt to learn new things. Any such new activity—whether solving puzzles, working mathematical problems, learning a new language, learning to play an instrument, learning a new sport, taking up painting, pottery making, or woodworking—will strengthen the brain and improve both its function and blood circulation within it. Activities that improve balance—dancing, yoga, or tai chi, for instance—also improve brain functioning. Even just listening to the music of Mozart, Beethoven, Haydn, or Bach can help to improve brain functioning and relieve stress. (See the Resources in the appendix for recommendations.) For the sake of your brain, we encourage you to continue to engage in new learning for the rest of your life.

In addition to working the brain, you must be certain to nourish it by eating a diet rich in good-quality fats—especially the omega-3 fats found in cold-water fish, such as sardines, salmon, mackerel, and herring, or in cod-liver oil—and some dietary cholesterol, which research has shown helps to forestall depression.

12

BORN TO BE FIT

You will never "find" time. If you want time,
you must make it.
—CHARLES BUXTON

The American obsession with fitness has led to a lifestyle that for many people may include miles and miles of running each day or hours spent pumping, rowing, stepping, and crunching in the gym—or to an overwhelming sense of guilt for not doing so. Sure it's sometimes a drag, but fitness is important, right? And all those hours of exercise pay off, don't they? The answer to the first question is yes, fitness is important, although clearly not as important as changing your diet. But surprisingly, the answer to the second question is a qualified maybe. The right kinds of exercise done properly can bestow tremendous rewards by restoring your youthfulness and strength, but the wrong kinds may reward you with precisely the opposite: a slowing, aging, and weakening of the body. Just as we did in *Protein Power,* where we stressed the importance of using resistance training to build lean muscle, strengthen bones, lose fat, and improve insulin sensitivity, we again want to emphasize the health benefits that the right kinds of exercise can add to those you'll realize from nutritional changes alone. That is not to say that you won't reap tremendous health rewards simply by altering your diet in the way that we recommend. You will. In fact, diet is a more effective tool to lose weight than exercise is by far, but the two methods complement each other. Even if you've not exercised in years—perhaps never enjoyed exercising—if you're like most of our patients, once you begin to feel the increase in energy that comes from regaining your hormonal balance and the lightness of movement that comes from reducing body fat, you will very likely discover a pleasure in exercising that you may never have experienced before.

For a hint at what we modern humans should be doing on the exercise front, let's look through that peephole into our Paleolithic past to see what kinds of activities our early ancestors engaged in. How did early humans stay in shape? Did they spend hours chest-pressing heavy rock barbells at the local Bedrock Gym, à la the Flintstones? Probably not. Mankind, like all free-living creatures, was simply born to be fit, naturally. Ah, you're saying, but those early people lived a hard existence just hunting and foraging for food; life itself was a daily workout for them. Not so for modern humans; we have to work at our fitness. And in some respects that assumption is true. Early humans sometimes did tremendous amounts of work, but according to some researchers not as much as you might think and not every moment of every day.

For instance, medical researcher Kerin O'Dea and her team of investigators in Australia performed a series of fascinating studies to investigate this point. By following along, recording, and watching, the team evaluated the number of hours per day spent in "work" in a contemporary hunter-gatherer population, the Australian aborigines, and compared this figure to similar measurements made on their aborigine counterparts who had left the traditional lifestyle of the bush and moved to the city to pursue modern, civilized existence. And the results? The city dwellers spent more time doing physical "work" than their bush-country cousins. Certainly, the hunter-gatherer lifestyle involves working to obtain food, but the workers become so efficient at the task that they spend far less of their time and energy doing it than most of us would imagine. And like Paleolithic humans, the contemporary hunter-gatherers stay lean, strong-boned, and fit. How? What's the secret? First and foremost, the hunter-gatherers, like their ancient ancestors, continue to eat a Paleolithic diet—high in protein and good fat and limited in carbohydrate foods. But beyond their better diet, what did our Paleolithic ancestors do that perhaps we should be doing to stay fit?

Exercise in the Paleolithic garden—if we can measure it by the contemporary hunter-gatherer yardstick—consisted of brief bursts of high-intensity output followed by long periods of relaxing, storytelling, and stretching. Envision a pride of lions on the savanna sleeping in the sun, grooming, stretching, contemplating the kingdom they survey. And then the hunt: stalking, crouching, and at the last moment the explosion of power to bring down the gazelle. Then they feast . . . then they rest. Although they may follow the trail of their prey slowly for some time—analogous to a brisk walk for you and me—the burst of high-intensity activity lasts only a few minutes. Not hours and miserable hours.

In order to survive in the garden, our early ancestors on occasion must have behaved much like their neighbors the lions, sprinting at high speed to corner and catch their prey. (Two crucial differences between the two, however, are that early humans also had to sprint or run full out—very high-intensity activities—to keep from becoming prey themselves, and evading predators must have demanded they be able not only to run but to climb and leap proficiently as well.) To be successful, when they finally sighted their quarry, early human hunters had to throw their javelins or spears great distances with accuracy. Accounts exist of contemporary hunter-gatherers actually hitting small game animals half a football field away with their thrown spears. Or of a band of five American Indians running buffalo into an 8-foot ravine to quickly kill them. Then this handful of men hauled the dead weight of the animals—some weighing more than a ton—up the steep sides of the ravine, expertly butchered them on the spot, and immediately headed back to camp, each man toting many pounds of buffalo meat. All these activities—sprinting, jumping, climbing, throwing spears, and power-lifting heavy loads—required short bursts of focused power, called high-intensity work. This kind of fitness, generating short bursts of maximum power, involves an anaerobic (without oxygen) type of energy production.

That's not to say that early humans weren't also aerobically fit. On occasion, survival for our early ancestors—like the lion on the hunt—involved exercise demanding great aerobic endurance as well. For instance, modern anthropology gives us accounts of contemporary hunter-gatherers, such as American Indian hunting parties, trotting after a big game animal or large bird for as much as a week before finally exhausting it. When the prey finally became too fatigued to flee, the human predator could more easily move in for the kill. Does this mean that it's good to jog for miles and miles many days a week? No, not really. In fact, by all accounts, although early humans could perform such feats when necessary, that doesn't appear to have been a daily or even regular occurrence. And as you'll see later, overtraining—repetitively performing too much of the same sort of exercise—can damage your health and happiness, impair your performance, increase your risk for severe injury, and leave you more susceptible to infections and possibly even cancers. Repeatedly performing the same type of exercise day after day after day doesn't promote whole-body fitness and is a far cry from the kind of exercise that the millennia of human adaptation left us best suited to do. Rather, our Flintstone anatomy and physiology would better benefit from varying the type of activity we choose—in a sense, cross-training—to keep us fit from head to toe with plenty of R and R and fun in the mix.

Our goal should be to adapt the benefits of Paleolithic exercise to our twenty-first-century lives. The same approach that kept early humans fit, lean, and strong can work for us today. We have but to train ourselves by doing short intervals of high-output work of a variety of types followed by periods of rest, recovery, relaxation, and stretching, with perhaps an occasional long-distance activity thrown in for good measure. Following the *Protein Power LifePlan* exercise prescription (which we'll describe shortly), you'll learn simple exercises designed to mimic the types of exercise your ancient ancestors would have naturally done in day-to-day living. These simple techniques will improve both your aerobic and anaerobic fitness, at home, in the gym, or on the road, without a large commitment of time. And by using these easy methods to improve your fitness, you'll take a step closer to the overall wellness that is your human birthright. But before we get into the how-tos of exercise, let's explore a little of the science of exercise, taking a look at where the energy comes from during specific kinds of activities.

The Nonstop Energy Machine

Did you ever wonder where the energy to move your body comes from? Every motion, from the blinking of your eyes to the beating of your heart to the push of your legs when you jump, has to be generated from within. Every cell in the body, but especially the heart and muscle cells, contains tiny energy plants called mitochondria, responsible for producing this energy as you need it in a form called ATP, which, although it sounds like a fuel additive, stands for the unwieldy name adenosine triphosphate. The muscles rely almost exclusively on ATP already manufactured and stored within them to generate instantaneous energy—for example, to jump out of the path of a runaway truck—or to perform brief intervals of maximum work, such as when a terrified mother lifts a 2-ton truck off her child. In the first few seconds of exercise, the body relies exclusively on ATP stores, which deplete quickly—there's only enough ATP for about ten seconds of strenuous work.

As the exercise or work continues, the muscle turns to other avenues to keep the energy coming, by calling on substances that help to recycle or regenerate the ATP. The chief player in this reprovisioning of energy is a substance called creatine phosphate. Steady dietary replenishment of creatine stores is one of the benefits of a meat-based diet. There's a ton of the stuff in red meat (almost twice as much as in chicken or other poultry), and at least in part it helps to explain the heightened energy and strength—the readiness to become involved in physical exercise—that usually accompanies the change to *Protein Power LifePlan* eating.

Creatine phosphate has recently received intense national attention as a supplement to enhance sports performance, thanks to the endorsements of a number of elite and professional athletes. Because of its reputation as a muscle builder, we're often asked (usually by teen- or college-aged young men) about whether the hype surrounding creatine is true. Indeed, research has clearly shown that creatine phosphate does help recharge the ATP battery and will keep the muscle able to do high-intensity work for longer periods of time without running out of fuel. Working the muscles harder (in the gym, for example, lifting heavier weights for more reps) supposedly brings about bigger muscle mass gains; those who swear by creatine supplementation say that it lets their muscles do just that. Does it work? The strength and muscular physiques of users of creatine seem to bear out their claim, as does a fair amount of scientific research. But is it safe in the long term? The scientific research needed to answer that question is as yet incomplete; however, that research indicates that use for the short term (thirty days or less) appears to be safe. There's great debate within the sports community as to whether use of the supplement, however efficacious, could increase the likelihood of injury by working the muscles beyond their natural fatigue point, as well as whether there might be any long-term consequences to its supplemental use. As yet, no clear answers have emerged in this debate, but time will surely tell. Until then, we feel more comfortable building up our own creatine phosphate through diet by eating red meat.

Beyond a minute or two, the muscles, if they're to continue their work, must turn to the burning of either carbohydrate (stored within the muscle as a substance called glycogen, or muscle starch) or fat to fuel ongoing energy needs. Research has shown that the muscle would prefer to burn fat or the breakdown products of fat for fuel, because, among other reasons, the burning of carbohydrate for energy can quickly lead to the buildup of lactic acid within the muscle in the aerobically unfit. In fact, when even the aerobically fit reach their point of muscle fatigue, it's the buildup of lactic acid from burning sugar that finally makes the muscle scream, "Enough, already!" and quit. If you've ever performed any exercise until your muscle felt like it was on fire—what's called the burn among athletes—you've felt the consequence of the buildup of lactic acid. The burn occurs quite readily if you're untrained athletically and eating a high-carbohydrate diet, because with insulin elevated (which it usually is in those who are out of shape and overweight) you can't effectively burn fat to fuel your exercise; elevated insulin blocks the entry of the fatty-acid fuel into the mitochondria. The readily available source for energy in people who eat a lot of carbohydrates is, quite naturally, stored carbohydrate. And burning it poorly can be a painful experience for your muscles.

When you eat the *Protein Power LifePlan* way, however, you'll keep your insulin low and your insulin receptors sensitive, and that means you can more easily shuttle fatty-acid fuel into those cellular energy plants. Instead of burning muscle starch for energy, which eating a baked potato or a bowl of linguine would quickly replace, you'll be effectively burning the fat within your muscles, the fat on your belly, the fat around your hips, and the padding packed around your heart, kidneys, and intestines as you exercise.

Putting More Energy Plants On-Line

Exercise places added demand on the muscles to do work, and the muscles respond over time by becoming more efficient at generating the energy to meet the extra demand. Since the number of mitochondria in a given muscle cell can produce only so much ATP, to generate more energy the cells must somehow build more mitochondria. And in fact, research has shown a substantial increase in mitochondrial density—that is, more power plants on line—in response to exercise, both endurance exercise (jogging or cycling) as well as the kind of high-intensity interval training we recommend. But the *Protein Power LifePlan* nutritional strategy also plays a role in this regard. By eating a diet richer in good-quality fats, you'll naturally increase the number of these tiny energy plants within each cell, which translates into more energy available to evade predators or to participate in whatever suits your fancy. Maybe like one of our patients you'll take up competitive country-western line dancing (in a good-looking pair of slim-fitting jeans), or, like others, you'll develop an interest in kickboxing or begin competing in martial arts. Or maybe, like many of our patients, you'll just enjoy being able to keep up with the kids or the grandkids in the park. The right diet coupled with the right kind of exercise can make that possible.

Making the Slow Ones Fast and the Fast Ones Better

And speaking of grandkids in the park, how many times have you heard it said of the unbounded energy of childhood, "If you could bottle it, you'd make a fortune!"? What is it about kids that they seem to be in perpetual motion all day long, nonstop running, hopping, fidgeting, talking, skipping, and never wearing out or slowing down? What makes them so? For one thing, it's the kind of muscle fibers that make up their muscles. The modern science of exercise physiology has elucidated multiple types of muscle fibers: fast-twitch, slow-twitch, and intermediate-twitch fibers. And while drawing a distinction between the types of muscle fibers may seem to be nothing more than a picayune bit of trivia from arcane medical research, it is a critically important one, and here's why. Young people in general and elite power athletes in particular (sprinters, power lifters, alpine skiers, and hockey, basketball, and football players) have substantially more fast-twitch fibers in their muscles than slow ones; it's probably what makes their special type of athletic prowess a cut above the rest. Nice for them, you might be thinking, but what's that got to do with the great normal mass of us in the middle of the bell-shaped curve? Plenty, because some research has shown that the right type of exercise can not only condition the fast twitchers you have, making them generate energy more abundantly and efficiently, but may actually alter the fiber type, converting some of the slow-twitch fibers to fast-twitch ones. While the slow-twitch fibers make for better endurance performance—marathoners and cross-country skiers have lots of these—fast-twitch fibers are better adapted for the quick release of maximal energy that you remember from your childhood and that was so much a part of our Paleolithic existence. Some of what's been termed the "normal" aging process involves the loss of some of our fast-twitch muscle fibers, and with it a loss of the explosive bursts of power during exercise that were a big part of the natural quickness and agility of our youth. Can we reclaim some of that burst energy through the right kind of exercise? The research certainly suggests that we can.

POWER UP: WORKING YOUR FAST-TWITCH FIBERS

Too busy to exercise? Just can't find the time? Those excuses won't work anymore. One of the benefits of exercising your body at its peak intensity is that you don't have to do it for long or all that often. In the world of power exercise, more isn't always better. For example, a recent research study compared two groups of weight trainers—one group trained the traditional way, performing three sets of eight to ten repetitions of each exercise, and the other group did only a single set, lifting a heavier weight only eight times. The researchers had expected the muscle gains to be substantially larger in the group doing more exercise; after all, they were working out three times as long. The results took them by surprise: there was virtually no difference in the muscle gains between the two groups. In fact, the intensity of the exercise seemed to have a greater benefit in building strength and lean muscle than the number of sets or the number of days a week spent doing it. The high-intensity exercises that we'll describe for you here build on that concept—like our ancient ancestors, you'll be doing brief bursts of maximum output with rests in between. We've even given some of our exercises names that will help you conjure up the image of why you would have been doing that sort of work had you lived way back then. Your workouts should be brief, varied, and fun—something you look forward to doing, not something you dread like the plague.

Paleolithic Exercising

Let's take a look now at some of these simple exercise techniques that you can do at home or on the road without a lot of fancy or expensive equipment. (In the Suggested and Related Readings sections of the appendix we've included a couple of helpful books devoted to this type of exercise for those who wish to know and do more.)

It's a good idea to stretch out before you begin your exercises, but stretching is something we hope you'll do every day as a part of greeting the world, just as lions, cats, dogs, or any other free-living creatures do—and as early humans most surely must have done as well. In the wild, stretching is usually the first order of business to shake the cobwebs out of the muscles and ready them for whatever may lie ahead; it should be no different for us in civilization. Here's how to do it.

STRETCH OUT AND TOUCH THE STARS

Certainly before you begin to exercise—and ideally also every morning as you wake to the new day—we recommend that you do at least a minimum amount of stretching. If you enjoy stretching, you may want to become involved in yoga, and we'd certainly encourage that interest, because stretching is good for you. But even if you don't like it at first, even if you're the stiffest and least flexible human on the planet, at least try each day to perform the following simple stretching exercises. You'll find that with time, your flexibility improves.

1. Sit up straight (either in bed or on the floor). Slowly drop your chin toward your chest, feeling the stretch of your neck and into your back. Breathe deeply in and out and hold the stretched position for a few seconds before returning to your starting position. Now tip your head backward as far as you comfortably can, resting the base of your skull between your shoulder blades. Hold the position, slowly breathing deeply in and out for a few seconds before returning to neutral. (If you're like us, not a teenager anymore, you may feel a few gentle cracks and pops as you do these exercises, but they should not hurt. If they do, stop! Go only as far as you *comfortably* can.) Now rotate your head to the right as though you were looking at someone over your right shoulder. Hold the position, breathing deeply in and out for a few seconds before returning to neutral. Now rotate toward the left, holding the position for a few seconds as you breathe deeply in and out, and then return to neutral.

2. Sitting on the side of your bed (or standing), reach your arms straight out in front of you, stretching as far as you can as though you would grab hold of an object just a few inches beyond your reach. Don't lean your body forward; just stretch with your arms. Inhale as you stretch. Hold the stretch for a few seconds,

breathing slowly in and out, and then exhale as you relax. (To receive the maximum release of muscles as you stretch them requires holding the stretch for about thirty seconds, but you can slowly build up to that goal.)

3. Still sitting on the bedside (or standing), raise your arms above your head, joining your hands, interlocking your fingers, and pointing toward the sky with your index fingers. Imagine pushing your index fingers higher and higher into the sky, elongating your back, stretching as tall as you can. Hold the stretch for a few seconds, breathing deeply in and out during the stretch and exhaling as you relax.

4. Now, either sitting or standing, wrap your arms around yourself, right arm across your chest and around your left shoulder, left arm across the chest and around the right shoulder—it's like giving yourself a big hug. Reach as far as your flexibility will allow, aiming to place your palms on your shoulder blades but coming as close as you can. Now take a deep breath in and use your hands to pull your shoulders toward the center of your chest. As you do, think of pushing your spine back at the same time to stretch the muscles of your mid back. Hold the stretch for a few seconds and slowly exhale and inhale as you continue to stretch. Exhale as you relax.

5. Now stand with your feet slightly apart, arms extended shoulder level to either side, thumbs pointing to the sky, palms facing in. Stretch your arms out, reaching with your finger tips as if to touch the walls on either side of you, breathing in deeply. Hold the stretch a few seconds, then exhale as you relax. Now with your arms extended as before, turn your head to the right, looking along your extended right arm as if you were sighting down the barrel of a rifle. Slowly twist your upper body from the waist, first going to the right. Try to keep your lower body facing forward, arms in the same position relative to your body, and continue to sight down your right arm as your turn, twisting around until you're looking as far behind you as you can. Hold the stretch, breathing slowly in and out, then exhale as you slowly return to the center. Now turn your head to the left to sight along your left arm, and turn your body to the left from the waist, continuing to sight along your left arm until you're again twisted

around looking as far behind you as you can. Hold the stretch, breathing slowly in and out, then exhale as you return to the center. Take a deep breath in and let it out slowly.

6. Now, standing with your feet slightly apart, inhale deeply and as you begin to exhale, slowly roll forward at the waist and hips, gently dropping your head and hands toward the floor. Go as low as possible, then take a slow deep breath in and relax as you exhale. Let the relaxation deepen the stretch, and drop your hands yet lower. Take another deep breath in, and as you slowly exhale, feel the tension in your low back begin to release as you relax into the breath. Let the relaxation slowly and gently stretch you a little farther. Hold that final stretch for at least a count of ten, breathing slowly in and out, before gradually returning to a standing position.

7. Now stand next to the wall or a chair if necessary for stability. Steady yourself with your left hand to perform a "runner's stretch" of the thigh. Lift your right foot, bending your right knee as if you were going to kick your own butt. Grab hold of your right foot with your right hand and gently pull your foot more tightly toward your buttocks. (Remember, you can use your left hand for balance on the wall or chair if you need to.) Feel the stretch along the front of your thigh (the quads). Hold it for at least a count of ten and then relax. Now repeat with the left leg, using your right hand for stability on the wall or chair. Bend the left knee, pull the left foot in to your buttocks with your left hand, and hold the stretch for at least a count of ten and relax.

8. (Optional) If you feel you can, you may want to stretch your pelvic and inner thigh muscles as well—particularly if it's before exercising. To do so, stand with your legs spread as widely apart as you can up to about 3 feet, toes pointing ahead or very slightly out. At first you may want to stand in front of a dresser, bathroom or kitchen counter, or the back of a sturdy chair or couch for stability as you do this. If you're able and your balance is good, just counterbalance by making a circle with your bent arms held shoulder high in front of you, pressing the loose fist of one hand into the open palm of the other. (Some of you may recognize that this exercise is an adaptation of the Kung Fu low stance.) Lean with your weight on your left leg, bending the left

knee as you lower yourself on your left leg. As you do, keep your right foot on the floor, right leg straight out to the right side, sliding your right foot a little farther out to the side if need be. You'll sort of be doing a squat on just your left leg—or a side lunge. (Ideally, you'll ultimately be able to take this stretch all the way down to a full squat that puts your butt resting right on your left calf, but begin where you comfortably can and attempt to gradually go lower over time.) Hold this stretched position for at least a count of ten, remembering to breathe slowly and deeply in and out as you do. Then, without standing back up, simply shift to the opposite side by gradually bending the right knee, moving through the center point to where you're squatting on both legs equally, and then finally pushing over to where you're squatting on the right side with the left leg extended straight on the left side—all in one smooth motion. Hold that position for a count of at least ten and then slide back to the left side, hold for at least a ten count, then back to the right, and hold for at least a count of ten. And you're finished!

HIGH-INTENSITY INTERVALS

The idea behind the exercises we're about to describe is to work big, powerful muscles—chiefly your shoulders, thighs, calves, and buttocks—at their maximum output for a short space of time to improve the vigor of the fast-twitch muscle fibers and the density of the mitochondrial power plants within the muscle cells. By doing so you'll train them to burn fat better and restore some of the quickness and agility of your youth. If you're already involved in a regular physical routine that works your whole body, then by all means continue it. But at least try to perform one of the high-intensity intervals one or two times a week, varying your selection from one session to the next. Just as we recommend that for good health you should eat a wide variety of foods, so for good physical conditioning you should perform a wide variety of exercises—aiming to condition *all* your muscles. For these exercises, you'll need comfortable clothing, a supportive pair of shoes, and a timer or a watch or clock with a second hand.

1. Sprint from the Lion

You can perform this exercise anywhere—on foot, on a bike, on cross-country skis, or probably even canoeing or sculling down a river, if that's what you like to do; you just have to imagine the lion could swim fast, or replace it with a large crocodile. Performing it outdoors in good weather is fun, whether you're home or on the road, but indoors you can use a stepping machine, a stationary bike, or a skiing or rowing machine, or simply jog in place; any of these will work fine. If you're outside, make sure you're on a reasonably level area—free of obstacles for the sprint portion. Also be certain you're wearing good supporting shoes and comfortable clothes.

Begin at a slow jog/ride/ski/row or fast walk for a minute or two. If you're outside, you may want to take a leisurely pace for a few minutes to warm up and enjoy being out in the sunshine. Once you feel warm and ready, imagine that you're walking across the open savanna when suddenly you see a lion, and it, unfortunately, sees you, too. SPRINT!! Go as fast as you can possibly go—as if your life depended on it—for ten to thirty seconds. (That's right, seconds; see, we told you it wouldn't take long to do this!) Now slow down to your comfortable pace for thirty seconds to one minute to catch your breath. Then, oh no, here he comes again! SPRINT!! Run for it as fast as you can for ten to thirty seconds, then drop back again to your slower pace. Repeat the cycle for five or six run-for-your-life sprints, each followed by the slow-down breather. When you've evaded the lion (i.e., finished your reps) stop briefly (if you're on your bike or stepper, get off) to release the tension of the chase. Take a deep slow breath in and stretch, reaching both hands toward the sky and holding the stretch for a five count. Then slowly exhale, bending at the waist, dropping your fingertips toward the ground to stretch your thighs and back. Repeat a time or two. All in all, the exercise will take less than ten minutes, but trust us on this: you'll know you've had a workout! If you're way out of shape or have cardiovascular (heart/blood vessel) problems, begin very slowly at the ten-second interval, stopping immediately if you feel breathless or have pain. No matter where you begin, as your conditions improves, slowly increase your sprint time—going up by literally just a second or two at a time—ultimately aiming for a total of one minute at each full-out sprint with a one-minute rest in between. Research has shown that you'll get a calorie-buring metabolic boost from this brief session that lasts for hours, and over the coming months, you'll improve both your aerobic and anaerobic conditioning and increase the density of the power plants in each muscle cell. Not bad for ten minutes of work a couple of times a week.

2. Leap to the Tree

When the occasion demanded, your Paleolithic ancestors surely must have used this technique, and so should you. It will work your buttocks, thighs, calves, and ankles. You can perform it indoors or out, but always opt for outdoors in good weather, so you'll get the benefits of sunshine and fresh air. Remember to stretch first.

Stand comfortably and relaxed, your feet a few inches apart, arms at your sides. Now imagine you're standing under a tree, when all at once a rhinoceros crests a distant rise, spots or smells you, snorts angrily, and charges. There's no time to run, but just a few feet above your head you spot a strong, low limb on the tree. If you could reach it, you'd be safe!

Crouch down now and, using the swing of your arms for added leverage, leap as high as you possibly can toward the branch, stretching as far as your arms will stretch to try to grab it. Oh no, you missed! Leap again, right away. Leap three to five times in a row—*bam, bam, bam.* (It should take about ten to fifteen seconds or so.) Take a breather for thirty seconds (you don't have long because he's closing on you). Leap again three to five times. Rest again for 30 seconds. Do four or five leap-rest cycles. Finally, you made it to the limb (i.e., you completed your reps!). Now you can rest there for a bit, and while you do, release the tension in your muscles. Stretch your arms up high above your head toward the treetop with a big breath in; hold the stretch for a five count; then, exhaling your breath, slowly drop forward at the waist, your fingertips aiming for the ground, to stretch your buttocks, thighs, calves, and back. If you're exceedingly overweight or have cardiovascular (heart/blood vessel) limitations, begin very slowly. Even a few leaps of 1 inch or just the deep squat and push-off without ever leaving the ground is a fine place to start if that's what you can do. As your conditioning improves, you'll leap for higher and higher branches and you'll add more leaps, aiming ultimately for eight to ten leaps in each attempt with thirty seconds to rest between. Also, for safety, at first, you might want to have someone spot you in case you become dizzy or lose your balance.

3. Crossing the River

This exercise also works the jumping muscles. To get your mind into the Paleolithic mode as you perform it, you should imagine that you and your Paleolithic band have decided to move your encampment closer to your food supply, which means, of course, that you must carry your belongings, such as they are, to the new location. On the way, you come to a broad stream dotted with five or six large boulders. Only their tips stick out above the rushing water. In order to cross the stream, you must leap from one boulder to another one (they're too far apart to merely step across) to ferry your things to the other side. It will take at least two trips to get it all.

Begin with both feet flat on the ground, on the edge of the riverbank, and prepare to leap to the nearest boulder on your right, making the biggest, highest hop you can. (If once you've mastered the exercise you'd like to make it a bit harder, weight yourself as you do this exercise with hand weights, ankle weights, dumbbells, a medicine ball held near your chest,[1] or even a pillowcase stuffed with your laundry.) To make the "crossing," you'll first jump to a boulder on your right: bend your knees and flex your hips, push off with your left leg, leaping upward and throwing your right leg up and outward to land atop the imaginary boulder with just your right foot. Balance there briefly on just your right foot, then leap to the next boulder, this time to your left.

---

1. A medicine ball is a large, heavy leather or vinyl ball, solidly filled. These balls usually weigh 7, 10, or 15 pounds and can be used in a variety of exercises at home. Check your local sporting goods retailer.

Your left knee and hip should already be flexed from your one-footed landing and ready to make the next leap. Leap to the left, flexing your hips and using the power of your right leg, throwing the left one upward and outward. As soon as you land on your left foot, prepare to leap to the next boulder on the right, then to the one on the left until you've done three leaps to each side.

To recap, you'll make a leap to the right (landing on just the right foot), one to the left (landing on just the left foot), back to the right, then to the left, then back to the right, and finally to the left. (Once you master the exercise, it should seem that you're almost bouncing back and forth from right foot to left foot to right foot to left with minimal time on the "boulder." Unless you've decided to add a "load," you should use your arms for balance and momentum.)

Rest on the far side of this imaginary riverbank for thirty seconds and then come back across to retrieve the remainder of your belongings, again making alternating leaps, three to the right, three to the left. Rest again and repeat, over and back with a rest in between. This should give you a total of four cycles of six leaps with breathers between them. (We realize that this puts you back on the same side of the river from which you started, but that's okay. If you're a stickler for realism, be our guest and hop back across once more . . . or as many times as you feel up for, within reason.)

When you've completed all the cycles, remember to stretch your jumping muscles. Reach your arms high above your head as you take a deep breath. Hold the stretch for a count of five, then as you exhale, drop slowly, bending at the waist with your legs kept straight, arms down, fingertips pointing toward the ground. Stretch as deeply as your flexibility will allow, holding for at least a five count, but up to thirty seconds. Repeat the stretch a few times.

4. Bringing Home the Buffalo

As an upper-body alternative exercise—and to mimic the upper-body work that our ancient ancestors would have done in carrying heavy loads, pushing, pulling, and dragging the carcasses of large animals—we want you to imagine you're among the band of native hunters that ran the buffalo over the ravine. You have to help, by pushing and pulling, using your strong back, buttocks, and shoulders to haul these beasts up onto the flat land for easier butchering. For this exercise all you need is your own weight and enough space to lie down on the floor. (You may want a mat for cushioning, but it's not necessary.) If you'd like to increase the load during the squats portion of the exercise, you can do so using two dumbbells, a couple of medicine balls, or a pair of plastic gallon jugs filled with water. The exercise has five parts and you'll do each of them to complete the workout.

(a) Begin by lying stretched out on your stomach, palms flat on the ground beside your chest. Keeping your body straight and using the strength of your shoulders, arms, buttocks, and back, lift as much of your own weight as you can, extending your arms fully—that's right, it's a simple push-up. Come back down to the floor briefly, hardly touching, and push back up. Try to do five as quickly as you can. Rest for thirty seconds and repeat. Aim at first for four or five cycles of five push-ups interspersed with the brief rest periods. After you've mastered sets of five, increase your sets to six, seven, and so on up to ten. If you can't do five full-body push-ups, do what you can (even if it's none or one), and for the remainder, drop your knees and lift just the top half of your body. Work from this position until you build up some upper-body strength. If you're extremely overweight or frail, try doing vertical push-ups against the door or wall. Stand about 2 to 2½ feet from the wall, lean into it with your arms in push-up position, and perform the same exercise, keeping your body straight, using your upper body to lower your chest and shoulders toward the wall and push away again. Work from this position until you're able to graduate to the knee push-ups on the floor. Remember to breathe in deeply as you push up and exhale as you lower yourself again. Don't hold your breath!

(b) Now stand up, spread your feet apart about three feet or so, toes pointing slightly outward. (If you're using dumbbells, medicine balls, or water jugs to increase your load, lift one up onto each shoulder to weigh you down equally. Alternatively, hold a single medicine ball clutched to the center of your chest, or hold one of the water jugs or dumbbells in each hand down at your sides.) Keep your back straight as you slowly squat down. Try not to lean forward. (At first, you may want to keep your hands free, forgoing the added weight, and stand near a sturdy table, counter, or couch that you can touch if need be to maintain your balance.) Go as low as you're able to, down to the point that your thighs are parallel to the floor—there's no need to go any lower. Hold the squat for a count of ten to start, but try to work up to a count of thirty. Breathe slowly in and out during the entire exercise. Slowly return to the standing position, using just the power of your abdomen, buttocks, and thighs. Immediately start slowly back down to your squatting position, hold the squat for the count of ten to thirty, then slowly rise. Try to do four or five squats.

(c) Next, lie down on your back, bend your knees, tuck your chin snugly against your chest, and extend your arms out in front of you alongside your knees. Keep your buttocks and low back firmly in contact with the floor as you curl your head, neck, shoulders, and chest toward your knees. Try to use only your abdominal muscles to do the work. Imagine you're standing on the edge of a ravine, helping to haul 2 tons of buffalo to the top. Reach your arms out, stretching them in front of you as you tighten your abdominal muscles against this great load you're helping to lift; slowly begin to curl yourself upward around a point just under the center of your rib cage. Hold the curl for a count of five and slowly let yourself back down. Repeat for a total of five curls.

(d) Flip back over onto your stomach, this time with your palms under your chest, thumb to thumb, index fingertip to index fingertip, making a small triangle of your hands that should fall just at the level of your breastbone. This hand configuration will more specifically strengthen the triceps muscles—on the back of your upper arms. Hold your body straight and lift your entire weight to full arm extension and back to rest, barely touching the floor, then push again. Aim at first to do five of these push-ups in quick succession. Then take a fifteen- to twenty-second breather and repeat. Do four or five cycles of five push-up sets with rest intervals between them. Again, if necessary, drop your knees or begin vertically against the door until you build up strength in your triceps muscles. Remember to breath in deeply each time you push up and exhale as you let your weight back down.

(e) Now flip back onto your back and repeat the set of 5 abdominal muscle curls, and you'll have gotten that buffalo up the hill. Take a breather and stretch out to relax. Lying on the floor, place your arms over your head, legs straight out, toes pointed. Now stretch yourself in both directions, hold the stretch for at least a ten count, then exhale and relax. Repeat the stretch.

5. Defending the Camp

In this exercise, imagine that your Paleolithic encampment has been attacked by a neighboring band or by a rampaging rogue mammoth. You use the weapons at your disposal to defend your spot, hurling the large rocks that are everywhere at your adversary. Instead of rocks, however, you'll use either a medicine ball, a heavy pillowcase filled with laundry, or a basketball or soccer ball. It's helpful to have a partner in this exercise to catch and return the "rocks" you'll hurl.

Hoist your "rock" high over your head, arms extended, and throw it with all your might either out onto the ground or in the direction of your partner. If you've got a partner, have them participate by hurling it back to you. (If you're working alone, the medicine ball or pillowcase full of laundry won't roll or bounce away like the basketball will.) However you're working, retrieve your "rock" quickly and "reload," hoisting it high above your head and hurling it as hard and as far as you're able. Hurl the "rock" five times quickly in a row to start, then rest for thirty seconds. Throw the "rock" again five times rapidly, hurl with all your might—after all, your encampment is being overrun and you must drive the interlopers away! Rest for thirty seconds. It will take you four or five cycles of repeated rock hurling and resting to save the day! When you're finished, remember to stretch your back and arms.

The same high-intensity philosophy can work in the weight room if that's your pleasure. To get this workout by lifting weights, however, requires a little different technique. You'll need to select a weight sufficiently heavy to permit you to correctly lift it for one set of eight to twelve repetitions with effort. By the last rep, the muscles you're working should ideally be fatigued and essentially unable to continue. It may take you a little experimentation to arrive at the correct weight.

When you're ready to go, you should lift the weight smoothly for the full number of reps you can manage (ideally eight to ten, no more than twelve), remembering to breathe in and out as you lift the weight and return it to the starting position. Rest for no more than thirty seconds to one minute as you move to the next exercise. Perform one high-intensity set of eight to twelve reps for each muscle group. If you feel that you could perform more reps in that set, instead try increasing the weight slightly. On any given day, work either your upper body—your chest (the pecs, or pectoralis muscles), your arms (biceps on the front, triceps on the back), your shoulders (deltoids on the outside upper arm and suprascapular muscles above your shoulder blades), and your back (the traps or trapezius muscles, the lats, or latissimus dorsi, and lower back)—or your lower body—your buttocks (the glutes, or glutei maximi), your thighs (the quads, or quadriceps femora in front and the hams, or hamstrings, in back), your calf muscles, and last but not least your abs (abdominal muscles).

It's sufficient to perform this kind of power and strength conditioning two times a week—once for the upper body and once for the lower body. The gains you'll see in muscle mass, according to recent research, should be as significant as if you had performed multiple sets of each exercise and had done them more frequently than once a week. Don't forget to breathe slowly and deeply as you exercise and to stretch out when you're finished.

When (and Why) More Isn't Better

If you've ever heard the expression "No pain, no gain!" we urge you to immediately forget it, to purge it forever from your memory banks. Pain is quite simply something to be avoided. Too often, in the quest for fitness, people buy into the mistaken notion that exercise has to hurt to help. If running thirty minutes is good for them, then running two hours must surely be better; if doing aerobics three days a week is beneficial, then seven days a week will be even more so; if one set of exercises in the gym helps build muscle, six sets will do it faster. More is not always better, and nowhere does that apply more clearly than with exercise. Moderate exercise relieves stress, but overexercising—too much or too often—adds stress, raises cortisol (the body's stress hormone), and with it increases insulin levels. With moderate exercise, researchers see a strengthening of the immune defenses, but with overexercise a dip in immunity. After an overly vigorous session of exercise, exercise scientists can record measurable falls in the levels of disease-fighting white blood cells in the blood. The dip lasts for several hours and doesn't fully return to normal for twenty-four to forty-eight hours. What that clearly means is that beating yourself up with heavy exercise day after day without taking a break can weaken your immune defenses—a consequence often seen in runners who almost become addicted to their sport, never taking a day off rain or shine, pounding out mile after mile. It's not unusual for these overtrainers to fall victim to frequent colds and sore throats and nagging injuries.

Our nurse, Debbie, an avid proponent of the active lifestyle and now a great example of how to do it right, became involved in running years ago, long before we knew her. At the time, she was a low-fat vegetarian, training to run marathons. In pursuit of her goal, she fell into the habit of long, grueling daily training runs without taking enough time off to rest—and without eating enough good protein and good-quality fat—to allow her body to repair and her tissues to rebuild. For her effort (or perhaps we should say her overeffort) Debbie's reward was a stress fracture of her femur, the big bone of the thigh—not an easy bone to break and not an injury easily overcome. She remembers being sick, tired, and troubled by nagging injuries during those years of nonstop running and low protein intake. Since she adopted *Protein Power LifePlan* nutrition, although she still runs, she takes sensible days of rest and varies her exercise patterns to avoid the overtraining that beat her down before. Clearly, more isn't always better.

Nor was more better for our patient Stan. He had been a running machine—cranking out a minimum of 30 miles a week, often more. And like many runners, he followed a low-fat, high-carbohydrate diet, with extra-carb-loading meals before races. (This was of course before he became our patient!) Stan, in his early forties at the time, tells us that during this period he suffered frequent respiratory infections and even contracted mononucleosis, a viral infection that finally put him to bed for a month. Sick and tired of being sick and tired, Stan finally gave up running and took up eating as a hobby. He decided he'd gladly trade his gaunt and haggard runner's physique for a very portly one (about an extra 70 or 80 pounds' worth of portly before it was over) if it meant he wouldn't feel sick all the time. When he finally became sick and tired of being overweight and out of shape, he discovered our *Protein Power* plan. With it Stan reduced his weight and took up resistance training—but this time with a good dose of common sense about the dangers of overtraining. He's in his mid fifties now and healthy, muscular and lean for the last eight or nine years; at last report, he was setting records for power lifting for his age. Less, in Stan's case, proved to be better.

We ask that you use common sense in your training to prevent the damage that can accrue with overdoing it. Moderate exercise brings tremendous health benefits by lowering insulin levels, improving insulin-receptor function, raising HDL (the "good" cholesterol) levels, lowering blood pressure, improving heart and lung function, and helping to detoxify your body by inspiring prolonged deep breathing and sweating—allowing two of the body's detoxifying organs, the skin and the lungs, to do their jobs.

We recommend that you do at least one, but ideally two, high-intensity interval sessions a week (if two, space them widely apart). Vary your routine, selecting from different exercises offered here or others you may devise, so you don't get into the rut of using only the same muscles each time and ignoring others. If you really love to exercise, add some upper-body or lower-body resistance work (weight training) a day or two a week. Remember to take time out at least once a week for something physical and fun. But, most important of all, plan to rest and do only some stretching and meditation at least one or two days each week to allow your body and brain to recharge and repair.

Modern Stress and the Meditative Mind

Modern life can be stressful. For many people, the days begin and end in a panicked rush of heart-thumping adrenaline: jumping out of bed to the jangle of an unpleasant alarm, getting the kids up, fed, dressed, and off to school, bolting down a cup of coffee with a breakfast roll (if there's even time for that), getting yourself ready, dashing to the car, bus, or train to make it to work, nerves frayed by traffic snarls and the shouts of equally frustrated and angry commuters, rush-rushing through a workday that's a series of brushfires to put out and problems to solve, pushing and shoving your way home again, dashing into the house, preparing dinner for the family, getting the kids to bed, finishing your day too exhausted to stand and too keyed up to rest. Sound familiar? If this hectic scene describes your life, it's time to take control and slow down. Not that you can necessarily alter the zillion things you may have to do each day or the dozens of hats you may have to wear, but what you can change are the physical and biochemical consequences of having to live in a hectic world— that is, you can learn to minimize the impact of a hectic life on your body and mind.

Humans weren't built for nonstop stress. Our physiology handles sudden brief stress very well—in fact, brief stress may even be good for us—but the chronic stress of modern life takes a measurable physiologic toll on our minds and bodies. To better understand what happens to a body under stress, let's take a look at how the stress system works normally. Each day our bodies produce varying amounts of the stress hormone cortisol in a rhythmic ebb and flow. Cortisol levels rise during the wee hours of the morning, reaching a peak designed to wake us up—in ancient times, that cortisol peak would have rousted us off the old cave-bear fur mattress to forage for our breakfast as the sun came fully up. (Depending on our work schedules, the jolt of our modern jangling alarm clocks may nor may not roust us out of bed in sync with that peak.)

As the day progresses, the cortisol level should naturally gradually fall, reaching its low ebb during the late evening hours and remaining low during the night until it begins to rise again in the

wee hours to wake us again the next day. That is, unless we receive a sudden stress during the day; in ancient times, encounter-
ing that predator we had to evade would have qualified. Then our
cortisol goes shooting back up to network with the other stress
hormones (such as adrenaline and insulin) to prepare us to fight
or flee by, among other things, raising our blood pressure, speed-
ing up our heart rate, and increasing the rate of our breathing.
Following such a sudden stress, cortisol levels may not drop back
to "normal" for that time of day for five or six hours.

Now imagine what happens if you're startled awake by your
unpleasant alarm (cortisol goes up), run at full tilt through your
morning preparations (cortisol goes up), shout angrily at the guy
who cut you off in traffic on the way to work (cortisol goes up),
have an unpleasant encounter with your office staff or your boss
(cortisol goes up), run desperately to catch the last bus or train,
anxious that you'll miss it (cortisol goes up), and arrive home to
find that your kids have spilled a quart of chocolate milk on the
ivory rug in the living room, where they weren't supposed to be
eating in the first place. Boy, does your cortisol go up! It's been
up all day, along with your heart rate, your blood pressure, and
your level of frustration, and it won't be back down for several
more hours. Your physiology simply wasn't designed for that kind
of stress, all day long, every single day.

But just as stress increases cortisol levels, the opposite of
stress—total relaxation—can reduce them. And the best means of
totally relaxing is to learn to meditate. Now, before you close the
book and say, "No way, not me!" let us hasten to add that meditation doesn't mean that you must sit cross-legged on the floor,
breathing incense and chanting om-om-om (unless of course
you'd like to do that, which is fine, too). It simply means getting
yourself into a comfortable position (a cushy chair, a favorite re-
cliner, even soaking in a hot Epsom salts or mineral bath—just
don't get too relaxed and go under!) in a peaceful, quiet place,
and completely letting your mind and muscles go for fifteen minutes or more. During your meditation, push away stressful
thoughts of the day; try to keep your mind open to whatever
pleasant thoughts may come, relaxed and free. Some people prefer to play soothing, soft music (classics such as Mozart, Haydn,

Bach, or Vivaldi, or even some of the mellower selections of Bee-thoven work well, and so do soft and mellow jazz, instrumental easy-listening music, or ocean sounds). It's best during meditation to have instrumental music only so that your brain doesn't get tied up listening to the words and singing along. Other people need a bit more direction, especially at first, to successfully relax into a meditation—for them, we recommend a guided medita-tion/relaxation exercise. There are a number of good audiotape and CD products available to help you through relaxation. We've listed a couple in the Resource section of the appendix.

Using whatever style of meditating seems comfortable to you, try to carve out at least a ten- to 15-minute section in the middle of the day (lunchtime or a mid-afternoon coffee break would work) to totally relax. If you're at work, block out sound and bright lights and meditate quietly to let your cortisol and stress hormones fall. If you've got access to a portable tape or CD player, you can plug into a guided meditation on your favorite relaxing music. If you've got access to a tape recorder, you can even make your own relaxing music tape of a specific duration, with a gentle prompting come-back-to-reality message at the end of the allotted time.

Begin your day gently. If you wake to an alarm, find one that will wake you gradually. A radio alarm equipped with a tape or CD player that wakes you to gentle music or a brief meditation exercise can provide a calmer start to your day, replacing the corti-sol and adrenaline jolt that may come from an unpleasant buzzing or ringing noise or even from blaring rock music or the news.

Following any stressful—particularly an angry—interchange, take five minutes to relax as totally as you can, blotting out the unpleasant thoughts, relaxing your tense muscles from head to toe to help bring your stress hormones back to more normal lev-els. Breathe slowly and deeply in and out, and as you do, imagine that you're breathing in a bright white cloud of calm, peaceful air, cleansing you of anger and frustration and that as you exhale, billows of dark, angry tension-filled air leave you. In a few min-utes, you'll feel more at ease, calmer, and ready to go at it again with less stress.

And at the end of the workday, when you return home worn

out, again, try to carve out fifteen minutes to totally relax with meditation before you dive into dinner or kid activities or work you brought home to do. Doing so will undo some of the damage of your hectic day, lowering your cortisol, reducing your blood pressure, relaxing tense muscles, slowing your heart rate, calming your mind. Research has shown that simply by regularly meditating—and making no other lifestyle change, such as altering diet or taking up exercise—people with hypertension can successfully reduce their blood pressure. It's a great way to keep your life in better balance and counteract the chronic stresses of modern living. Take our advice and make time for a fifteen-minute chill break once or twice eacy day. We suggest thinking of it as "doctor's orders" for your health.

Pleasure Is a Nutrient

As much as we'd like to take credit for describing this simple notion with so succinct a phrase, we must give the credit to our dear friend and colleague Robert Crayhon, author of *Robert Crayhon's Nutrition Made Simple* (M. Evans & Co., 1996) and *The Carnitine Miracle* (M. Evans & Co., 1998). Pleasure is indeed an essential nutrient for humans today, as we feel sure it was during the millennia of our development. And the pleasure we derive from activities that make us feel good—as long as they're not harmful in and of themselves—can by extension be said to be nutrients as well. We benefit, both physically and emotionally, from the laughing, smiling, hugging, joking, and camaraderie that occurs as a natural byproduct of recreational sport with friends and family. Whether it's hiking, biking, canoeing, waterskiing, snow skiing, swimming, beach play, tennis, basketball, volleyball, vigorous dancing, or wrestling with the kids on the lawn, we encourage you at least once every week to do something just for the fun of it. If you can manage it more often, so much the better. You'll find that it doesn't seem like exercise when you're playing and having fun.

And occasionally you may want to engage in some sort of activity of longer duration as an exercise in pushing your endurance, just as your ancient ancestors must have done in tracking game, on long gathering expeditions, or in moving an encampment. We recommend that this exercise, too, be a fun one. For example, a few years back we were visiting friends who live on the Hawaiian island of Maui. While there, several of us decided to make the hike across Haleakala Crater, a thirteen-mile trek that takes you from about 10,000 feet altitude down shifting sandy trails to the crater base 2,000 feet below, then across a lunarlike landscape that becomes grassy and verdant again as you climb the steep 1,000 feet out. Hiking Haleakala is a physically wearing experience, sure, but we had a blast, getting to see specimens of the Silver Sword plants that grow nowhere else on earth and the endangered Hawaiian goose, the nene. We look back on it as an adventure, not as exercise. And so we encourage you once in a while to plan a long amble. It doesn't have to be remote sightseeing down a volcanic crater; it could just as easily be striking out on foot to see the sights of any great city from Manhattan to Milan, or taking a leaf-peeping hike through the New England woods in autumn. And there's sure to be plenty of opportunity closer to home; perhaps there are nature trails in a state or national park near you. Call your state's Department of Parks and Tourism to find out what's available, then head out into the beauty of the outdoors with family or friends for a nature hike. Whatever you love to do, plan to do it! Make the time to nourish yourself regularly with the pleasure of playful exercise—your body and your spirit will appreciate it.

The Real Reason

Regular exercise of the types we recommend here will help to improve both your ability to perform the short bursts of maximal power needed to jump, spring, throw, lift, and carry, as well as your capacity for longer-duration exercise of lower intensity, such as a hike through the autumn woods or across a field of summer wildflowers. We recommend that you exercise not just for the metabolic benefits but also for the enhanced quality of life it can bring. Although we hear regularly from readers telling their stories of how our regimen has improved their quality of life, no story comes close to the one we heard from a reader who was able to shed 150 pounds with *Protein Power* nutrition. She wrote to tell us of what happened on a recent vacation trip she'd taken with her family. As a group they'd climbed more than 800 feet to the top of a towering Caribbean waterfall and taken pictures of the view—and of each other to record their feat for the family album. She wanted to express to us her delight in being able to make that climb. (And let us add that her delight became ours; even though we hear them all the time, we still honestly love to hear the success stories of people our regimen has helped!) Before she had lost the 150 pounds, she never would have been able to tackle such a climb; she wouldn't even have tried. As she put it, while everyone else participated, she'd have been on the sidelines, where she'd been most of her adult life. But now, there she was, at the top of the falls, smiling and waving at the camera. That's why you want to exercise and eat properly: to live your life to the fullest and enjoy the health and vitality you were born to have.

BOTTOM LINE

▼

T he American obsession with fitness has led to a lifestyle that for many people may include miles and miles of running each day or hours spent pumping, rowing, stepping, and crunching in the gym—or to an overwhelming sense of guilt for not doing so. Fitness is important, right? And all those hours of exercise pay off, don't they? The answer to the first question is yes, fitness is important. But surprisingly, the answer to the second is a qualified maybe. The right kinds of exercise done properly can bestow tremendous rewards by restoring your youthfulness and strength, but the wrong kinds may reward you with precisely the opposite: a slowing, aging, and weakening of the body.

For a hint at what we modern humans should be doing on the exercise front, let's look through that peephole into the Paleolithic garden to see what kinds of activities our early ancestors engaged in. How did early humans stay in shape? Although early humans sometimes did tremendous amounts of work, according to some researchers it proved not to be as much as you might think and not every moment of every day. Sure the hunter-gatherer lifestyle involves working for food, but based on time-motion studies of modern hunter-gatherer tribes, the workers become so efficient at the task that they spend far less of their time and energy doing it than most of us would imagine. And like Paleolithic humans, the contemporary hunter-gatherers stay lean, strong-boned, and fit.

How do they do it? First the hunter-gatherers, like their ancient ancestors, continue to eat a Paleolithic diet, high in protein and good fat and limited in carbohydrate foods. But beyond their better diet, what do these people do to stay fit? Exercise in the Paleolithic garden—if we can measure it by the contemporary hunter-gatherer yardstick—consisted of brief bursts of high-intensity output followed by long periods of relaxing, storytelling, and stretching.

Brief high-intensity exercises of varying type (cross-training) that work large-muscle groups—those involved in jumping, sprinting, and lifting—coupled with a nutrient-dense, higher-fat diet encourage the muscles to increase the numbers of mitochondria, the tiny "furnaces" or power plants, within the cells, where the body burns fuel for energy. More mitochondria means more energy production, better fat-burning potential, and greater benefit from and performance during exercise. High-intensity intervals help to rapidly improve insulin sensitivity, lower blood sugar, and increase HDL, the "good" cholesterol.

In this chapter, we've designed a regimen of high-intensity exercise, stretching, and stress-reducing meditation that mimics the kinds of activities our ancestors would naturally have done. Maximum benefit from minimal time investment is what we're after. The exercises are intended to be fun and fanciful, so you won't get bored, and fruitful, so you'll keep at them. You'll find them and instructions for their use outlined on pages 285 through 296.

How much should you do? In short, begin where you can and build from there. But at no time should you become obsessed with hours of work; at that point, exercise ceases to be fun. While accounts attest that ancient people could perform amazing feats of intense strength and endurance, they apparently did so only when necessary and not day after day. We discourage overtraining—repetitively performing too much of the same sort of exercise—because it can damage your health, impair your performance, increase your risk for severe injury, and leave you more susceptible to infections and possibly even cancers. The simple techniques we describe here will help to improve both your aerobic and anaerobic fitness, at home, in the gym, or on the road, without a huge commitment of time. And by using these techniques you'll take a step closer to the overall wellness that is your human birthright.

LifePlan Nutrition

One of the secrets of life is continuous small treats.
—Iris Murdoch

Reading this book may change your mind about nutritional truth, but it will not change your life. Applying its concepts will. You should now be well armed with all the nutritional and lifestyle information you'll need to rehabilitate and preserve your health or to wring all the potential from an already healthy body. But it is by living the plan day to day that you will reap the health and vitality that should be—and indeed, is—your birthright as a human being. Our new *Protein Power LifePlan* offers a blueprint not just for lowering your cholesterol, triglycerides, and blood sugar and not just for losing weight and feeling fit again, but also for living in a way that is designed to help you reclaim your wellness and to fulfill your genetic potential. As the army would say, to "be all that you can be." While the first part of the book told you *why,* in this part of the book, you'll learn the *how-tos* for overhauling your lifestyle and being well again. Finally, we'll pull the whole plan together and you'll be able to see what really living this comprehensive plan day by day looks like. A graphic representation of such a plan might look something like figure 13.1; you'll

FIGURE 13.1

The Overlapping Circles of Health

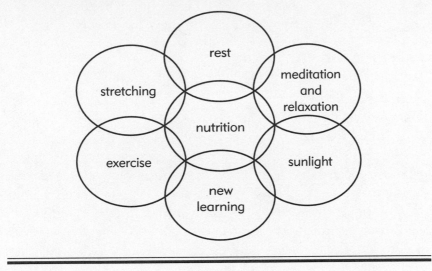

notice the circles overlap, as do the integrated benefits of these facets of your life. Ignore one and they all come apart. Strive to find a balance in your life and you'll be well on the way to health and fitness.

You'll notice, too, in the overlapping circles of health in figure 13.1 that the center, the focus, the cornerstone of a healthy life is good nutrition. Without it, none of the other facets reach their full potential. And, to be fair, in accordance with the 80/20 philosophy, 80 percent of the benefit of this plan will derive from the nutritional changes you'll make, the other 20 percent from the ancillary facets. However, if you want to live your life to the fullest, to extract every ounce of wellness you can wring from your life and drink it in, work the plan in its entirety. But since you build a strong body from the foundation up, and proper nutrition is the cornerstone, let's turn our attention there.

The Nutritional Cornerstone

For many of you, it's now time to begin the work of recovering your health, of undoing the damage of years of nutritional and physical abuse. That process begins with a period of fairly intense nutritional and lifestyle changes that we've termed Intervention. The period of time you'll spend at the Intervention Level will vary, depending on your current state of health. It might be as little as a few weeks to alter cholesterol, triglycerides, blood sugar, or blood pressure, for example, but it could last several months or more if your goal is to lose a substantial amount of weight (say, 50 pounds or more). Once you've completed the intervention process, you'll enter a slightly less stringent level we call Transition, and then finally you'll graduate to Maintenance, where you'll remain (most of the time) for years to come—we hope, forever.

We've spent more than a dozen years helping thousands of patients recover their health using our nutritional strategies, and during that time our patients and readers have taught us a thing or two about how best to do that. One of the most important things we've learned is that different people bring different levels of commitment to their health care. Some people will undertake with an almost fanatical zeal a lifestyle they believe in. No regimen is too stringent; no sacrifice too much to ask; no hardship too great to bear to reap the maximum reward possible in health and fitness. Others may be willing or able to make only modest changes in nutrition or lifestyle and will be content to accept commensurately less improvement in life and health. Most people probably fall somewhere in the middle most of the time. We say *most of the time* because the same individual may bring a different degree of commitment to the life plan under different circumstances or at different times throughout life. For this reason, we have refined the original nutritional regimen we presented in *Protein Power* to accommodate these differences. We've developed the nutritional rules of the game for the following three levels of commitment to healing:

1. The Hedonist. This plan incorporates only those changes that will bestow the greatest rewards with the least effort and the fewest nutritional adjustments.

2. The Dilettante. This is a middle-of-the-road plan for those who wish to achieve certain additional health benefits without sacrificing all the pleasures of the Hedonist regimen.

3. The Purist. This is the strictest regimen, one that closely mimics the diet our ancient ancestors thrived on and therefore bestows the maximum health and fitness rewards.

The main difference in these three regimens involves the progressive elimination of certain foods or groups of foods that were unavailable to our Paleolithic ancestors (such as grains and dairy products) and with which, consequently, we have had relatively few years' experience when measured against the time line of human existence. In some instances we've eliminated specific foods, such as wheat and corn, that research has shown may disrupt the intestinal barrier (see chapter 6, "The Leaky Gut") and may commonly cause and perpetuate autoimmune problems. All three regimens still have the same requirements for protein, the same need for good-quality fats, and the same limitations on grams of carbohydrate, depending on which level you're in, Intervention, Transition, or Maintenance. The biochemical rules—that excess carbohydrates increase insulin and promote the diseases of insulin resistance in susceptible people—remain the same; regardless of which level of commitment to change you choose, overeating sugars and starches will still carry the same detriment to your health. As you'll see, we offer three tiers of carbohydrate restriction (the Intervention, Transition, and Maintenance levels) superimposed on three degrees of commitment to Paleolithic purity in food choices (the Hedonist, Dilettante, and Purist regimens).

We don't want you to get the mistaken notion that, despite its name, the Hedonist approach means you can throw caution to the wind and eat everything you might want in any amount anytime and still reap any health benefit. That would be nutritional utopia, for sure, but as far as we know, it doesn't exist in the real world. Rather, nutritional Hedonism means you're free to enjoy more food choices than on the other two regimens, but not necessarily greater amounts. You'll have fewer restrictions on the *kinds* of carbohydrates you select—for example, unlike under the stricter plans, you'll have access to corn, pasta, breads, tortillas, muffins, and the like—but only in the amounts permitted by the carbohydrate restriction of the level of rehabilitation you're on. If you're just getting started on the plan, at the early Intervention

Level, you'll have 7 to 10 grams of effective carbohydrate available in each of your three meals (and an optional snack), and you can use virtually any source of carbohydrate to meet that allotment. Be aware, however, that foods rich in concentrated starches and/or sugars, such as pasta, bread, potatoes, corn, rice, and most desserts will chew up your small Intervention allotment in a hurry. But it's still your choice; if ¼ cup of cooked corn would make your meal, you can certainly elect to use up 8.5 effective grams of your 10-gram carbohydrate allotment to have it along with, for instance, a couple of cups of salad greens and a chicken breast, steak, or piece of salmon. Over the years we've had many patients who would make that choice for a little taste of the starchier foods they love. And (for those who tolerate grains) it works just fine—as long as the measured ¼ cup doesn't turn into an eyeballed ¾ cup (which it does for many people).

In addition, our many years of experience with our patients has taught us that people differ in how much direction and guidance they want (or need) in adopting a new nutritional regimen. Many people prefer to make their own food choices, delighting in and thoroughly enjoying the creative experience of culinary innovation, of seeking out new twists on favorite recipes. For those of you who fall into this group, we've provided a set of basic nutritional rules to follow for each of the three levels of commitment. But we recognize also that there are others of you who want step-by-step guidance in making your food choices; for you, we've included specific mix-and-match meals to help guide you effortlessly from Intervention through to Maintenance at whichever level of commitment feels right for you and your health needs. Let's see how it works.

The Corner of the Cornerstone:
Your Minimum Protein Requirement

For a nutritional regimen to work properly, it should be tailored to meet the specific needs of the individual using it, and that means one size simply won't fit all. It will come as no great revelation that the nutritional requirements for the NFL's Brett

Favre differ significantly from those of the waiflike model Kate Moss. And yet as different as they are, the basic premise is the same: for good health Mr. Favre and Ms. Moss must both eat a diet that provides enough complete protein to maintain their respective lean body masses. The difference in protein requirement will naturally be dictated by the number of pounds of lean body being maintained and the wear and tear being placed on those pounds. The huge lean body mass of a Brett Favre will require an enormous amount of protein per day to replace just the wear and tear of living, let alone the demands placed on it during the grueling NFL season. The diminutive, willowy Ms. Moss will require a fraction as much, but she, too, will have a minimum amount that she must eat if she's to be healthy.

Most of us fall somewhere between the Brett Favres and Kate Mosses of the world, but the rules are the same: if we're to be optimally healthy, we must eat a diet that provides us with enough complete protein for growth, maintenance, and repair of our tissues—whatever our size, whatever our age, whatever our level of physical demand. How can you determine how much protein your body will need? It's really very simple.

In our previous book, *Protein Power,* we provided a means of calculating lean-body mass and body-fat percentages that we had used ourselves in our medical clinic for years with good results. The procedure required only a few simple measurements, use of a few densely numbered tables, and some relatively simple mathematical steps, and voilà, out came the answer, with accuracy within a percentage point or two of expensive computerized fat/lean analysis (bioimpedence) machines. While most readers found it fairly easy and straightforward, others found it impossibly difficult and daunting, judging from some of the letters we've received. And because it's important to your health that you eat a sufficient amount of protein, we went to work to make the process simpler and essentially foolproof. As you can see from table 13.1 (for women) and table 13.2 (for men), there are no calculations involved at all. If you know your gender, your height, and your weight, the table will tell you your recommended minimum protein requirement per meal. If you eat at least this amount of protein three times per day, you'll automatically get enough pro-

TABLE 13.1

Minimum Protein Requirement per Meal (Women)

HEIGHT	5'0"	5'1"	5'2"	5'3"	5'4"	5'5"	5'6"	5'7"	5'8"	5'9"	5'10"	5'11"	6'0"	6'1"	6'2"	6'3"
WEIGHT																
100	20	20	20	20	20	20	20	20	20	27	27	27	27	27	27	27
105	20	20	20	20	20	20	20	27	27	27	27	27	27	27	27	27
110	20	20	20	27	27	27	27	27	27	27	27	27	27	27	27	27
115	27	27	27	27	27	27	27	27	27	27	27	27	27	27	27	34
120	27	27	27	27	27	27	27	27	27	27	27	27	27	27	34	34
125	27	27	27	27	27	27	27	27	27	27	27	27	27	27	34	34
130	27	27	27	27	27	27	27	27	27	27	27	34	34	34	34	34
135	27	27	27	27	27	27	27	27	27	27	27	34	34	34	34	34
140	27	27	27	27	27	27	27	27	27	27	27	34	34	34	34	34
145	27	27	27	27	27	27	27	27	27	27	27	34	34	34	34	34
150	27	27	27	27	27	27	27	27	34	34	34	34	34	34	34	34
155	27	27	27	27	27	27	34	34	34	34	34	34	34	34	34	34
160	27	27	27	27	27	34	34	34	34	34	34	34	34	34	34	34
165	27	27	27	27	34	34	34	34	34	34	34	34	34	34	34	34
170	27	27	27	34	34	34	34	34	34	34	34	34	34	34	34	34
175	27	27	34	34	34	34	34	34	34	34	34	34	34	34	34	34
180	34	34	34	34	34	34	34	34	34	34	34	34	34	34	34	34
185	34	34	34	34	34	34	34	34	34	34	34	34	34	34	34	34
190	34	34	34	34	34	34	34	34	34	34	34	34	34	34	34	40
195	34	34	34	34	34	34	34	34	34	34	34	34	34	34	40	40
200	34	34	34	34	34	34	34	34	34	34	34	34	34	40	40	40
205	34	34	34	34	34	34	34	34	34	34	34	34	40	40	40	40
210	34	34	34	34	34	34	34	34	34	40	40	40	40	40	40	40
215	34	34	34	34	34	34	34	34	40	40	40	40	40	40	40	40
220	34	34	34	34	34	34	34	40	40	40	40	40	40	40	40	40
225	34	34	34	34	34	34	40	40	40	40	40	40	40	40	40	40
230	34	34	34	34	34	40	40	40	40	40	40	40	40	40	40	40
235	34	34	34	34	34	40	40	40	40	40	40	40	40	40	40	40
240	34	34	40	40	40	40	40	40	40	40	40	40	40	40	40	40
245	34	34	40	40	40	40	40	40	40	40	40	40	40	40	40	40
250	40	40	40	40	40	40	40	40	40	40	40	40	40	40	40	40
255	40	40	40	40	40	40	40	40	40	40	40	40	40	40	40	40
260	40	40	40	40	40	40	40	40	40	40	40	40	40	40	40	46
265	40	40	40	40	40	40	40	40	40	40	40	40	40	40	46	46
270	40	40	40	40	40	40	40	40	40	40	40	40	40	40	46	46
275	40	40	40	40	40	40	40	40	40	40	40	40	40	46	46	46
280	40	40	40	40	40	40	40	40	40	40	40	40	46	46	46	46
285	40	40	40	40	40	40	40	40	40	40	40	46	46	46	46	46
290	40	40	40	40	40	40	40	40	40	40	46	46	46	46	46	46
295	40	40	40	40	40	40	40	40	46	46	46	46	46	46	46	46
300	40	40	40	40	40	40	46	46	46	46	46	46	46	46	46	46

Note: Women under 5'0" or 100 pounds use 20 grams; women weighing more than 300 pounds use 46 grams.

TABLE 13.2

Minimum Protein Requirement per Meal (Men)

HEIGHT / WEIGHT	5'4"	5'5"	5'6"	5'7"	5'8"	5'9"	5'10"	5'11"	6'0"	6'1"	6'2"	6'3"	6'4"	6'5"	6'6"	6'7"	6'8"	6'9"	6'10"
125	27	27	27	27	27	27	27	27	27	27	34	34	34	34	34	34	34	34	34
130	27	27	27	27	27	27	27	27	34	34	34	34	34	34	34	34	34	34	34
135	27	27	27	27	27	27	27	27	34	34	34	34	34	34	34	34	34	34	34
140	27	27	27	27	34	34	34	34	34	34	34	34	34	34	34	34	34	34	34
145	34	34	34	34	34	34	34	34	34	34	34	34	34	34	34	34	34	40	40
150	34	34	34	34	34	34	34	34	34	34	34	34	34	34	34	40	40	40	40
155	34	34	34	34	34	34	34	34	34	34	34	34	34	34	34	40	40	40	40
160	34	34	34	34	34	34	34	34	34	34	34	34	34	34	40	40	40	40	40
165	34	34	34	34	34	34	34	34	34	34	34	34	34	34	40	40	40	40	40
170	34	34	34	34	34	34	34	34	34	34	34	34	40	40	40	40	40	40	40
175	34	34	34	34	34	34	34	34	34	34	34	34	40	40	40	40	40	40	40
180	34	34	34	34	34	34	34	34	34	34	40	40	40	40	40	40	40	40	40
185	34	34	34	34	34	34	34	34	40	40	40	40	40	40	40	40	40	40	40
190	34	34	34	34	34	34	34	40	40	40	40	40	40	40	40	40	40	40	40
195	34	34	34	34	34	34	40	40	40	40	40	40	40	40	40	40	40	40	40
200	34	34	34	34	40	40	40	40	40	40	40	40	40	40	40	40	40	40	40
205	40	40	40	40	40	40	40	40	40	40	40	40	40	40	40	40	40	40	40
210	40	40	40	40	40	40	40	40	40	40	40	40	40	40	40	40	40	40	40
215	40	40	40	40	40	40	40	40	40	40	40	40	40	40	40	40	40	40	40
220	40	40	40	40	40	40	40	40	40	40	40	40	40	40	40	40	40	40	40
225	40	40	40	40	40	40	40	40	40	40	40	40	40	40	40	40	40	40	40
230	40	40	40	40	40	40	40	40	40	40	40	40	40	40	40	40	40	46	46
235	40	40	40	40	40	40	40	40	40	40	40	40	40	40	40	40	46	46	46
240	40	40	40	40	40	40	40	40	40	40	40	40	40	40	40	46	46	46	46
245	40	40	40	40	40	40	40	40	40	40	40	40	40	40	40	46	46	46	46
250	40	40	40	40	40	40	40	40	40	40	40	40	40	46	46	46	46	46	46
255	40	40	40	40	40	40	40	40	40	46	46	46	46	46	46	46	46	46	46
260	40	40	40	40	40	40	40	46	46	46	46	46	46	46	46	46	46	46	46
265	40	40	40	40	40	40	46	46	46	46	46	46	46	46	46	46	46	46	46
270	40	40	46	46	46	46	46	46	46	46	46	46	46	46	46	46	46	46	46
275	40	46	46	46	46	46	46	46	46	46	46	46	46	46	46	46	46	46	46
280	46	46	46	46	46	46	46	46	46	46	46	46	46	46	46	46	46	46	46
285	46	46	46	46	46	46	46	46	46	46	46	46	46	46	46	46	46	46	46
290	46	46	46	46	46	46	46	46	46	46	46	46	46	46	46	46	46	46	46
295	46	46	46	46	46	46	46	46	46	46	46	46	46	46	46	46	46	46	46
300	46	46	46	46	46	46	46	46	46	46	46	46	46	46	46	46	46	46	46

Note: Men weighing less than 125 pounds should eat at least 20 grams per meal; men weighing more than 300 pounds or taller than 6'10" should eat at least 46 grams per meal.

tein to meet your needs. If you get a little more in a snack or two, that's gravy! Remember, the protein requirement you calculated is a *minimum* requirement. If you feel hungry, you can have a little more lean protein (as long as it's relatively free of carbs) anytime.

It's important to understand, however, that in streamlining the calculating process, we've taken a method involving numerous body measurements and activity variables and compressed them into a two-variable table based on slightly above-average activity levels and average body-fat percentages for a given height and weight. By doing so, we've sacrificed a little refinement and accuracy for ease and expedience. There's no doubt that the convoluted calculation method is more accurate, and those of you who wish to use it should pick up a copy of *Protein Power* and go for it. But rest assured, these average numbers we've worked out will provide you with plenty of good-quality protein to ensure your health and success on whichever *Protein Power LifePlan* regimen you select, and without all the hassle. They're close enough—as they say—for guv'ment work. (Because of the use of average numbers, you may want to make some commonsense adjustments. For example, if you find that your height and weight place you on the border between two levels of protein requirement and you'd rate yourself as sedentary, you might want to drop the lower of the two requirements. On the other hand, if you fall on the junction and you'd rate yourself as very active physically, you might want to step up to the higher number of grams of protein per meal.

So to begin you'll just need an accurate measure of your height and your weight. We prefer that you not guess, that you actually measure, since your health depends on your eating enough protein, and eating enough protein depends on your height and weight. Once you've got your numbers, take a look at table 13.1 (ladies) or table 13.2 (gentlemen) and find your weight on the left-hand side and your height across the top. Where the weight row and the height column intersect you'll find a number. For example, in the women's table, where 160 pounds meets 5'4", you'll see the number 27. That means that a woman of that height and weight requires 27 grams of protein per meal. By the simple maneuver of finding the number at the end of the weight row and height column that best describes you, you've just calculated your minimum protein requirement per meal. Simplicity itself! Henceforth, you should strive to eat at least this many grams of protein at each of your three meals—breakfast, lunch, and dinner—every day. *Note:* If your goal is to lose a significant amount of weight, you'll want to periodically return to these tables as your weight declines to "recalculate" your new protein needs as you shrink.

Since the protein requirement is a minimum, you can add a snack or two of protein throughout the day. Although snacks aren't required—you'll meet your minimum protein requirement with your three meals—anytime you feel hungry you can enjoy a protein snack, such as lean meat, chicken, fish, or jerky without disrupting your metabolic harmony or interfering with your metabolic rehabilitation.

When shopping for or cooking protein foods, most of us don't think in grams of protein, however.[1] What most people want to know is not how many grams of protein they should eat but how much chicken or fish or steak or eggs. And, we've made that easy, too. In table 13.3 you'll see various kinds of mainly protein foods (meat, fish, poultry, eggs, cheeses, tofu, and combinations of these foods) for the different grams-per-meal protein requirements in tables 13.1 and 13.2. Below each grams-per-meal number (e.g., 27g/meal) is the appropriate portion size of each of these foods. For example, in the 27-grams-per-meal column the proper portion of meat, fish, or poultry is about 4 ounces. (And for those of you around the world who do measure the weight of your food in grams, 1 ounce is about 30 grams, so a 4-ounce portion of chicken would be about 120 grams by weight and would provide 28 grams of protein—that's close enough to 27 for us.) Easy as pie—no, make that easy as beef tenderloin!

We encourage you to measure portions at first or to purchase them already weighed, but based on our own years of doing this,

1. For those readers who do think in grams, let us clear up a misconception that arose for some readers of *Protein Power.* When we say *grams of protein,* that does not refer to the total weight in grams of a particular food; it refers to the weight of the protein content in that amount of a particular food. For example, 1 ounce of chicken—which is 30 grams of total weight—contains only about 7 grams of protein. The remainder comes from water and/or fat.

TABLE 13.3

Protein Portions

Meat (beef, pork, poultry, fish)	= about 7 grams per ounce
Eggs	= about 6 grams whole; about 4 grams egg white only
Hard cheeses (cheddar, Gouda, Muenster, Swiss, Edam, blue, mozzarella)	= about 6 to 7 grams per ounce (and 1 gram carb)
Soft cheeses (cream cheese, Neufchâtel)	= 3 to 4 grams per ounce (and 1 gram carb)
Curd cheeses (cottage, ricotta)	= about 7 grams per 1/4 cup (and 2 grams carb)
Tofu	= about 5 grams per ounce

FOOD	20g/MEAL	27g/MEAL	34g/MEAL	40g/MEAL	46g/MEAL
Meats	3 ounces	4 ounces	5 ounces	6 ounces	7 to 8 ounces
Poultry	3 ounces	4 ounces	5 ounces	6 ounces	7 to 8 ounces
Fish	3 ounces	4 ounces	5 ounces	6 ounces	7 to 8 ounces
Shrimp	11 large*	13 large*	15 large*	17 large*	20 large*
Oysters	6 medium	8 medium	10 medium	12 medium	14 medium
Eggs	3 or 2 + 2 egg whites	4 or 2 + 4 egg whites	5 or 2 + 6 egg whites	6 or 3 + 6 egg whites	7 or 3 + 6 egg whites
Curd cheeses (cottage, ricotta)	3/4 cup	1 cup	1 1/4 cups	1 1/2 cups	1 3/4 cups
Tofu	4 ounces	6 ounces	7 ounces	8 ounces	9 ounces
COMBINATIONS OF FOODS	20g/MEAL	27g/MEAL	34g/MEAL	40g/MEAL	46g/MEAL
Eggs + Meat	2 or 1 + 2 egg whites + 1 ounce meat	3 or 2 + 2 egg whites + 1 ounce meat	4 or 2 + 3 egg whites + 2 ounces meat	5 or 2 + 4 egg whites + 2 ounces meat	6 or 3 + 4 egg whites + 2 ounces meat

Combination					
Eggs + Hard cheese	2 or 1 + 2 egg whites + 1 ounce cheese	3 or 2 + 2 egg whites + 1 ounce cheese	4 or 2 + 3 egg whites + 2 ounces cheese	5 or 2 + 4 egg whites + 2 ounces cheese	6 or 3 + 4 egg whites + 2 ounces cheese
Eggs + Soft cheese	2 or 1 + 2 egg whites + 2 ounces cheese	3 or 2 + 2 egg whites + 2 ounces cheese	4 or 2 + 3 egg whites + 2 ounces cheese	4 or 2 + 4 egg whites + 2 ounces cheese	6 or 3 + 4 egg whites + 2 ounces cheese
Eggs + Curd cheese	2 or 1 + 2 egg whites + 1/4 cup cheese	3 or 2 + 2 egg whites + 1/2 cup cheese	4 or 2 + 3 egg whites + 1/2 cup cheese	4 or 2 + 4 egg whites + 1/2 cup cheese	6 or 3 + 4 egg whites + 1/2 cup cheese
Eggs + Tofu	2 or 1 + 1 egg white + 2 ounces tofu	3 or 1 + 2 egg whites + 2 ounces tofu	4 or 2 + 2 egg whites + 2 ounces tofu	4 or 2 + 3 egg whites + 3 ounces tofu	6 or 3 + 4 egg whites + 4 ounces tofu
Meat + Curd cheese	2 ounces meat + 1/4 cup cheese	3 ounces meat + 1/4 cup cheese	3 ounces meat + 1/2 cup cheese	4 ounces meat + 1/2 cup cheese	5 ounces meat + 1/2 cup cheese
Meat + Tofu	1.5 ounces meat + 2 ounces tofu	2 ounces meat + 3 ounces tofu	2 ounces meat + 4 ounces tofu	3 ounces meat + 4 ounces tofu	4 ounces meat + 4 ounces tofu
Tofu + Hard cheese	3 ounces tofu + 1 ounce cheese	4 ounces tofu + 1 ounce cheese	5 ounces tofu + 1 ounce cheese	7 ounces tofu + 1 ounce cheese	8 ounces tofu + 1 ounce cheese
Tofu + Soft cheese	3 ounces tofu + 2 ounces cheese	4 ounces tofu + 2 ounces cheese	5 ounces tofu + 2 ounces cheese	7 ounces tofu + 2 ounces cheese	8 ounces tofu + 2 ounces cheese
Tofu + Curd cheese	3 ounces tofu + 1/4 cup cheese	4 ounces tofu + 1/4 cup cheese	4 ounces tofu + 1/2 cup cheese	5 ounces tofu + 1/2 cup cheese	6 ounces tofu + 1/2 cup cheese

*Figure 16 to 22 large shrimp per pound.

it won't be long until you'll be an old hand at sizing up portions and gauging the correct portion size of any food just by using the eyeball method. Until then, feel free to make a copy of your protein portion chart and stick it up on the refrigerator door or take it with you when you go to the grocery store, out dining, or on vacation. Although the protein portion of your meal should become the cornerstone, there are two other important macronutrient classes to think about: fats and carbohydrates. Let's see how they fit in.

How Much Fat Should You Eat?

The better question would be *what kind* of fat should you eat, since the quality of fat more clearly determines good health than the quantity does. After having read chapter 3 (or at least its "Bottom Line" summary), you should be well acquainted with the concept of good fats and bad fats and know that good fats are important both as a source of metabolically neutral calories (that is, calories that don't inspire major shifts in insulin) and as structural raw materials for fat-dependent structures within the body—chief among them the brain, the immune system, and the cell membranes of every one of the billions of cells that make you you! And you'll no doubt remember that bad fats lead to disastrous health problems, just as poor-quality construction materials lead to disastrous collapses of bridges and buildings.

So we ask that you first concern yourself with eating the kinds of fats that promote health: omega-3 fats, found in cold-water fish, wild game, and flax seed oil; monounsaturated fats, found in nuts, seeds, olives, avocados, and their naturally pressed oils; and naturally saturated fats, found in eggs, meat, poultry, and dairy. The next concern is keeping a rein on amounts of the omega-6 fats you eat. These you'll find in small amounts in vegetables and grains but in excessive amounts in corn oil and vegetable oils—items that you'll naturally want to avoid. By so doing, you can improve on the all-important omega 3–to–omega 6 ratio—critical to good health and optimal functioning of the cell membranes throughout your body (see chapter 3, "The Fat of the Land," and chapter 11, "Calisthenics for the Brain").

And at all costs, no matter which level of commitment you select, we urge you to avoid eating processed polyunsaturated fats, such as margarine, vegetable shortening, vegetable oils, corn oil, and any product that lists as an ingredient "partially hydrogenated" oil of any kind. The manufacturing process for these kinds of fats, which are called trans fats, involves heating polyunsaturated oils (corn, soybean, cottonseed, safflower, and others) to a high temperature with a metal catalyst to force hydrogen molecules into their structure. This process alters the configuration of the oil molecules, leaving them bent and rigid. Remember, the fats you eat become a part of each and every cell membrane within your body—the normally shaped "healthy" ones as well as the misshapen trans ones. The difference, however, is that the trans ones interfere with the functioning of the cell membranes and consequently of the organs and tissues those cells make up. Eating good-quality fat is of paramount importance to reclaiming and preserving your health. To make the selection easier, we've provided you with table 13.4, "Good Fats vs. Bad Fats."

But back to the original question: How much fat should you eat? The answer is both simple and complex. If you're not trying to lose weight (body fat), then you can eat as much good-quality fat as it takes to satisfy your appetite and to maintain your weight—even if that means you munch on nuts, seeds, nut butters, cheeses, jerky, guacamole, and olives all day long. The more calories you expend in exercise or work, the more calories from good-quality fat you'll need to eat to stay in energy balance. Conversely, if you're carrying too much fat weight, although you must still stick to only good-quality fat for your health, during your period of weight loss, you'll want to keep a rein on the amount of it you eat in order to create a calorie deficit to lose. That way you'll burn your own body fat stores for energy, not the fat you're eating. So, in a nutshell, if you're trying to lose weight and you're stuck—even though you're keeping your carbohydrate intake within the recommended Intervention Level guidelines (described in next section) and being sure to get the important vitamins, minerals, and other micronutrients necessary for good health (see Micronutrient Roundup in the appendix)—you're probably eating too much fat (that is, too many calories) for you to be able to lose. So

TABLE 13.4

Good Fats vs. Bad Fats

Good Fats and Oils

For Cooking or Panfrying
Butter
Ghee (clarified butter)
Olive oil
Sesame seed oil
Coconut oil
Lard
Fat that occurs in natural meats and poultry*

For Baking
Almond oil
Butter
Canola oil
Ghee
Lard (natural or organic if you can find it)

For Salads
Avocado oil
Almond oil
Canola oil
Hazelnut oil
Macadamia nut oil
Olive oil
Sesame seed oil
Walnut oil
Flax seed oil

Good Supplemental Oils
Flax seed oil (should be kept light protected and refrigerated and never be heated)
Sardine oil (and other fresh marine oils if you can find them)
Cod-liver oil (should be kept light protected and refrigerated and never be heated)
Capsules of fish oil, flax, DHA, EPA. If you use any of these highly unstable oils in capsule form, be aware that oxygen can penetrate the capsule and cause rancidity of the contents and the formation of lipid peroxides. You must bite a test capsule every few days to see if the oil is still fresh. A fishy taste means you must throw the bottle out! Rinse your mouth thoroughly afterward with a bit of wine or distilled spirits if you find a rancid capsule.

Bad Fats

Corn oil
Vegetable cooking oils
Margarine
Vegetable shortening
Partially hydrogenated oils of any kind

*Fat from lot-fed or grain-fed animals is not as healthy as that of free-range animals.

cut back a little on the nutrient-dense foods that can wipe out your calorie deficit in a snap. For example, while a 1-ounce portion of nuts containing 160 calories and only 3 or 4 grams of carbohydrate won't have much of an adverse impact on your weight loss, munching eight 1-ounce portions of them throughout the day will pile on an extra 1,300 calories and 24 to 32 grams of carbohydrate. We've seen just this scenario in numbers of patients who stopped losing weight and couldn't figure out why. During your weight-loss period, if you're not losing well, either watch the portions of nuts, seeds, nut butters, butter, cheeses, and oils or increase your calorie output with more exercise and you should begin to lose. Once you've gotten to your weight goal, you won't have to worry about limiting your intake of good-quality fats anymore as long as you keep your insulin controlled. You simply cannot store fat—and add on fat pounds—unless you turn your insulin loose. But to keep a rein on insulin output, most people will have to limit carbohydrate intake, at least to some extent, most of the time. Let's look now at this critical third player in the nutritional shell game and the adjustments you'll need to make in your carbohydrate intake to restore your health and to preserve it.

How Much Carbohydrate Should You Eat?

In deciding how much carbohydrate you can tolerate—and how much restriction you should place on this part of your diet—consider the following factors: your current state of health, your level of physical activity, and whether or not you need to lose a significant amount of fat.

Take a moment to envision the government's famous USDA Food Guide Pyramid. What do you see at its base? That's right: six to eleven servings of bread, cereal, and/or pasta a day for good health! A base made of cereal-grain foods. Now put on your Paleolithic glasses and review a little of the ancient history you've learned. How long have humans existed as humans on planet Earth? By recent estimates over a million years for *Homo habilis* and more than three million years for our protohuman ancestors. And when did the agricultural revolution occur (that is, when did we adopt the habit of cultivating, storing, milling, and eating ce-

real grains)? About 10,000 years ago by the most generous estimate—and for some ethnic groups, as little as 1,000 years ago. So
for at least 990,000 years, what did a poor human do without his
six to eleven daily servings of bread, cereal, and pasta? As you've
already discovered, he lived in better health than he did after the
advent of farming, that's what! So where do the luminaries of
modern nutritional wisdom get off recommending such non-
sense? We're not sure, but certainly not from any basis in biochemical or historical fact. Avoid the government's pyramid
scheme: limit your carbohydrates.

So what are the facts regarding carbohydrates? First and foremost, they're totally nonessential to your health and well-being.
Although you'll hear from nutritional "authorities" all the time
that you "must have carbohydrates for energy," that's simply not
true. The body has all the machinery it needs to manufacture its
own carbohydrate out of protein or fat. If you ate zero carbohydrates (which traditional Eskimos do much of the year, since at
their high latitude there isn't any edible vegetation to speak of),
you'd do fine as long as you got enough good protein, good fat,
water, and minerals. We know that may sound like nutritional
heresy, but it's the plain truth, and you should know it. You don't
need them at all, but that doesn't mean that you can't tolerate
some in your diet. Remember, your foremost goal in reclaiming
your health is to control your insulin levels—in effect, to become
more insulin sensitive, so that it takes less insulin to do the job.
And clearly the most effective way to accomplish that goal is by
restricting carbohydrate intake. So what does that mean in terms
of food?

Any food that contains simple sugars, starches, or fiber contains carbohydrates. That means virtually anything that came from
the plant kingdom or any dairy product contains some amount of
carbohydrates. What we're interested in is controlling blood sugar
rise and insulin release that carbohydrates inspire. And that means
it's better to eat the lower-starch and lower-sugar fruits and vegetables that have a more moderate effect on your insulin level than
the potatoes, bread, corn, rice, pasta, and sugars that will send it
through the roof. In short, we encourage you to eat those foods
that give you the most nutrient bang for the carbohydrate buck

with the least metabolic impact. Let's look at the effective carbo-hydrate content (ECC) of foods in a bit more detail.

WHAT IS THE ECC?

The total carbohydrate content of any food is the sum of sim-ple sugars, the starches, and the fibers (and any other nonabsorba-ble sugars, such as sugar alcohols) that the food might contain. But, metabolically speaking, only the absorbable forms—the sug-ars and the starches—can have a metabolic impact on insulin and blood sugar. Fiber is sugar, too. Fiber, just like starch, is simply many molecules of glucose hooked together into long chains. The difference between starch and fiber lies in the fact that the human digestive tract doesn't have the enzymes needed to break the links of the fiber chain and turn it into glucose. Based on this differ-ence, we developed our concept of the effective carbohydrate content, or ECC, of foods, a new and more accurate means of counting carbohydrates that widely expands your food choices on a restricted-carbohydrate program. If the body can't turn a food substance into glucose, that food component can't cause a rise in insulin, and therefore can't perpetuate the insulin-resistance cycle. Fiber falls into this category. It passes through the digestive sys-tem intact, and far down the intestinal pathway in the colon, bac-teria act upon it, digest it there, and produce short-chain fatty acids from it that "feed" the cells that line the colon. And that means that fiber—or any carbohydrate that can't be broken down and absorbed by the digestive machinery, such as a sugar alco-hol—doesn't count in your daily effective carbohydrate gram total. If it doesn't have an *effect* on your insulin, it's not an *effective* carbohydrate.

It's easy to determine the EEC of any food; you need only know the total amount of carbohydrate it contains and the amount of fiber or unabsorbable sugar alcohols, if any. Then by this simple formula you can calculate the ECC:

Total Carbohydrate − Dietary Fiber = Effective Carbohy-drate

By subtracting the grams of dietary fiber (as well as those of sugar alcohols, if the food contains them) from the total grams, you'll know what's left to have an effect. It's this number—the ECC—not the total grams of carbohydrate, that makes up your 7 to 10 grams per meal at the intervention level, for example. Let's turn now to look at some specific food choices.

Vegetables, Beans, and Grains. Veggies vary widely in the amount of starch they contain. A 2-cup serving of broccoli, for example, is at least half fiber and contains only about 4 effective grams of carbohydrate, whereas an equal serving of corn (which, although it does have some fiber, has a load of absorbable starch, too) provides a whopping 68 grams of usable carbohydrate. If you're at the Intervention Level and have only 7 to 10 grams of EEC to spend at a meal, a large serving of broccoli would fit in easily with room for servings of other vegetables as well; a serving of corn, however, would have to be scaled back considerably—to the 8.5 grams of ECC in about ¼ cup—to qualify for Intervention, and even this meager portion would take up most of your allotment all by itself. When you're putting together a meal, appropriate-size portions of any allowable vegetable will work, but you'll find that if you stick to the lower-starch vegetables, such as salad greens, asparagus, artichokes, cauliflower, cabbage, celery, carrots, broccoli, garlic, green beans, mushrooms, onions, peppers, tomatoes, radishes, turnips, squashes, and the like, you'll get a much larger portion for fewer of your allotted carbohydrates. You'll be able to enjoy ½ cup to 1 cup of most any of these individual vegetables and still have room for 1 or 2 cups of salad greens, without exceeding an Intervention limit. However, if you select starchier vegetables, such as white potatoes, sweet potatoes, and legumes (cow peas and dried beans), and grain products, such as corn, rice, oats, bread, crackers, and pasta, you won't get as much of them for your allotment. At the Intervention Level, a meager ⅛ cup to ¼ cup of most of these higher-starch foods will take up the lion's share of your 7-to-10-gram allotment: a half slice of regular sandwich bread or one slice of most varieties of light bread will contain 6 or 7 grams of EEC; four saltine crackers will cost 8 grams; half of a regular hamburger bun contains 12 or 13 ECC grams; a light bun about 7. To make sense of it all, you may find it helpful at first to make a list of the foods you especially enjoy (particularly the vegetables, fruits, and grains) and jot down their ECC values using our new book, the *Protein Power LifePlan Gram Counter,* or any complete food count book. Remember though, if you don't use our counter, the one you choose must list fiber grams as well as carbohydrates—otherwise the ECC cannot be calculated. For a list of common foods and their ECC, see table 13.5. In making your carbohydrate choices, we'd urge you not to focus simply on quantity but also bear quality in mind. Be sure you've read chapter 6, "The Leaky Gut" (or at least its Bottom Line summary) to learn about the damaging potential of legumes and grains to the gastrointestinal tract and the risks these foods may pose to certain people.

The Fruits of the Field. Many fruits and berries are carbohydrate bargains. Among the best are melons (cantaloupe, honeydew, watermelon), which contain only about 5 to 8 grams of ECC per ½ cup, and most berries (strawberries, blueberries, blackberries, and raspberries), which contain about the same or even less. A half cup of strawberries contains only about 3.3 grams and is a nice sweet complement to any meal. Fresh grapes offer another bargain, at only about 7.5 ECC grams in ½ cup—great for a snack with some jerky or cheese. Whole pieces of fruit can fit in, too, even in Intervention, the most restrictive phase of the rehabilitation; a medium peach has but 8.3 grams ECC and a Valencia orange a little over 10. You can enjoy either one with a grilled chicken salad or a couple of burger patties and greens. Difficulties arise in trying to incorporate the starchier fruits, such as bananas, papayas, mangos, and other tropical fruits, which have much higher ECC levels, into your plan; a medium banana has about 25 grams, a medium pear or apple, about 20. Does that mean that you can never enjoy these fruits on Intervention? No. But it does mean that you'll have to split them; enjoy half an apple or pear or a third of a banana and save the remainder for a future meal or share it with a friend.

Remember that in the Paleolithic world fruits were wild and seasonal. Early humans couldn't go down to the market and buy whatever fruits they wanted anytime of the year. In much of the Paleolithic world, what wild fruit trees there were bloomed in the spring; the fruit ripened in the summer and provided our ancestors with concentrated sugars at the end of summer to raise insu-

TABLE 13.5

Effective Carbohydrate Content of Basic Foods

FOOD	PORTION	ECC (IN GRAMS)
Vegetables		
Alfalfa sprouts	½ cup	0.4
Amaranth, boiled	1 cup	5.4
Artichoke, boiled	1 medium	6.9
Arugula, raw	1 cup	0.8
Asparagus, boiled	4 large spears	2.9
Bamboo shoots, boiled	½ cup	0.6
Beans (black), boiled	½ cup	16.8
Beans (butter), boiled	½ cup	12.2
Beans (Great Northern), boiled	½ cup	15.6
Beans (green), boiled	½ cup	7.6
Beans (kidney), boiled	½ cup	16.8
Beans (lima), boiled	½ cup	12.9
Beans (navy), boiled	½ cup	20.7
Beans (pinto), boiled	½ cup	18.6
Beans (red), boiled	½ cup	12.0
Beans (wax), boiled	½ cup	9.0
Beans (white), boiled	½ cup	22.5
Beets	½ cup	5.7
Bok choy, raw	1 cup	0.8
Broccoli, raw	1 cup	2.2
boiled	1 cup	4.0
Brussels sprouts	10 sprouts	8.6
Cabbage, raw	1 cup	3.0
boiled	1 cup	3.6
Carrots, raw	1 medium	3.3
boiled	½ cup	4.3
Cauliflower	1 cup	1.8
Celery, raw	1 stalk	0.9
boiled	½ cup	3.0
Chard, boiled	½ cup	3.6
Chickpeas, boiled	½ cup	20.0
Chives, raw	1 tbsp.	0.1

TABLE 13.5 (Continued)

FOOD	PORTION	ECC (IN GRAMS)
Coleslaw (no sugars)	½ cup	7.5 (variable per recipe)
Collard greens, boiled	1 cup	7.8
Corn, boiled	½ cup	17.0
Cowpeas (black-eyes), boiled	½ cup	17.0
Cucumber, raw	1 medium	6.0
Eggplant, boiled	1 cup	6.4
Garlic, raw	1 clove	1.0
Ginger root, raw	¼ cup	3.6
Hominy, boiled	½ cup	15.0
Kale	1 cup	7.6
Leeks, boiled	½ cup	4.0
Lentils, boiled	½ cup	16.0
Lettuce, raw	1 cup	0.8
Mushrooms, raw	1 cup	2.2
boiled	1 cup	4.6
Mustard greens, boiled	1 cup	3.0
Okra, boiled	½ cup	5.8
Onions, raw	½ cup	5.6
Onions (green), raw	½ cup	2.5
Parsley, raw	½ cup	1.9
Peas (green), boiled	½ cup	10.3
Peas (split), boiled	½ cup	21.2
Peppers (bell)	1 cup	4.8
Peppers (hot chili), roasted	½ cup	4.2
Peppers (sweet, yellow), raw	1 large	11.8
Pimientos, canned	1 tbsp.	0.6
Potato (french fries)	5 fries	10.0
Potato (sweet w/skin), baked	1 medium	24.0
Potato (white w/skin), baked	½ medium	25.5
mashed	½ cup	15.0
Pumpkin, boiled	1 cup	12.0
Radicchio, raw	½ cup	0.9
Radishes, raw	½ cup	1.3
Rhubarb, boiled	½ cup	3.5
Rutabaga, boiled	½ cup	6.6

TABLE 13.5 (Continued)

FOOD	PORTION	ECC (IN GRAMS)
Sauerkraut, canned	½ cup	5.1
Shallots, raw	1 tbsp.	1.7
Spinach, raw	1 cup	0.6
boiled	1 cup	3.1
Squash (summer: yellow crookneck, scallop, zucchini), raw	1 cup	4.0
boiled	1 cup	5.2
Squash (winter: acorn, butternut, hubbard, spaghetti), boiled	1 cup	8.5
Tomatillo, raw	1 medium	2.0
Tomato (green), raw	1 medium	6.2
Tomato (red), raw	1 medium	4.1
Tomato (sundried)	¼ cup	7.5
Turnip, boiled	1 cup	4.4
Turnip greens, boiled	1 cup	2.8
Water chestnuts, canned	1 whole	1.0
Fruits		
Apple, raw	1 apple	18.0
cooked	½ cup	10.0
Applesauce, unsweetened	½ cup	12.0
Apricots, raw	1 medium	3.2
Avocado	½ medium	3.7
Banana, raw	1 medium	25.0
Blackberries, raw	½ cup	5.9
Blueberries, raw	½ cup	8.6
Boysenberries, raw	½ cup	8.0
Cantaloupe, raw	½ cup	5.7
Casaba, raw	½ cup	10.5
Cherries (sour), canned	½ cup	10.9
Cherries (sweet), raw	5 whole	5.1
Crab apples, raw	½ cup	11.0
Cranberries, raw	½ cup	6.0

TABLE 13.5 (Continued)

FOOD	PORTION	ECC (IN GRAMS)
Cranberry sauce	1 tbsp.	7.0
Currants (black), raw	½ cup	5.6
Dates, dried	1 whole	6.0
Elderberries, raw	½ cup	13.5
Figs, raw	1 medium	9.6
dried	1 whole	12.2
Gooseberries, raw	½ cup	7.7
Grapefruit, raw	½ whole	8.8
Grapes, raw	½ cup	7.6
Guava, raw	1 medium	10.7
Honeydew, raw	½ cup	7.8
Kiwi, raw	1 medium	8.7
Kumquat, raw	1 medium	3.1
Lemon, raw	1 medium	5.4
Lime, raw	1 medium	7.1
Mango, raw	½ cup	16.5
Nectarine, raw	1 medium	13.8
Orange (Valencia), raw	1 medium	11.5
Orange (Mandarin)	½ cup	11.9
Papaya, raw	½ medium	13.5
Passion fruit, raw	1 medium	2.3
Peach, raw	1 medium	8.3
Pear, raw	1 medium	20.8
Persimmon, raw	1 medium	8.4
Pineapple, raw	½ cup	8.7
Plantain, cooked	½ cup	24.0
Plum, raw	1 medium	8.6
Pomegranate, raw	1 medium	26.4
Quince, raw	1 medium	14.0
Raisins	¼ cup	27.8
Raspberries, raw	½ cup	4.2
Strawberries, raw	½ cup	3.3
Tangerine, raw	1 medium	9.4
Watermelon, raw	½ cup	5.5

TABLE 13.5 (Continued)

FOOD	PORTION	ECC (IN GRAMS)
Breads and Cereals		
Amaranth flour	1 cup	99.4
Bagel	1 medium	30.0
	1 mini-bagel	13.2
Biscuit	1 small	
	(³/₄ ounce)	9.7
	1 medium	
	(1 ounce)	12.0
	1 large	
	(2 ounces)	32.0
Bread (pita)	1 medium	
	pocket	20.0
Bread (raisin, regular)	1 slice	13.0 (variable)
Bread (sandwich, regular)	1 slice	12.0 (variable)
Bread (sandwich, light)	1 slice	6.0 (variable)
Bun (hot dog/hamburger, regular)	1 bun	27.0
Bun (hot dog/hamburger, light)	1 bun	14.0
Cornmeal	1 cup	84.0
Crackers (saltine)	1 cracker	2.0
Croissant	1 medium	25.0
Couscous, cooked	1 cup	34.0
English muffin	1 whole	26.0
Melba toast	1 slice	3.5
Oats, dry	1 cup	86.0
Oat bran muffin	1 medium	25.0
Pasta (egg noodle)	1 cup	26.0
Pasta (spaghetti)	1 cup	37.0
Pie crust	¹/₈ of 9" pie	9.0
Quinoa, dry	1 cup	101.0
Rice, cooked	1 cup	42.0
Taco (corn)	1 medium	
	shell	7.3

TABLE 13.5 (Continued)

FOOD	PORTION	ECC (IN GRAMS)
Tortilla (wheat, regular)	1 whole	25.0
Tortilla (La Tortilla whole wheat low-fat)	1 whole	3–7.0
Waffle	4" square	12.7
Wheat flour, dry	1 cup	92.0
Nuts and Seeds		
Almonds, dry roasted	1 ounce	1.8
Cashews, dry roasted	1 ounce	8.4
Macadamia nuts, dry roasted	1 ounce	1.3
Peanuts, dry roasted	1 ounce	2.2
Pecans	1 ounce	3.0
Pistachios	1 ounce	4.7
Pumpkin seeds	1 ounce	14.0
Sunflower seeds	1 ounce	4.2
Walnuts	1 ounce	3.8
Dairy Products		
Cheese, hard	1 ounce	1.0 (average)
Cheese, soft	1 ounce	1.0 (average)
Cottage cheese	¼ cup	2.0
Cream (half and half)	½ ounce	0.6
Milk (skim)	8 ounces	12.0
Milk (whole)	8 ounces	11.0
Sour cream	1 tbsp.	0.6
Yogurt (low-fat)	8 ounces	17.0
Yogurt (whole milk)	8 ounces	12.0

lin and increase fat storage—potentially important for their winter survival. But bear in mind that the wild fruits that early humans enjoyed seasonally hadn't been Luther Burbanked and bore little resemblance to the huge, sweet, hybrid apples, pears, peaches, and plums you'll find in markets today. And for that reason, particularly if a part of your rehabilitation is losing body fat, you should not overeat fruits. We encourage you to enjoy reasonable servings of a wide variety of different fruits daily for their nutrient benefits, such as their antioxidants and cancer-fighting chemicals, but to eat them along with salad greens and other colorful low-starch vegetables in your complete diet.

Sweeteners. We've devoted an entire chapter to the discussion of sugars and the use of artificial sweeteners. If you have not done so, please read chapter 7, "How Sweet It Is . . . Not!" or at the very least its Bottom Line summary to familiarize yourself with the facts about sweeteners, both real and artificial. For our purposes here, let us simply remind you that real sweeteners, such as sucrose (table sugar), fructose (concentrated fruit sugar), corn syrups, and honey, all carry the same metabolic burden—about 4 grams of readily absorbable carbohydrate and 16 calories per level measuring teaspoon. Please also note that a level measuring spoon teaspoon is substantially smaller than a level flatware "teaspoon"—in fact, it's about half the size. And a heaped up flatware coffee- or teaspoon of sugar probably has about 12 grams of carbohydrate, not 4 grams. You'll need to count every one of these grams in your day's total, which means that you'll actually be able to use only limited quantities of any real sweetener.

Artificial sweeteners aren't really a perfect solution, either, for many reasons (see chapter 7), among them that intense sweetness blunts your taste receptors for sweet and makes you crave sweetness all the more. If you can strive to reduce your intake of highly sweetened foods, you'll find in a few weeks that your craving for added sweetness diminishes markedly. It's truly better in the long run to try to avoid artificial sweetners; however, when you occasionally feel you must use sweetener, we'd give lukewarm recommendations to saccharine and the newly approved Canadian product sucralose (see Resources in the appendix if you cannot locate it in your area) as the lesser of evils. Although by itself the artificial sweetener acesulfame K is no worse than saccharine or sucralose, we've learned that in products it's often blended with aspartame, and when it is, we don't recommend it. We can no longer recommend aspartame as safe. We now feel that the weight of scientific evidence indicts this sweetener as harmful for some people. We hope that you'll try to avoid it as an added sweetener and avoid consuming foods already sweetened with it.

From Intervention to Maintenance

If you currently suffer from any of the insulin-related disorders—high blood pressure, high triglycerides, high total cholesterol, low HDL cholesterol, heart disease, erratic blood sugar (hypoglycemia or type II diabetes), elevated serum ferritin, sleep apnea, gout, gall bladder disease, gastric reflux, or obesity—then you must first reclaim your health. To do so, you should begin at the Intervention Level of carbohydrate restriction. *If you're currently under a doctor's care for these disorders or taking medications to control them—especially if you're a diabetic on insulin or oral medications to control blood sugar or on diuretics to control blood pressure—you must consult with your physician before beginning this plan!* This nutritional strategy is potent and will rapidly cause changes in blood pressure and blood sugar that will make your current doses of medication far too high. Continuing to take the medication while adhering to this plan could have serious health consequences—not from the plan, but from overdosing on your current medication. Your physician will have to work with you to taper your medication doses; quite probably he or she may soon be able to discontinue some or all of them. (If your doctor is willing to work with you to do this and would like to contact our office for more information, please feel free to ask him or her to write, fax, e-mail, or call us. Immediately we'll send a packet of information containing the bibliography of medical research upon which we based our plan, along with medical abstracts of the most crucial articles and explanatory text as to why they support our position. We'll also send information about the basics of managing your medication changes in concert with the diet. And lastly, we'll be happy to arrange to answer any specific questions your physician might have about your condition with regard to our nutritional strategy. While medical and legal limitations preclude our diagnosing or treating specific medical conditions of individuals whom we have not seen personally in our clinic, we can consult with their physicians, professional to professional. We're delighted to teach our nutritional treatment methods to any physician who wants to learn them. And we can answer general questions that you may have pertaining to the diet itself and your use of it.)

The Intervention Level is where everyone should begin—even those already pretty fit and healthy—at least for a few days to a week to quickly induce the metabolic shift to fat burning as the main energy source. If you're out of shape or have serious medical problems to conquer, you'll be here for a while—a few weeks, several months, or longer. But hang in there; in the great scheme of things, it really won't seem so long. Besides, however long it takes, what's the hurry? You've got the rest of your life to be lean and healthy!

At this level of restriction—termed Phase I Intervention in *Protein Power*—you will limit your intake to 7 to 10 grams of effective carbohydrate per meal or snack. Remember that by *effective carbohydrate* we mean that which has an effect on your blood sugar and insulin. The total carbohydrate gram content of any food is the sum of all the sugars, starches, and types of fiber in the food, but all you need concern yourself with are those grams that can have an effect on your blood sugar and your insulin—that is, the absorbable sugars and starches. When you use our concept of ECC, or effective carbohydrate content, 7 to 10 grams goes a pretty long way. For example, you could have 2 cups of broccoli, ½ cup of fresh mushrooms, a couple of cups of mixed salad greens, *and* half a fresh tomato in a single meal and not exceed your ECC limit. You'll find guidelines to help meet the appropriate level of carb intake for the Purist, the Dilettante, and the Hedonist later in the chapter and mix-and-match meal suggestions in chapter 15. Those folks who want to create their own meals should consult table 13.5 for a list of common foods and their ECC. As we mentioned earlier, for a more complete listing, pick up a copy of our new book the *Protein Power LifePlan Gram Counter*.

When will you know that you've completed the Intervention process? You'll want to stay at the Intervention level of carbohydrate intake until you solve your underlying health problem—that is, until a repeat of your blood tests shows that your triglycerides, cholesterol, HDL, blood sugar, uric acid, etc., have returned to normal levels; until your weight or fat percentage approaches your desired goal (we recommend you normally shoot for 20 to 25 percent body fat in women and 15 to 20 percent body fat in men);

until your symptoms of gout or gastroesophageal reflux have disappeared; or until your physician feels that your sleep apnea has improved sufficiently to allow you to safely discontinue use of assisted-breathing devices. Again, that may mean a few weeks for some, many months for others. But however long it takes, once you've conquered your problem and reclaimed your health, then it's time to move to the Transition Level for a month or two. If at that level of carbohydrate intake everything remains stable—that is, your lab values don't begin to creep up, your fluid retention or reflux symptoms don't recur—then you're ready to move to Maintenance for the long haul. Please don't be in a hurry; keep reminding yourself that you've got the rest of your life to be healthy, so what's a few weeks or months in the great scheme of things? (For recommended carbohydrate allowances during the Intervention, Transition, and Maintenance levels, refer to table 13.6.) We can't stress enough that this is a life plan, not a diet; we

TABLE 13.6

Carbohydrate Intake Guidelines

LEVEL	ECC PER MEAL OR SNACK* (IN GRAMS)	ECC PER DAY (IN GRAMS)
Intervention	7 to 10	< 40
Transition	15	< 60
Maintenance†		
Week 1	20	< 80
Week 2	25	< 100
Week 3	30	< 120

*You may have up to 10 ECC grams each day in optional snacks in Intervention *if you desire*. That could be a single snack of 10 ECC grams or two snacks of 5 ECC grams or three snacks of 3 ECC grams apiece each day. During Transition, you can have up to 15 ECC snack grams—a single snack of 15 grams, two of 7.5 grams each, or three snacks of 5 ECC grams apiece each day. During Maintenance, you can spend up to 25 total ECC snack grams all at once or divided throughout the day.

†Proper Maintenance levels of carbohydrate can vary from individual to individual. To determine your level, gradually move up the carbohydrate ladder until you begin to retain fluid, gain weight, develop your old symptoms, or see your lab values begin to climb again. At that point, move back down to your last stable level and remain there for the long haul. Recognize that some people will tolerate no more than 15 or 20 grams per meal; others will do fine with 35 or even 40. And remember that the more active you are, the more carbohydrate you'll be able to tolerate. Conversely, if your activity declines because of injury or other circumstance, you must decrease your carbohydrate intake per meal and per day to prevent a regain.

urge you to undertake it as a new and better way of living, not as something you'll do for a few weeks to reach some artificial, short-term goal.

If your blood pressure, blood sugar, blood fats, and body fat are currently within the normal range, congratulations! You can spend a few days to a week at the Intervention Level of carbohydrates to allow your body to adapt to the new regimen and then quickly move through Transition to Maintenance. (If you're already a *Protein Power* devotee, simply continue your Maintenance Level of carb intake and fine-tune your program, if you like, using the new information you'll find in the Purist or Dilettante approaches below. If, Heaven forbid, you've fallen off your plan, then dive right back in at the Intervention Level and get back with the program, get yourself fit, and move on to Transition and Maintenance once again.)

Are You a Purist, a Hedonist, or a Dilettante?

But first things first. Before you begin to intervene, you'll need to decide how much effort and commitment you're willing to bring to bear in living this plan. Be aware that your current selection is not chiseled in stone; you may move to any of the three commitment levels whenever you choose and for as long as you choose. Today a Purist, next week a Hedonist. In the dozen-plus years since we developed and adopted this nutritional regimen ourselves, we have wended our way in and out of each of these three levels as the occasion demanded—and we continue to do so.

In the next sections, you'll find a set of food-selection guidelines that specify the types of foods permitted for the Hedonist, the Dilettante, and the Purist. They are intended to help you in shopping, cooking, and ordering in restaurants. The guidelines, you'll notice, say nothing about portions of these foods permitted. Consult table 13.3 for the approximate portion of various mainly protein foods that you'll need to meet your body's minimum protein requirement. For the mainly carbohydrate foods, check the ECC listings in table 13.5 or your ECC gram counter for portion sizes appropriate to your level of rehabilitation, as outlined in table 13.6. For simplicity, we've divided the foods in these guidelines into categories of mainly protein foods and mainly carbohydrate foods. We recognize that food categories aren't pure; there is some protein in certain grains and vegetables and a bit of carbohydrate in some shellfish and egg yolks, for example, but we've chosen to ignore these minimal amounts. You'll also find listings of the fats, oils, sweeteners, and beverages allowed. Take a look now at the three commitment levels and see which one seems to fit your current needs best.

The Hedonist's Approach

The Hedonist's regimen offers the least restriction of the three plans. Its premise is simple: always get enough good-quality protein to meet your body's needs, keep the total amount of carbohydrate per meal within the prescribed limits, eat good-quality fats, drink plenty of water, and replace potassium and magnesium. By making just these minimal adjustments you can reap 80 percent of the health benefits possible with the *Protein Power LifePlan* strategy. That's why we say this approach follows the 80/20 rule: 80 percent of the benefit comes from 20 percent of the effort. By far and away, the most potent force in health rehabilitation comes from controlling your insulin and improving your insulin sensitivity, both of which come from simply controlling your carbohydrate intake and eating enough protein, two very simple and easy-to-accomplish measures.

We designed the Hedonist's plan for those people who wish to better their health, lower their cholesterol and triglycerides, improve blood sugar control, sleep more soundly, and trim their waistlines by making only a few changes in nutrition, in most cases without veering much from the diet they currently eat—or would like to eat. It's ideal for those who, while they may wish to do more to benefit their health, feel that their current life situation will permit them to make only a few alterations in diet. Remember the words of the Greek god Apollo chiseled into the stone above the doorway at his temple at Delphi: "Know thyself!" Know what you'll stick to given your current situation in life; don't bite off more than you can reasonably chew, or you may set yourself up for disappointment with a plan that is more rigid than your lifestyle can accept at present. Our nutritional Hedonism—despite its name—is a reasonable place to begin your health rehabilitation, allowing you to make the nutritional changes gradually and still reap great rewards; it's essentially the plan that well over two million readers have used with great success already. And even if you choose to begin with a more stringent plan—the Dilettante or even the Purist regimen—you can adopt a Hedonist's approach if the occasion demands—for a party, out with friends, on vacation—without feeling that you've abandoned your commitment to health. Regardless of the plan you choose, you'll still be reaping great rewards. If you feel the Hedonist's nutritional strategy best suits your current health and lifestyle needs, here are the guidelines you'll need to follow:

GENERAL FOOD-SELECTION GUIDELINES FOR THE HEDONIST

PROTEIN

In meeting your protein requirement at each meal, you may select from any of these "mainly protein" foods in portions suitable to your lean body size:

- *Beef, pork, lamb, or poultry.*
- *Wild game.* (For mail-order sources, see Resources in the appendix.)
- *Fish, seafood, or shellfish* (fresh, frozen, or canned).
- *Eggs.* Pasteurized egg whites or egg-substitute products are also acceptable.
- *Jerky* (if possible without MSG).
- *Seeds or nuts* (almonds, Brazil nuts, cashews, hazelnuts, filberts, macadamia nuts, peanuts, pecans, walnuts) *and their butters.*
- *Soy products* (tofu, miso, texturized vegetable protein, or TVP).
- *Dairy products* (milk, yogurt, cheeses).
- *Protein powders* made of egg white, soy, milk solids, or microfiltered whey protein.
- *Protein bars.* (See Resources in the appendix.)

Protein sources not allowed: None.

Required protein amounts: The actual amount of protein needed per meal or per day depends on the size and activity level of the individual. Please consult tables 13.1 or 13.2 to determine your daily minimum protein requirement and table 13.3 to determine the protein serving size (per-meal portion) that is appropriate for you.

CARBOHYDRATE

You can select from among these "mainly carbohydrate" foods in portions *up to* the number of effective grams allowed per meal or snack on your level of rehabilitation. Consult a good gram counter or see table 13.5 for specific serving sizes:

• *Fresh, frozen, or canned vegetables.* Best (lowest-carbohydrate) choices are asparagus, avocado, broccoli, cauliflower, celery, cucumbers, garlic, greens, green beans, leeks, lettuces, mushrooms, olives, onions, peppers (red, green, yellow, and hot), radishes, summer squashes (crookneck, scallop, zucchini), tomatoes, and turnips. Slightly higher in starch are beets, carrots, eggplant, jicama, and winter squashes (acorn, butternut, spaghetti, pattypan). Highest-carbohydrate vegetables* include white potatoes and yams.

• *Fresh, frozen, or unsweetened canned fruits.* Best carbohydrate bargains include blackberries, grapes, strawberries, raspberries, lemons, limes, melons (cantaloupe, Crenshaw, honeydew, watermelon), and rhubarb. Modestly higher-carbohydrate fruits include grapefruit, blueberries, kiwi, nectarines, oranges, and peaches. Highest-carbohydrate fruits* include raisins and other naturally dried fruits (without preservatives), apples, apricots, bananas, papaya, pears, pomegranate, coconut (fresh or unsweetened dried), and mango and most other tropical fruits.

• *Legumes in small amounts.* Legumes within the carbohydrate limit of the plan include dried beans, lentils, peas, and peanuts.

---

*Foods marked with an asterisk (*) may contain significant numbers of carbohydrate grams. During the Intervention and Transition levels of the diets, be very careful to measure portions of these higher-starch, higher-natural-sugar foods.

- *Grains,* their meals or flours, and products made with them in small amounts.* Within the carboydrate limit of the plan these include amaranth, barley, corn, millet, oats, rice, rye, spelt, and wheat.

- *Seeds and nuts.** Be aware that these foods contain significant numbers of carbohydrate grams (from 2 to 4 per ounce) and many calories (about 150 to 160 per ounce). During the Intervention and Transition phases of the diets, nuts and seeds should be consumed only in modest quantities, particularly if weight loss is a part of the overall health goal.

- *Soy products.* These include tofu, miso, texturized vegetable protein (TVP), protein powders, and soy milk or soy cheese. Amounts vary from product to product, so check the labels. Soy milk is acceptable, but beware the number of carbohydrates in soy beverage products—many of them are sweetened. To our knowledge, only the White Wave company's soy-milk product called Silk contains as few carbohydrate grams as regular cow's or goat's milk.

- *Whole eggs, shellfish, and some seafood.* The amount in these foods is so small that it doesn't really count.

- *Dairy products.* Fluid dairy products (milk, plain yogurt) contain about 1.5 grams of usable carbohydrate (as milk sugar) per ounce; cottage cheese, about 2 grams per ¼ cup; hard cheeses, about 1 gram per ounce; and soft cheeses, about 2 grams per ounce on average. Low-fat and nonfat dairy products in general contain slightly more carbohydrate per ounce than higher-fat varieties.

Carbohydrate sources not allowed: None, although amounts of beans, grains, potatoes, and other starchy fruits and vegetables will naturally be limited by the carbohydrate allotment of the plan.

Allowed carbohydrate amounts: The amount of carbohydrate allowed per meal and per day will vary as you work your way through the plan. The greatest restriction comes during Interven-

---

*Foods marked with an asterisk (*) may contain significant numbers of carbohydrate grams. During the Intervention and Transition levels of the diets, be very careful to measure portions of these higher-starch, higher-natural-sugar foods.

tion, increasing modestly during Transition, and finishing with a still higher Maintenance level of carbohydrate intake designed to keep insulin controlled for the long term. Please see table 13.6 for actual grams allowed for each phase of the plan.

SWEETENERS

In very limited quantities, you can use the following sweeteners on your plan:

• *Honey, corn syrup, rice syrup, cane or beet sugar, maple syrup, or sorghum molasses.* These products contain about 4 grams of quickly absorbable carbohydrate per measured teaspoon. If you choose to use them, do so only in small amounts that will keep you within the carbohydrate limits of your rehabilitation level.

• *Fructose or high-fructose corn syrup.* Use it in small amounts within the carbohydrate limits of the plan—if at all. (Reread chapter 7, "How Sweet It Is . . . Not!," for details on the dangers of concentrated fructose.)

• *The sweet herb stevia.*

• *Artificial sweeteners,* including sucralose, acesulfame K, and saccharine in moderation. Be aware that some products sweetened with acesulfame K contain aspartame (in a half-and-half blend). We've found that this fact may not always be correctly listed on the labels. We used a small amount of it in protein shake products we've designed but made sure through independent analysis that the sweetener the manufacturer used didn't contain aspartame before we approved the formula. (For sources of sucralose, marketed in Canada as Splenda, see Resources in the appendix.)

Sweetener sources not recommended: Aspartame and products made with it.

Required sweetener amounts: None.

FATS AND OILS

You should select fats and oils from the following sources:

• *Cold-pressed oils* from the nuts, seeds, olives, avocados, as well as the foods these oils came from.

- *Fresh flax seed oil* (refrigerated and light protected).
- *Fresh marine oils,* found in "wild" cold-water fish (salmon, mackerel, herring, sardines, tuna), in sardines canned in their own oil, olive oil, or water, or in bottled cod-liver oil. (We think Carlson's Cod Liver Oil in the glass bottle tastes best. Keep it refrigerated after opening and use it within two weeks.)
- *Raw or roasted seeds or true nuts* (almonds, Brazil nuts, cashews, hazelnuts, filberts, macadamia nuts, pecans, walnuts) *and peanuts and their butters.*
- *Egg yolks.*
- *Butter or clarified butter (ghee).*

Fats not allowed: Trans fat sources (including processed fats and oils, margarine, vegetable shortening, corn or vegetable cooking oils, partially hydrogenated oils) and potentially rancid oils, such as fish oil and flax oil in oxygen-permeable capsules. Be aware that processed fats and oils occur widely in most prepackaged foods.

Allowed fat amounts: You should look upon good-quality fats as sources of metabolically neutral calories. By that we mean that although they're rich in calories (about 100 calories per tablespoon), they don't have any effect to speak of on your insulin levels. The actual amount you eat will depend on your daily calorie needs, and once you're at the Maintenance Level, you'll eat foods higher in good-quality fat to maintain your energy balance. Much of the fat you eat will inevitably accompany the protein you eat; the two quite commonly occur together in foods. If you are getting the right amount of protein, you need not be concerned about the amount of fat; it will pretty much take care of itself. And if you are not overweight, you needn't restrict your fats, so long as they are good fats from the sources specified above. If you are overweight, however, it is best to limit your consumption of high-calorie foods as we've previously discussed. (See "How Much Fat Should You Eat?" above, for complete details.)

BEVERAGES

You should consume plenty of liquids from the following beverage sources on your plan:

- *Good tap water or filtered water.*
- *Bottled water* (still or naturally carbonated).
- *Coffee* (regular or decaffeinated).
- *Tea* (black, green, or herbal).
- *Alcohol* (beer, wine, distilled spirits) in moderation—that is, a 5-ounce glass of wine, a 12-ounce beer, or 1 ounce of distilled spirits per day.

Beverages not recommended: Soft drinks (since they contain far too much sugar, corn syrup, and high-fructose corn syrup to be of any use) and diet soft drinks containing aspartame.

Required Beverages Amount: A minimum of 64 ounces of liquid per day.

The Dilettante's Approach

Many people—ourselves included—opt for this middle-of-the-road approach most of the time, choosing to adopt some of the more stringent guidelines of the Purist without giving up all the joys of dietary Hedonism. For example, while we can live without sugars, sweeteners, and wheat or corn most of the time, we would just as soon not forgo our wine with dinner or our good "fully leaded" coffee with half-and-half to start the day. The Dilettante option incorporates the same restriction in carbohydrate amount and the same prohibition against trans fats and aspartame as the Hedonist does, but certain additional health benefits derive from its slightly more stringent strategy. For example, the Dilettante will strengthen the "leaky" junctions of the gut by avoiding the most problematic cereal grains (corn, millet, rye, and wheat), thereby preventing the influx of molecules that can mimic our own tissues and trigger any of a host of autoimmune disorders (see chapter 6, "The Leaky Gut"). By eliminating most sucrose and added fructose, the Dilettante strategy places less of a burden on the immune system (not to mention improving blood lipids and insulin sensitivity). Because many conventionally produced foods may contain toxins (such as pesticides on fruits and vegetables), antibiotics, and growth factors and other hormones used to increase animal size, egg production, or milk output that may interfere with the body's hormonal harmony, adopting the Dilettante strategy further reduces the potential burden of toxicity by opting whenever possible for organic produce, organic dairy products, and natural meats and eggs. These refinements seem small, but for many of us, the rewards we reap from making these extra efforts are great in terms of better health.

Who should consider adopting the Dilettante's approach to nutrition at least to start? Certainly people at risk for (or suffering from) any of the autoimmune disorders—MS, rheumatoid arthritis and related arthritic conditions, systemic lupus, psoriasis, scleroderma, inflammatory bowel disorders (ulcerative colitis and Crohn's disease)—and perhaps those suffering from Parkinson's and Alzheimer's diseases. Those people who have or are at risk for cardiovascular diseases, have elevated blood fats, high blood pressure, type II diabetes, sleep apnea, or gout also reap additional health benefit beyond the Hedonist's approach. Does this mean that people with these disorders *must* abandon Hedonism and opt for a more stringent plan? No, it doesn't. Remember that 80 percent of the health reward of *Protein Power LifePlan* eating comes from controlling insulin and improving insulin sensitivity, and in large measure you'll accomplish that simply by controlling your intake of carbohydrates and getting enough protein—the small changes we outlined in the Hedonist's regimen. But for many people the added benefits to health outweigh the burden of further restriction. The Dilettante and the Purist are further refinements to the original plan that has already helped over two million people reclaim their health, and these refinements add additional health benefits for those who decide to adopt them. If you feel that the Dilettante's plan best suits your current level of health and commitment to change, here are the *added restrictions* beyond the Hedonist's plan that you'll need to follow:

ADDITIONAL FOOD-SELECTION GUIDELINES
FOR THE DILETTANTE

1. Where possible, try to use natural meat and poultry products, but standard meats are acceptable occasionally if necessary. The term *natural* denotes range-fed animals (or cage-free in the

case of chickens) that have not been grain-fed on a feed lot and were never treated with antibiotics or hormones. Opt for wild game when you can. (For sources of wild game and natural beef products, see Resources in the appendix.)

2. Avoid processed meat products containing nitrites or MSG. Monosodium glutamate, like aspartame, may be damaging to your brain. (See chapter 11, "Calisthenics for the Brain," and chapter 7, "How Sweet It Is . . . Not!" for more information.)

3. Although standard eggs are acceptable occasionally if necessary, try to use eggs from cage-free naturally raised chickens. The Gold Circle Farms brand is an excellent choice, because their chickens have been enriched with essential fats and vitamin E.

4. When eating canned fish products (sardines, tuna, salmon, mackerel) select only those canned in their own oils, in olive oil, or in spring water. Avoid those canned in soy oil (an added source of omega 6 that you don't need).

5. If you cannot abide fish, you must take either Carlson's Cod Liver Oil (1 to 2 tbsp. daily) or, if you're in reasonably good health, fresh flax seed oil (1 to 2 tbsp. daily) as a source of omega-3 fats.

6. If possible, purchase organically grown fruits and vegetables, preferably fresh but organic canned or frozen (in either case without sugar) will work, too. If you must purchase fresh conventionally grown fruits and vegetables, we encourage you to triple wash them and to use a commercially available product to enhance the removal of pesticides and other surface chemicals. (See Resources in the appendix for information about one of these products.)

7. Avoid the following grains: wheat, corn, millet, and rye, their meals, their flours, and any product made with them, because of their potential to mimic certain body proteins and their possible connection to some autoimmune disorders. (You may have rice, oats, spelt, barley, and amaranth within the limits of your level of carbohydrate restriction.)

8. Eliminate crystalline fructose, high-fructose corn syrup, and regular corn syrup and foods made with them. In very limited amounts, you may have honey (the best choice), table sugar, and rice syrup occasionally.

9. Use, wherever possible, only organic dairy products. Occasional use of conventionally made products is acceptable when dining out or when organic products are unavailable.

The Purist Approach

We designed a third regimen for those people who wish to approximate a Paleolithic eating pattern in a modern world. Although it doesn't mean you have to hunt your food with a pointed stick or gather it from the natural fields and forests around you, it's a good idea to think in those terms: *Could* you have done so? Is this a kind of food that would have been available to you forty thousand or more years ago? Did early humans make use of it before the advent of the plow and the hoe? If so, it's probably one that your Fred Flintstone physiology and biochemistry can handle fully even if it comes in a George Jetson wrapper. By adopting the Purist approach, you'll maximize your insulin sensitivity, improve gut function, minimize autoimmune triggers, and optimize nutritional healing.

Who should adopt this most natural—and without doubt most stringent—of the three *Protein Power LifePlan* approaches? Those people who wish to eat a diet that is maximally in sync with their ancestral nature; those people who suffer from serious complications of the diseases brought on by modern diet and life-style (diabetes, elevated blood cholesterol and triglycerides, heart disease, peripheral vascular disease, and especially the autoimmune diseases, such as MS, rheumatoid arthritis, ulcerative colitis, Crohn's disease, and others); those people whose symptoms have not fully resolved on one of the less restrictive plan options; those people who wish to reverse the diseases that afflict them as quickly and as fully as possible; and those people who when they approach change like to do so all the way, without compromise and without cutting corners for convenience or expedience. Have we done it ourselves? Yes, we have. Is it the optimal nutritional strategy for reaping the maximum degree of wellness possible? Yes. Do we maintain this degree of restriction at all times? No, we don't. We choose to accept a little less wellness for a little more pleasure most of the time, occasionally tightening up to the

Purist ideal and always feeling better for having done so. If you feel that at this point in your life the Purist's nutritional strategy best suits you and your health needs, here are the added rules of your game. Although these additional steps may not seem like many, they place quite a restriction on your dining and shopping options. On this plan, you'll go beyond the Dilettante's level, aiming to avoid all modern nutritional adaptations to make the following *additional restrictions.*

ADDITIONAL GUIDELINES FOR THE PURIST

1. Avoid *all* cereal grains and products made from them, which can act as autoimmune mimics to imitate modern afflictions (see chapter 6, "The Leaky Gut"). That means no wheat, oats, rice, corn, amaranth, rye, barley, or spelt.

2. Eat *only* organic fruits and vegetables, always opting for fresh foods.

3. Eat *only* natural meat and poultry products or game. (See Resources in the appendix for where to obtain natural beef and game products.)

4. Avoid *all* legumes (dried beans, including soybeans, dried field peas, and peanuts).

5. Avoid *all* dairy products (milk, yogurt, cheeses, butter solids), since, in the first place, there's no evidence that ancient man ever made use of these foods in the preagricultural world, and, in the second, there's at least some evidence that milk proteins (particularly if they've been heated, which they are in cooking and in the pasteurization process) may promote heart disease and may be mimics for initiating autoimmune damage to the insulin-producing cells in the pancreas in some people. The single exception is whey powder. If it's a cross-flow microfiltered product, it appears that most of the immune-damaging power has been eliminated, and in fact, whey may boost the immune system.

6. Avoid *all* processed foods, again, since they're modern contrivances, but also because they're filled with trans fats, sugars, and grain-based carbs.

7. Avoid *all* sugars but honey, since it's the only source that early man had access to. And even then, avoid consuming regular large quantities of it.

8. Eliminate *all* artificial sweeteners, except the sweet herb stevia.

9. Eliminate *all* sources of caffeine, drinking only herbal teas and decaffeinated coffee. (This exception for decaf coffee is actually a bit of a stretch, since early humans, except possibly in certain areas of the world, did not have access to coffee beans.)

10. Eliminate *all* forms of alcohol: beer, wine, and distilled spirits.

Fill 'er Up!

As you begin your nutritional rehabilitation, within the first day or two your insulin level will begin to fall. You'll know that it's happening—even without taking another blood test—because of insulin's potent effect on the kidneys. Insulin stimulates the kidneys to retain sodium, and where sodium goes, water follows; in other words, excess insulin makes you retain fluid. As insulin levels plummet, your kidneys will get the signal that it's now okay to get rid of all that excess salt and water, and consequently you'll spend a fair amount of time in the so-called little room during the first few days on the plan. But once your new nutritional regimen has brought your fluid balance back to a normal level, your trips to inspect the plumbing facilities will subside. You'll reach a balanced state such that what goes in comes out, and relatively soon. If you drink a large glass of water, within just a few minutes, you'll need to get rid of a large glass of water. And that's how it's supposed to be, a constant inflow and outflow of fluid to keep your body cleansed and your urinary tract healthy.

And so from day one on this regimen, we request that you drink, drink, and drink your fluids, aiming for a goal of at least 64 ounces of water (or other allowable calorie-free beverages) a day. Keep a bottle of water at your side, in the car, on your desk at work, when you travel. Every time you think of it, fill 'er up! In the hot summertime or when you've had a hard, sweaty workout, drink even more. Since you'll be drinking so much of it, it's a good idea to check the quality of your water (see chapter 9, "The Magnesium Miracle," for more details), and if it's full of chlorine and/or impurities, filter it or drink a good bottled water (see table 9.1).

What About Vitamins and Minerals?

Given the cornucopia of foods available to you at even the most restrictive level of the plan (Intervention), you can get every essential nutrient the "authorities" recommend and more. Let's take a look at the official list of what the RDA recommends and at where on this plan you could find it in adequate (or, usually, more than adequate) amounts. In table 13.7 we've listed the richest sources of these nutrients you'll find on this plan—ones that will exceed the RDA with reasonable and allowable servings.

As you can easily see, if you eat a varied diet within the confines of this plan as we've outlined it, you can meet the requirements set forth in the RDA in every category. (Not, as you know, that that means much as a level that will promote optimal health.) However, we've noticed in the nearly fifteen years we've been helping patients correct their health with this plan that just because sardines are chock full of important nutrients and they're freely permitted on this program doesn't necessarily mean you'll eat them. Like former President George Bush with his famous aversion to broccoli (incidentally, a food filled with nutrients and freely allowed on this plan), most of us have certain foods we don't like and won't eat no matter how good they might be for us. Perhaps you're different. Maybe you're obsessive about carefully selecting a combination of foods that will always provide an ideal balance of vitamins and minerals every day. If so, that's great; keep up the good work. But if you're like most folks, you eat mainly what you like, not particularly paying attention to or even knowing what's in it as far as vitamin and mineral content goes.

If the latter description fits you—and believe us, it fits most everyone we've ever seen in twenty years of clinical practice—we recommend that you take a complete multivitamin-and-mineral supplement every day. That's not because you're following this plan; we'd recommend the same whether you elected to follow the dreaded low-fat Food Guide Pyramid or any other nutritional plan that allows you the freedom to select your own foods. That

TABLE 13.7

Nature's Vitamin Shop

VITAMIN / MINERAL	RDA	WHERE YOU'LL FIND THAT ON THE PLAN
Vitamin A	800 to 1,000 mcg	carrots, spinach, cantaloupe
Vitamin D	400 IU	dairy products, sunshine
Vitamin E	10 mg	almonds, sunflower seeds, nut butters, olive oil, canola oil
Vitamin K	45 to 80 mcg	eggs, beef, strawberries, cabbage, broccoli, asparagus, greens, tomatoes
Vitamin C	50 mg	tomatoes, red cabbage, oranges, avocado, strawberries
Thiamin (B$_1$)	1.5 mg	pistachios, sunflower seeds, meats, poultry, bread and tortillas (H only), rice (D and H only)
Riboflavin (B$_2$)	1.8 mg	meat, mushrooms, asparagus, spinach, calamari, almonds, roasted soybean nuts
Niacin (B$_3$)	20 mg	chicken, beef, salmon, mackerel
Vitamin B$_6$	2.0 mg	chicken, beef, turkey, sunflower seeds, almonds
Folate	200 to 400 mcg	spinach, asparagus, seaweed, greens
Vitamin B$_{12}$	2 mcg	eggs, meat, poultry, game, fish
Calcium	800 to 1,200 mg	dairy (D and H only), sardines, spinach, salmon, trout, almonds, sunflower seeds
Phosphorous	800 to 1,200 mg	fish, seafood, meat, poultry
Magnesium	280 to 400 mg	almonds, cashews, sunflower seeds, blackberries, meat, poultry, cheese (D and H only)
Iron	10 to 15 mg	beef, game, spinach
Zinc	15 mg	beef, game, poultry
Iodine	150 mcg	seafood, eggs
Selenium	50 to 75 mcg	sardines, other seafood, meat, nuts, seeds

freedom of choice also gives you the leeway to leave out a few foods that you're not so fond of. Although food is the best source of vitamins and minerals, taking a good supplement allows you the peace of mind to make your food choices without worrying about getting each and every vitamin and mineral in sufficient amounts.

What constitutes a good vitamin-and-mineral supplement? To make it easier for you, we've included a profile of a good one in the Micronutrient Roundup in the appendix. You should be able to find one with a similar profile in a health food store in your area. Don't get all tied up trying to find one that hits the recommended amounts of every nutrient precisely on the head; just come close and you'll do fine. The only absolute prohibition is to find one without added iron (unless you have a documented iron deficiency). If you have trouble finding an acceptable product in your area, see Resources in the Appendix for some suggestions.

There are two specific areas where we do want to be sure you have enough of a critical nutrient, even if it means regularly taking an extra supplement: magnesium (see chapter 9), of which you'll want to be sure to get 400 to 600 mg a day; and four antioxidants—vitamin E (for most people 400 IU mixed tocopherals and tocotrienols a day), alpha-lipoic acid (at least 100 mg per day), vitamin C (about 200 mg per day), and coenzyme Q10 (about 100 mg a day). As you'll recall from chapter 5, "Antioxidant Use and Abuse," we don't recommend the wholesale gobbling of individual antioxidants, preferring instead that you get the whole network from the berries, nuts, seeds, and colorful vegetables in your diet. However, these four are so critically important to your health in such a broad way that we'd rather you not leave their intake to chance.

Potassium, Potassium, Potassium. In public speaking classes, instructors always impart this advice: "If you want your audience to remember something, you must say it three times!" And thus the title of this section. In the initial stages of this regimen, you absolutely *must* take a daily supplement of potassium. Why? Because, unfortunately, as your kidneys waste the excess sodium and fluid they've been so busily accumulating when your insulin was high, they'll waste some potassium as well. Potassium, like magnesium, resides inside the cells of the body, meaning that the levels of it in the blood don't really tell you much about total body levels. In general, people with insulin-related disorders—particularly those who have been on diuretic medications for fluid retention or blood pressure—may be deficient in potassium at the start of their rehabilitation. And the loss of excess fluid that occurs in the first week or so will only compound that problem. Low potassium will make you feel like—as they say in the South—"something the cat drug up." Too tired to climb the stairs, too tired to even breathe. And low potassium can cause your muscles to cramp and, more important, can put you at risk for disturbances of heart rhythm. Take your potassium, take your potassium, take your potassium (again, we've said it three times so you'll take note of its importance). One way to incorporate more potassium into your diet is by using salt-replacement products, such as NoSalt Salt Alternative or Morton's Lite Salt or Salt Substitute on your foods. Just a sprinkle on salads or hot foods can help to keep your potassium levels in the normal range. In the early weeks of the plan, however, that addition may not suffice, so before beginning the program, we recommend purchasing an over-the-counter potassium supplement (each tablet will contain 99 mg) and taking four each day for the first several weeks you're at the Intervention Level. After that you can probably taper off to a couple a day plus what's in the varied diet you're sure to be eating.

One important word of caution here: *If you currently take medications for your heart, migraine headaches, fluid retention, or blood pressure, be sure to check with your pharmacist before supplementing with potassium.* Certain medications for these conditions (but by no means all) can block the potassium loss that usually comes with ridding the body of excess water. Taking potassium along with these medications might lead to a buildup of too much potassium—a condition just as dangerous as too little is. Your pharmacist will know if your medications could cause this. Ask to be sure.

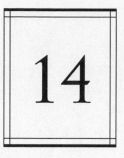

The *Protein Power* Kitchen and Other Practical Pointers

Make everything as simple as possible, but not simpler.
—ALBERT EINSTEIN

For any plan to work, however good it might sound in theory, you have to be able to live it in the real world. It must be flexible enough to meet the demands of family, friends, work, and entertaining, or what good is it? We've been living the *Protein Power* lifestyle for nearly fifteen years now and on it have been able to accommodate rigorous work schedules, entertain, travel, and raise three handsome, smart, healthy sons. Once you get the hang of it, you'll find it both easy and satisfying. In this chapter, you'll learn the tricks, tips, and pointers that we've gathered from nearly a decade and a half of living this plan. They will put you way ahead of the game in being able to quickly incorporate these changes into a healthy, happy lifestyle. Since the plan hinges first and foremost around nutrition, let's head to the kitchen and start with the changes there that will make living a *Protein Power*ed life a little easier for you and your family. If you don't cook, it's time you learned at least the basics, because for the money you absolutely can't beat the quality of nutrition you can provide for yourself at home. That's not to say you can't easily find *Protein Power LifePlan*–compatible meals dining out; you can, but you'll get more cluck for your buck and be certain of what it is you're getting when you develop a habit of eating more meals at home. In the Resources section of the appendix, we list several cookbooks we've found helpful over the years.

Remodeling the Kitchen—A Protein Power *Kitchen Makeover*

In this case, remodeling the kitchen doesn't mean we want you to rip out cabinets and countertops to improve your kitchen's function or aesthetics. (Although if you don't already have them, you might want to be on the lookout for a good price on a few inexpensive appliances to make things easier—a food dehydrator for making inexpensive jerky, a heavy-duty blender, and a water filter, for example.) Our main concern is rather what's *in* your kitchen cabinets, pantry, freezer, and refrigerator. Those are the areas you'll want to go through carefully, purging them of unhealthy foods.

First, search out all foods that contain trans fats. Doing this will mean critically reading the labels of whatever is there, looking for the words *partially hydrogenated* in the ingredients list. When you locate items containing partially hydrogenated fats—you'll find these especially in prepared or packaged foods—remove them from your kitchen. Put the unopened cans, boxes, sacks, and jars of food containing trans fats into a large cardboard box and donate them to your local food bank. Even though they're not the healthiest foods in the world, some food is better than no food to those who are hungry, and there's simply no need to waste it. Opened items you should discard. Throw out margarine, vegetable shortenings of all types, and cheap cooking oils, such as corn oil, vegetable oil, or any oil that has those dangerous words on its label: *contains one or more of the following* partially hydrogenated *oils,* followed by a list of the possible suspects.

If you're planning to adopt a Purist or Dilettante approach, you'll want to discard (or move to the freezer) all products containing wheat, corn, or other grains not permitted on those plans. This would include products made with these grains—such as pasta, bread, cereal, crackers, chips, pastries, pies, cakes, or cookies—as well as their ground meals or flours. Unless you're convinced that you'll never eat these items again—which may or may not ultimately prove to be the case, and that's okay—it's a good idea to bag them in double zip-closure freezer bags and store them away if you've got room rather than discard them. (That's where we store ours for those times we choose Hedonism.)

Place bags or boxes of sugars of all types in zip-closure bags or tight-seal plastic canisters (or put the contents of less airtight canisters into zip-closure bags), since you won't be using these items much on any form of the plan, and not at all if you're aiming for the Purist approach. Bagged, they'll stay fresher without clumping for longer periods of time. Our entire family probably doesn't use a pound of sugar in five years—except, of course, at Thanksgiving and Christmas—so we always store the small amounts of these items that we keep around tightly zipped in the back of the pantry.

Now you're ready to begin to add to the shelves some of the things you'll want to keep on hand at all times for healthy eating and easy preparation at home. This list will get you going—it's pretty much what we keep on hand at our house—but it's certainly not exhaustive. For more information, see the Food-Selection Guidelines for Hedonists on page 337 and the additional restrictions for Dilettantes and Purists on pages 343 and 346.

THE PANTRY STAPLES

• *Canned goods* (organic products for Dilettantes; Purists don't use canned fruits or vegetables but can use canned stocks and broths). Several cans each of chicken, beef, vegetable, and/or mushroom broth; several cans of stewed tomatoes with spices; several cans of mushroom pieces (or packages of dried mushrooms); several cans of low-starch vegetables (for example, green beans, green peas, carrots, asparagus, turnip/mustard greens, zucchini, water chestnuts, bean sprouts, bamboo shoots; black and green olives; roasted green chili peppers or other hot peppers you like.

• *Canned meat/fish.* Several cans of tuna and salmon (packed in spring water or their own oil or olive oil); several cans of sardines (packed in sardine or olive oil, water, or mustard or hot sauce); a can or two of kippered herring if you like it; a can or two of boned chicken breast (it now comes in single-serving cans, too).

• *Condiments* (organic products for Dilettantes and Purists). Canola mayonnaise (Purists may wish to make their own); spicy/grainy mustard; horseradish; crushed garlic or garlic paste; low-sugar ketchup (Purists may wish to make their own); several types of vinegar (sherry, red wine, raspberry, white wine, and balsamic, for example); dill pickle relish; dill pickles; reconstituted lemon juice (for emergencies); Worcestershire (or similar) sauce; soy sauce (wheat-free for Dilettantes and Purists).

• *Oils* (organic products for Dilettantes and Purists). Extra-virgin, virgin, or pure cold-pressed olive oil; canola oil; avocado oil; and/or any other cold-pressed oil from a true nut or seed that you like (walnut, almond, sesame, etc.).

• *Nuts and nut butters* (organic products for Dilettantes and Purists). A vareity of true nuts (almonds, walnuts, pecans, macadamia, and pine nuts, etc.) and seeds (pumpkin, sunflower, sesame, for example). You can buy them in bulk and raw to roast yourself or buy them dry-roasted, salted or unsalted. And nut butters: although peanut is the cheapest and hands-down favorite for most people, almond and cashew butters have better fat profiles and less likelihood of allergic reaction. If you like peanut butter, buy a variety that has no or little added sugar.

• *Spices* (organic if possible for Dilettantes and Purists). Salt (kosher and/or sea salt if possible), potassium salt (NoSalt Salt Alternative or Morton's Salt Substitute or Lite Salt, for example), coarsely ground black pepper or mixed peppercorns, dried basil, cilantro, rosemary, sage, and tarragon—and any of the zillion others you like—and dried onion (for emergencies).

• *Sweeteners.* Only honey or stevia for Purists, and it's helpful to find a honey made locally if possible; Splenda (Canadian sucralose) if you can find it (see Resources in the appendix); saccharine's a compromise if you can't (see chapter 7, "How Sweet It Is . . . Not!," for more information), and a bit of sugar for the Hedonists.

• *Crunchy things.* This category is tough once you get past pork rinds—and even there, you have to worry about what kind of oil they were fried in—but there are a few things. Hedonists can have Wasa Fiber Rye Crispbread (which has a low ECC and makes a great substitute for bread) or other types of melba toast or crackers; chips as long as they contain no trans fats—carefully read the labels, because any fat in these is likely to be polluted with trans molecules—in servings that fall within the carb limit of their plan, which won't be many chips (each has about 2 grams). Dilettantes stick to fat-free brown-rice crackers (this is one place where fat-free comes in handy: if there's no fat at all, you'll know there are no trans fats). There are a variety of them in different seasoning tastes available at many stores. Purists, of course, avoid all grains and grain products.

• *Protein powders.* For quick breakfast shakes or power yogurts (see recipes on page 363), keep a product that you like the taste of, that mixes well, and that contains few carbohydrates. You'll get the best form of biologically active protein from whey, but depending on your preference, it might also contain egg white or casein or soy. (There are literally dozens of such products in the stores, and we've listed a few good ones in the resources section.)

THE FREEZER

• *Meats* (natural products for Dilettantes and Purists). To make dollars go farther, stock up on what goes on sale and freeze it. A good variety of meats that freeze well might include packages of stew meat (for soups and stir-frys), lean ground beef, steaks, roasts, pork chops, chicken tenders, chicken breasts, chicken thighs/legs/wings. Buy the extra-large family-size packages and divide them into meal-size portions suitable for your needs, seal in a zip-closure bag, label the date and contents, and store. And don't forget fish and seafood, bacon and sausage (natural and nitrite-free for Dilettantes and Purists), and wild game if you like it. (See Resources in the appendix.)

• *Fruit* (organic products for Dilettantes; a true Purist opts for fresh and organic). Keep a variety of berries on hand—buy sacks of frozen blueberries, raspberries, and sliced strawberries, all without sugar, for snacking, side dishes, desserts, breakfast protein shakes, and Paleolithic Punch and Pops (page 366).

• *Vegetables* (organic products for Dilettantes; a true Purist opts for fresh and organic). Although fresh is always better, for convenience it's helpful to have a variety of low-starch veggies on hand for throwing together quick soups, stews, stir-frys, omelets, or quiche. Keep a bag or box or two of spinach, broccoli, cauliflower, green beans, peppers, and mixed veggies.

• *Breads* (for Hedonists only). Since you won't be eating as much, you might like to keep a loaf in the freezer, taking out only what you'll use that day. Look for low-carbohydrate "lite" varieties, preferably ones made without any trans fats (although that may be tough to find). And you'll surely want a supply of La Tortilla Factory whole wheat, low-fat tortillas (and low-carb, according to the maker, with only 3 effective grams in each tortilla). They can be great for burritos, as "toast" with breakfast, for enchiladas, fajitas, or quesadillas, and they freeze well. See Resources in the appendix for where to get them.

THE FRIDGE—FRESH MEAT, FISH, AND PRODUCE

Whenever possible (and always for those opting for the Purists approach) use fresh, whole food. There's an inescapable nutrient loss in canning, drying, or freezing, and you'll get more of what you pay for in fresh foods. We understand that always using fresh food isn't feasible for many people; with our hectic lives, it isn't always feasible for us either. When we drag back home at midnight from some airport or other after a stint on the road, you can be sure there's not a fresh thing in the house (or if there was when we left, it's not fresh anymore). So frozen, canned, and dried foods have come to the rescue more times than we can count. Still, as soon as we can we head for the store (or the farmers' market in the summer and early fall) to replenish our supply of fresh foods. Fresh tastes better and provides more nutrition, so opt for it when you can.

• *Meats* (natural products only for Dilettantes and Purists). When you shop for fresh meat or poultry, look for what's on special and buy the large economy size. For instance, it's okay to eat chicken three or more times in one week if the price is right—just ask our kids! But try also to use fresh items to add variety. Select from chops, roasts, or pork tenderloin (these will often make dinner and several lunches), chicken, turkey, and lamb. Buy only enough fresh meat to use in the next few days. And don't forget deli meats and poultry for a quick bite, even okay occasionally for Purists as long as they are prepared naturally without MSG or nitrites. Pick out several kinds you like and ask the counter person to weigh them in the portion suitable for you, wrap them, and label them. Then they're ready when you're ready for something to eat or to pack a quick lunch for yourself or the kids. Ask the butcher to weigh out 1-pound portions of inexpensive flank steak or hanger steak to use in making your own jerky. If the price is right, have several one-pound portions done and freeze a few to use later.

• *Fish and seafood.* Fresh is the absolute best way to have fish! If your store has a good fish counter, you may be able to find fresh (although often previously flash-frozen) salmon, trout, shrimp, scallops, tuna, snapper, mussels, crab, lobster, and more. Mix up your selections, but try to have at least one or two fish meals each week for the good fats they contain—breaded fast-food fish fillet sandwiches don't count. Remember: Fish, like houseguests, should leave after three days! (After that, they both can start to stink!)

• *Eggs* (cage-free, antibiotic-free and hormone-free for Purists and serious Dilettantes). Keep a couple of dozen on hand at all times. They're a good, cheap source of protein and good-quality cholesterol, and they'll keep for several weeks in the fridge if you leave them in the container they come in.

• *Dairy* (organic products only for Dilettantes; Purists don't "do" dairy and can skip on down). Keep on hand ultrapasteurized half-and-half or cream (if you like it in coffee or tea and also to use in cream sauces and soups), milk (for the kids and to make protein shakes), plain yogurt (cow's or goat's milk), butter, cottage cheese, hard cheeses, soft cheeses, and sour cream, if you like. (Although it's fine to use low-fat and fat-free dairy products, bear in mind that this generally means they'll be slightly higher in carbohydrates per ounce.)

• *Vegetables* (organic produce only for Dilettantes and Purists; thoroughly washed to remove pesticides otherwise). Choose the low-starch veggies you prefer. We always try to keep a variety of the following kinds of low-starch veggies in the crisper: mixed salad greens, spinach, broccoli, asparagus, cauliflower, summer squashes (zucchini, yellow crookneck, scallop), carrots, spaghetti squash (a winter variety), cucumbers, peppers, brussels sprouts, artichokes, mushrooms, and perhaps a couple of ripe avocados (for salads and guacamole). Tomatoes are stored on the counter, *never* in the crisper; refrigeration ruins the taste and texture of a good fresh tomato!

• *Herbs* (organic only for Dilettantes and Purists; well washed otherwise). If you don't have your own sunny kitchen window to grow a pot of fresh herbs (and it's so easy you should do so if you can), you'll want to grab one or two fresh varieties at the market when you shop. Fresh basil, Italian parsley, cilantro, chives, rosemary, thyme, oregano, and dill can make the most mundane dish sparkle—and they're good for you, too.

• *Fruits* (organic produce only for Dilettantes and Purists; thoroughly washed to remove pesticides otherwise). Go for what's seasonal and lowest in sugar/starch, selecting from such fruits as strawberries, raspberries, blackberries, blueberries, melons, small oranges, grapefruit, kiwi, peaches, or small apples or plums. Small amounts of tropical and exotic fruits are okay, too, especially to add to fruit mixtures with lower-sugar varieties. Keep some fresh lemons and limes on hand for adding zip to water, for fish and seafood, and to make guacamole and fresh vinaigrettes.

NOW YOU'RE COOKIN'

This isn't a cookbook, and although we've included a few recipes, it doesn't contain a ton of them—the Resources section in the appendix mentions some good cookbooks that do. What we want to do is give you some general food preparation tips to make living this *Protein Power LifePlan* simpler for you and your family. Let's begin as the day does, with breakfast.

QUICK AND EASY BREAKFAST IDEAS

In our household, when the boys were growing up and in school, the early morning could have been chaos—we had to get to the office and get three boys up, dressed, fed, and off to school with *Protein Power* lunches packed. We've been there and know exactly how tough this can be to do. Even though breakfast may not be a meal to linger over (with everybody moving at high speed, there's no time), it's a critical meal. Studies have shown that what you (or your kids) eat for breakfast sets the tone of what you (or they) will want to eat the rest of the day. Recent studies have proven that a higher-protein, higher-fat breakfast, lower in sugars and starches, will prevent overeating later on and may be a big factor in preventing the rising epidemic of childhood and adolescent obesity, a problem that has doubled in the last ten years! On days when you do have time (weekends or vacations) for a more luxurious breakfast, you'll be delighted to rediscover foods you've been told to shun: eggs, cheeses, bacon, sausages. Now you can enjoy those things again without feeling a pang of guilt. But such lazy days come all too rarely in this rush-rush world, so here are some suggestions for protein on the fly:

• *Eggs on the Run.* Although you may think eggs would take too long, that's often shortsighted thinking. While you may not have the time to bring poached, fried, or even scrambled eggs to the table every single day, you can still have eggs. One easy way to do that is by precooking them. The night before, hard-boil as many eggs as you'll need for the next morning (a couple per person at least). Peel them and stick them in the fridge in a zip-closure bag. The next morning, they can either be eaten cold as you run out the door, or you can quickly chop them in a bowl, add a pat of butter for each egg, salt and pepper them, cover, and heat in the microwave until the butter's melted and they're hot. Stir them around and enjoy. You can even teach older kids how to do their own as they come to the kitchen in shifts in the morning. They're delicious and full of good protein.

• *Perfect Eggs in Minutes.* If you've got time to "make" an egg meal—and it honestly won't take you more than about 10 minutes; the problem is getting the whole family to the table at one time, while the eggs are hot—here's an easy way to do it. Heat the skillet on medium and in it melt 1 or 2 pats of butter (or 1 or 2 tablespoons of bacon drippings) to coat the bottom. Break two to six eggs (more if it's a very large skillet) into the hot melted butter or fat, let them sizzle as the whites begin to set (about 30 to 45 seconds), then pour 2 to 4 ounces of water into the skillet—it will pop and bubble, so be careful—and cover with a tight-fitting lid. Let the eggs steam for a minute or two, until the whites are totally set and opaque and the yolks are as "done" as you like them. Lift them out with a perforated spatula, gently draining off the liquid, and serve. They won't stick, won't look "wallered," as our fathers would have said, and as a bonus, the water deglazes the skillet, so even cleanup is quick and easy. The whole operation takes less than 10 minutes—you could even microwave bacon or sausage while you're cooking the eggs and make up a batch of Paleolithic Punch (page 366) in the blender to boot! In fact, this is exactly the breakfast we have many mornings.

• *The Crustless Quiche.* Another good make-ahead egg meal is Crustless Quiche. In the morning just open the fridge, pull out the number of slices you need, cover them with waxed paper or plastic wrap, microwave, and enjoy. While you're at it, make two quiches! The quiche could have any of a number of wonderful additions, such as mushrooms, zucchini, asparagus, cheeses, spinach, tomato slices, onion, garlic, fresh herbs, ham, turkey, sausage, bacon, shrimp, crab—the list could go on and on. (Yes, we know, cooking broken yolks may cause damage to the cholesterol in them, but occasionally, it won't hurt Dilletantes or Hedonists.) The basic rules of quiche making are this: Melt a pat or two of butter in a quiche or pie plate in a 375° oven. Beat 8 to 10 eggs until they're pale yellow and frothy. Add salt and pepper to taste. Add ½ cup half and half or ½ cup shredded cheese and salt and pepper to taste. Pour into quiche plate. Now put in your additions. Add lightly cooked fresh veggies (sauté or briefly microwave them to soften), thawed frozen veggies or spinach (press the water out first), drained canned veggies, meats, and/or cheeses—be creative and arrange the additions artfully if you want, but it's not necessary. Pop the quiche into the oven and bake for 35 to 40 minutes or until set. Serve immediately, or cool, cover, and store up to three days in the fridge for future breakfasts.

• *Shake It Up.* When there's little time and/or a big group to feed, the morning *Protein Power* Shake is often a good plan; it's simple and doesn't require much cleanup. Use milk or water (about 8 ounces per person) and enough protein powder to provide the minimum-gram requirement for each person. Add ¼ fresh berries for flavor, 1 tablespoon of fresh flaxseed oil, some lecithin if you like, and blend. For each batch/person, it won't take even 2 minutes—bigger kids can learn to make their own! There's always time for a quick shake, and it makes a good, healthy high-protein, low-sugar start to the day.

• *Yogurt Power Cup.* Another quick option is to use plain yogurt (8 ounces has about 12 grams of carb, 4 ounces only 6), to which you add 1 tablespoon fresh flaxseed oil or Carlson's Cod Liver oil plus enough protein powder to make a minimum protein serving. If you use a smaller yogurt serving, you'll have carbohydrate room to add ¼ cup fresh berries or mixed seeds and nuts for variety. Stir well, and eat! (For Dilettantes and Hedonists only; Purists, of course, don't indulge in dairy products.)

• *Leftovers Are Ready Now.* If you've got cold steak, roast, meat loaf, burgers, chops, chicken breasts, legs, or thighs in the fridge, you've got a quick breakfast. It's a good idea to always cook more than you'll need of these kinds of foods, because they can so easily turn into breakfasts and lunches later. Even deli meat or jerky can serve as a good high-protein breakfast on the run. Just add half an apple, some hard cheese, some berries, or melon and you've got a quick, filling breakfast that won't take a minute! Blueberries, roasted almonds, and turkey jerky have made more than one breakfast for us in a pinch.

• *Curds and Whey.* In literary circles, there may be some debate about whether Miss Muffet was eating cottage cheese or yogurt. We decree it was cottage cheese, which you can eat straight (especially if your protein requirement is pretty large, since at 2 grams of carb per ¼ cup, just the serving of curds may eat up your carb allotment by itself) or mixed with fruit, nuts and seeds, or tomatoes with salt and pepper. It makes a quickie breakfast that's a winner for Dilettantes and Hedonists alike.

THE LITTLE BROWN BAG LUNCH

In the years that we were packing multiple school lunches each morning, we used our fair share of little brown lunch sacks. Nowadays, it's more likely to be Barney or Mulan insulated sacks or boxes, but whatever the container, the idea is the same: you want your kids to eat a decent meal at lunch. Recognizing that all you can do is pack it—it's up to them to actually eat it—here are some portable lunch ideas that will work for school lunches (or even for your own):

• *Deli meat roll-ups.* Chicken, turkey, beef, ham, pastrami— whatever they like. Take a couple of slices of meat, spread with good canola mayonnaise or mustard if desired, top with a thin slice of good cheese, and roll up, jelly-roll fashion. Secure with toothpicks. Send three or four or more in a plastic sandwich bag or waxed paper sack along with some pickles if they like them.

• *Fresh carrot, celery, cucumber, bell pepper, or zucchini sticks.*

• *Deviled eggs*—made with good canola mayonnaise, mustard, garlic, salt, pepper, and dill pickle relish if that's their pleasure. Wrap two halves together in plastic wrap—they can pull them apart like a cream sandwich cookie!

• *Low-carb bread sandwiches.* Fill them with deli meats, cheeses, chicken salad, tuna salad, egg salad, and good mayonnaise, mustard, lettuce, tomatoes, sprouts, and/or seeds, or with nut butter and a little all-fruit spread (no added sugar).

• *Low-carb tortilla wraps.* Fill them with deli meats, cheeses, chicken salad, tuna salad, egg salad, lettuce, tomatoes, sprouts, and seeds. If your kids have access to a microwave (and they're old enough to use it safely), send quesadillas made with low-carb tortillas, chicken or beef, and cheese.

• *Leftover chicken, steak, burgers, or chops.* These can be reheated in a microwave, too.

• *Boneless, skinless chicken breasts.* For smaller kids, cut boneless, skinless chicken breasts into shapes with a sharp metal cookie cutter, and sauté them in butter, salt, and pepper. Do enough for several lunches at once. Pack several chicken shapes into a bag or plastic container for reheating if a microwave is available. Works great for dinner, too!

• *Homemade soup, chili, or stew.* Send a small thermos filled with homemade chicken/beef/wild game and vegetable soup or chili or stew. It's easy to make a huge pot that will last all week for lunches.

• *Fresh fruit.* Send a plastic bag filled with whole berries, chunks of melon, grapes, apple slices (dipped in lemon juice to prevent browning), or a peach or small orange. Or fill a plastic reusable container with a fresh fruit "cocktail" of sliced berries, kiwi, grapes, orange slices, peaches, melon, etc.

• *Roasted mixed nuts or seeds.*

• *Natural or homemade jerky.*

• *Sardines.* If your child is really a hard-core *Protein Power* kid, send a can of sardines and a plastic fork! Be prepared; it will probably cause a stinky stir at the lunch table. Some kids will relish the hoopla, others won't ever take them again.

PALEOLITHIC SNACKS

Having high-quality *Protein Power*–style snacks handy can often mean the difference between eating properly and breaking your commitment. We encourage you to keep these kinds of foods readily available at home and work (as far as it's possible), to help you fend off hunger and maintain balance. One of the biggest problems that nutritionally committed parents face is the presence of "kid snacks" in the house. Our advice is to keep the good stuff around so that neither you nor the kids will be tempted to go face over in a bag of chocolate chip cookies or nacho chips. If you've got kids at home—or like us have had, but now they're grown—you can attest to the fact that they're always hungry. They come home from school ravenous and go through half the pantry as a warm-up to dinner. It's natural that they should need and want to eat often—after all, they're busy building a bigger, stronger body; the problem is rather what they snack on. Sadly, most kids today snack on carbo junk: candy bars, soda pop, cereal, cookies, fries, ice cream, and chips. And unfortunately, many parents give in to the sweet tooth—especially since many of these nonstop eating machines don't seem to gain weight from this horrendous diet—excusing it with the mistaken notion that they're kids and they can get away with it. Unfortunately, it's becoming much more obvious that many of them *do* gain weight.

What you feed your kids or teens today determines the adult they will become, as we reminded our own boys when they whined that they didn't regularly get the junk that their friends got to eat. "This isn't a popularity contest," we told them. "We're not simply raising kids, we're building grown men. You'll thank us when you're cutting your tennis match short to visit your friends in the hospital with their heart attacks!" Remember that just because you can't see the damage doesn't mean your kids escape unscathed from carbo junk. If you're struggling with any of the insulin-related problems, from high cholesterol or triglycerides to blood pressure to being overweight, don't forget that your kids have your genes and may have inherited the tendency for those disorders as well. You can't begin too early to prevent the damage to their metabolic systems that eating a lousy diet can cause. So it's important to have healthy snacks and quick foods around for them to eat when they hit the house "starving." Here are a few easy snack ideas—and one sweet selection—(for them or for you):

• *Paleolithic Punch and Pops.* We've mentioned this treat already, but it's worth reminding you of again. Use ½ cup each frozen low-sugar berries (blueberries, raspberries, sliced strawberries) plus ½ to 1 cup water and 1 teaspoon honey (optional, if the berries aren't very sweet). If all other berries are frozen, you can use fresh strawberries for easier blending and it will still turn out frosty and thick. Place the frozen berries and water in a heavy-duty blender and process until smooth and thick. This makes one large serving containing about 15 grams of effective carbohydrate or two smaller portions of 7.5 grams each (a far cry from the 48 grams in a single 12-ounce soda pop). Pour the slush into popsicle molds and freeze overnight for Paleolithic Pops, a fun, frosty, fruity treat. One recipe should make three or four small pops with 4 or 5 grams carb each.

• *Hot Nuts.* Put 1 cup raw whole almonds in a microwave-proof bowl, top with half a pat of good butter, sprinkle with a potassium salt substitute (such as NoSalt Salt Alternative or Morton's Salt Substitute or Lite Salt). Cover loosely with a lid or waxed paper and microwave for 30 seconds on high, shake bowl, microwave for another 30 seconds, shake, microwave for 30 seconds, shake, and after a final 30-second microwave blast, shake and allow to cool slightly. The roasted, buttery almonds will smell as delightful as hot buttered popcorn but pack a much better nutrient punch. (Works well with pecans, walnuts, and seeds, too.) Preroasted nut mixtures (again, look for dry-roasted nuts to avoid trans fats) can also make good quick snacks.

• *Jerky.* Whether you make it yourself or purchase bags of premade jerky, this snack treat goes anywhere—to work or school, on a hike, traveling, skiing, or into the backyard to play. If you make your own—a really easy proposition with a simple home food dehydrator—you can control what goes in. If you're buying ready-made, be sure that it doesn't contain MSG (an excitotoxin that can be bad for the brain) or nitrites (potential cancer-causing chemicals). Ask your butcher to thinly slice flank steak or hanger steak for jerky. Most dehydrators will accommodate about 1 to 1½ pounds at a time. We marinate our jerky meat in about 1 cup pepper-blend steak sauce plus a little chopped fresh garlic and salt and pepper. (Although Worcestershire or soy sauce will work well, don't forget that sweeter sauces, like teriyaki, may have a fair amount of carb in them.) Lay the thin slices of meat onto the dehydrator trays, leaving room for air to circulate, and dry overnight (at least 8 hours). Store in a zip-closure bag—although if our house is any example, a batch won't hang around for long.

• *Trail Mix.* You can also dry berries (blueberries, raspberries, strawberries) in your dehydrator to add to a mixture of roasted nuts, seeds, unsweetened coconut flakes, and small pieces of jerky. We cut the jerky into bite-sized pieces with kitchen shears for easy munching on the trail. The carb cost won't be extremely high if you just perk up the saltiness of nuts, seeds, and jerky with the tang of the dried berries and the sweetness of the coconut, perhaps adding ¼ cup of dried berries and ¼ cup coconut to ½ cup jerky pieces and ½ cup nut/seed mixture. Be aware, though, that drying concentrates the sugars in the berries, so a given volume will have substantially more carb dried than fresh.

• *Frozen Kiwi on a Stick.* Peel kiwi fruit and skewer them on wooden skewers or popsicle sticks. Wrap tightly in plastic wrap and freeze for several hours or overnight. They will freeze solid overnight, but allow them to thaw slightly and you'll have a delicious, tangy, frozen treat. An alternative is to slice the kiwi and freeze the slices on a waxed paper–covered tray, then store in the freezer in a zip-closure bag for finger-food snacks.

• *Frozen Fruit.* Grapes, blueberries, raspberries, or strawberries (slice if very large) can be frozen, too, though you can buy berries prefrozen in bags at the grocery for a lot less work. For grapes, spread out the fruit in a single layer on a waxed paper–lined tray, freeze, and bag in a zip-closure bag for finger-food snacks. There's only about 7.5 grams of effective carb in ½ cup. The carb cost for blueberries is about 8 effective grams per ½ cup, for raspberries about 3, and for strawberries about 3.3 per ½ cup.

• *Protein Power Shake.* Instead of a carbo junk shake or malted milk after school, why not treat kids to real nutrition. Bigger kids can make this themselves—and budding athletes will love it. Use 8 ounces fresh milk and a scoop or so of low-carb protein powder (in any flavor) to provide another 15 to 20 grams of good protein (see Resources in the appendix for product information); if you like, add ¼ to ½ cup fresh berries, peaches, or tangerine or orange slices, or use flavoring extracts to create more flavors than Jelly Belly jelly beans. Blend until thick and smooth. Enjoy a glass of high-protein nutrition without a ton of wasted carb! You'll get 10 to 12 grams in the milk, 2 or 3 in the protein powder, and, if you elect to add it, 3 to 7 grams from the fruit. So at around 20 ECC carb grams for the works, it's fine for active growing kids or adults at the Maintenance level.

• *Nutrition Bars.* Here you'll have to be a bit more careful in reading labels, because often what's touted as a "nutrition" bar may not be much different from a candy bar. Many of these bars claim to contain "explosive carbo energy" and often tip the carb counter at 30 or 40 or more grams per bar. Most don't have much protein, either, and may contain trans fats galore. Still, there are some products out there that we'd recommend, and we've listed them in the Resources section of the appendix.

• *Veggie Sticks.* Low-starch, low-sugar veggies make good crunchy snacks, especially coupled with a little natural pimiento cheese, herbed cream cheese, herbed cottage mock cream cheese, or nut butters. Try celery sticks filled with any of these. Crunchy veggies such as carrots, jicama, radishes, snap peas, or zucchini make good dippers for these spreads, too. To make Mock Cream Cheese, blend ½ cup cottage cheese with ½ cup plain yogurt and a shake or so of whatever herbs or spices you like (garlic, onion, basil, tarragon, salt, and pepper). Line a large strainer with a paper coffee filter and suspend it over a bowl. Pour the mixture into the filter, cover with plastic wrap or waxed paper, and let all the liquid drain from it. Refrigerate after 3 hours. It will develop the consistency of cream cheese but will be higher in protein! It's great for spreading on veggies or low-carb toast—or, when Maintenance time comes, half a bagel (if you're adopting a Hedonist approach) with smoked salmon.

• *NB and J.* Instead of the standard peanut butter and jelly sandwich, try tempting the kids with a variety of other nut butters (almond, cashew) and a little no-sugar-added jelly, jam, or preserves on crunchy, thin brown rice crackers. Or start with LaTortilla Factory whole wheat low-carb tortillas (warmed slightly over the burner or in the microwave to make them pliable) to make an NB and J quesadilla! Spread the warm tortilla with nut butter, top with a little jam, fold over, cut into wedges, and enjoy.

• *Mini Lemon Cheesecakes.* For a sweet treat with only 5 to 6 ECC grams per serving (and only 2 to 3 if made with an artificial sweetener), try these muffin cup-size cakes. Finely chop 1 cup pecans or walnuts and mix them with 2 tablespoons melted butter, 1 teaspoon salt, and 1 tablespoon honey (or 4 packets of any artificial sweetener except aspartame). Divide the mixture evenly in the bottoms of twelve mini muffin cups (lined with cup liners). Combine 1 jumbo egg, ¼ cup artificial sweetener or honey, 1 teaspoon vanilla extract, ½ teaspoon lemon extract, and one 8-ounce package cream cheese, softened, and blend until smooth. Fill muffin cups two-thirds full and bake for 15 minutes, or until the filling sets at the edges (center may still be moist). Sprinkle the tops with grated lime or lemon zest when cool and store in the refrigerator in a tightly sealed container.

DINNER—THE OLD-FASHIONED WAY

The word *dinner* once conjured up images of warm, delicious smells emanating from the kitchen as everyone gathered around the table not just for nourishment but for family conversation as well. Dinner in this fast-paced world has often become a catch-as-catch-can proposition, grabbed on the run from whatever fast-food haven lies in your traffic pattern or the one the kids seem to prefer. It too often comes in recyclable polyfoam boxes or paper bags, eaten between stoplights on the way to or from this practice or that meeting. And unfortunately, most fast food falls short as far as healthy nutrition goes; on most menus the items consist of starch, sugar, and trans fats that take various forms, with numbers for names. For many people the traditional family dinner, with the whole bunch (whether friends or family) sitting down together and enjoying a leisurely meal and talking to one another, has slipped into history. And with it, one of the great joys of life—the social aspect of a meal. Too often people bemoan its passing but say there's just no time for that nowadays. We say, Baloney!

At our house, when the boys were growing up, we were both working from early in the morning until at least eight o'clock in the evening. The kids were all involved in sports, in school plays and clubs, in scouting, in fund-raisers, and all the other activities that kids want to participate in. Yet it was a rare night that we didn't all five sit down for a family dinner of real food, usually cooked at home. It may have been late—often, as is the European fashion, dinner didn't begin until 9 P.M.—but at no other point in the day could we really visit with each other. Dinnertime was family time, when we could each share the victories and frustrations of our day and tell stories and jokes. As often as not, it ended with picking up the guitar (always at hand in our kitchen) and singing familiar songs. Sharing joys with family and friends over a meal resonates deeply within the human consciousness, tracking all the way back to the days when our ancestors gathered around the cooking fires, eating, laughing, telling stories, and reveling in the pleasure of human companionship. Europeans understand; in France, Italy, Spain, and Greece, for example, people linger over meals, not only relishing good food but also recognizing that meals should be enjoyed at many levels. In our fast-paced world, even though you may not be able to do so every evening, we urge you to make time, as often as possible, for the joy of family, good friends, and good food. Here are a few tips that can make it a bit easier. (You'll find many more dinner ideas in the next section, General Food Preparation Instructions.)

• *Roast extra meats when you cook.* Bake enough chicken or chops for a large family, even if there are just two or three of you. It doesn't take much longer to prepare ten or fifteen chicken thighs than it does to cook four or five, but with the leftovers, you've got the basis for another lunch or dinner or two. The same applies when you're preparing meat patties—hamburger, lamb-burger, or turkey burger—or even fish or shrimp. Grill or broil a large batch, then wrap the extras tightly in plastic wrap and/or foil or zip-closure bags when cool enough to handle.

• *Make a pot of soup, stew, or chili large enough to last several meals.* Refrigerate in serving-sized portions or freeze in zip-closure freezer bags or snap-top plastic freezer containers for future meals.

• *Carefully evaluate available ready-to-eat takeout foods so you can let someone else do the work.* Ask the deli counter or restaurant takeout about their food—what kinds of oils, cheeses, meats, and vegetables they use. Once you find a source that meets your standards, then takeout isn't a bad option when you're pressed for time. For example, you can create a great dinner around rotisserie-grilled whole chicken, rounded out with a salad and some low-starch sautéed vegetables.

General Food-Preparation Instructions

These guidelines are simply designed to help you start cooking the *Protein Power LifePlan* way, not as a comprehensive cookbook. We hope they will get your creative juices flowing and spur you on to new, innovative, protein-rich, low-carbohydrate creations based on your own favorite dishes.

MEATS, POULTRY, AND SEAFOOD

• *Meats.* You can use a variety of seasonings or marinades to spice up the taste of meats. Here's a marinade we use for steaks: ¼ cup virgin olive oil, 1 or 2 cloves garlic finely chopped and crushed, ¼ cup Worcestershire sauce, ¼ cup red wine (optional), 1 teaspoon salt, 1 teaspoon black pepper. Put steaks and marinade into a zip-closure bag and marinate in refrigerator overnight (or at least 30 minutes at room temperature) prior to grilling or broiling. For medium rare, grill or broil about 4 to 5 minutes per side (add 30 seconds to 1 minute per side for medium and medium well). For pork chops, try using olive oil, 1 or 2 cloves garlic, 1 teaspoon salt, 1 teaspoon pepper, about 1 teaspoon rubbed sage, and ¼ cup white wine. Grill or broil about 5 minutes per side—until juices run clear and meat is no longer pink. For pork or beef tenderloin, try 1 to 2 teaspoons of kosher salt and 1 tablespoon each of coarsely ground black pepper and garlic powder as a rub prior to roasting. Mix the spices and distribute evenly on waxed paper. Roll the tenderloin in the spices to coat all sides. For easiest cooking, preheat oven to 500°, put rubbed meat in a roasting pan, and place uncovered in the oven. For beef, close door and immediately turn oven off. Leave undisturbed for 4 hours. It will be perfectly cooked to medium rare when you pull it out. For pork, roast at 500° for about 10 minutes (put ¼ broth or water into the roasting pan to prevent smoking). Then turn over off and leave undisturbed for at least 4 hours. It will be cooked through at the end of that time. (This can be done in the morning and left until you return from work or school if it's at least 4 hours.) To serve hot, slice tenderloin and gently reheat (so as not to overcook the beef) in a hot skillet, a microwave, or a slow oven. It's delicious right away but also great left over. Eat cold for snacks or lunches or reheat (gently) for dinner. Cook two pork tenderloins at once and slice up one for future lunches or dinners to save time. (You could do the same with beef tenderloin, but it might break your budget.)

• *Poultry.* A simple way to cook chicken pieces is to wash them thoroughly first, pat them dry, rub them with salt and pepper, and place them in a roasting pan (coat it with olive oil or butter or line with aluminum foil to make cleanup easier). Dot each piece with butter or drizzle with olive oil, sprinkle ½ teaspoon dried rosemary per piece on top, and bake uncovered for 30 to 45 minutes at 375°. Or try the chicken with the butter or olive oil, lots of black pepper, and the juice of several lemons, scattering the spent lemon peels and a cut-up yellow onion over all. Any number of spices will work well. Try paprika, or garlic and basil, or garlic and onions, or garlic, diced tomatoes, and cilantro, or simply poultry seasoning, salt, and pepper. The variations are endless.

• *Fish.* Most fish, whether salmon, mahi-mahi, snapper, tuna, sea bass, roughy, or even freshwater varieties (trout, crappie, or panfish), respond nicely to simple seasonings, such as a marinade of olive oil, garlic, cilantro, lemon or lime juice, and salt and pepper. Mix about ¼ cup oil, 1 or 2 cloves finely chopped or crushed garlic, ¼ cup chopped cilantro, the juice of a lemon or lime, and salt and pepper to taste and place marinade and fish into a zip-closure bag. Marinate in the refrigerator overnight (or at least 30 minutes) prior to cooking. Grill or broil for about 10 minutes per inch of fish at the thickest point (with half the time spent on each side). Adjust time to cook only until fish flakes easily with a fork but doesn't dry out. Overcooked fish is no joy to eat. To panfry small fish or thinner fillets, melt butter in a hot skillet, season fillets as above, and quickly panfry about 3 to 4 minutes per side—again until the flesh flakes with a fork but isn't dry. To give some peppery heat to your fish, top with a tablespoon or so of salsa made from 1 fresh tomato, seeded and diced; ½ red onion, peeled and diced; 1 small bunch fresh cilantro leaves, chopped fine; ¼ cup medium to hot canned green chili peppers, roasted, peeled, and chopped; the juice of 1 lime; and salt and pepper to taste.

• *Shellfish.* Broiling shrimp is easy. Simply oil a baking dish, then place peeled or unpeeled shrimp (thawed if frozen) on the dish in a single layer. In a small saucepan or in the microwave, melt some butter to which you have added crushed garlic, pepper, and cilantro, oregano, or basil. Pour this over the shrimp and run shrimp under the broiler for 3 to 5 minutes. Shake dish to turn shrimp over and move them about, then broil again for a few minutes, until the flesh of all the shrimp is opaque. Sprinkle with fresh lemon or lime juice and a bit of whichever herb(s) you used in the cooking. Try this method with scallops, crabmeat, lobster meat, or oysters, too. To grill the shrimp, marinate in the same sort of marinade used above for fish, skewer on metal skewers, and grill for 3 to 5 minutes a side, until the flesh of all the shrimp is opaque.

Preparing Vegetables

• *Sautés.* Coarsely dice or chop any of your favorite low-starch veggies—zucchini, yellow crookneck squash, broccoli, cauliflower, bell peppers of any color, asparagus, or mushrooms, for example—allowing ½ to 1 cup raw vegetable per person. It's lovely to mix several together. Heat a couple of tablespoons of olive oil in a slope-sided skillet or wok, add 1 to 2 cloves garlic sliced or diced, and, if you like, ¼ onion sliced or diced. Before the garlic (and onion) browns, add the vegetables and sprinkle with salt, pepper, and any herb that appeals to you. Toss and stir until vegetables are crisp-tender. Another delicious and quick option is to sauté greens—fresh spinach, for instance—in a little olive oil, garlic, and onion. Cook until the greens wilt and darken slightly.

• *Grilling or broiling.* Place chunks of low-starch vegetables, whole mushrooms, or pieces of bell pepper in a zip-closure bag with ½ cup olive oil, 1 or 2 cloves crushed garlic, the juice of one lime or lemon, 1 tablespoon fresh or 1 to 2 teaspoon dried herbs, 1 teaspoon salt, and 1 teaspoon pepper, and marinate for at least 30 minutes prior to grilling or broiling. Skewer or use a grill basket, and cook the vegetables for a few minutes per side, being careful not to overcook and dry them out.

• *Pan-roasting.* To save time, roast vegetables along with meats in the oven. When cooking a roast, chops, or chicken, for example, sprinkle the chunks of low-starch veggies in the pan over the meat. Add about 1 cup of broth—vegetable, chicken, beef, or mushroom—to keep them moist, and cover with foil during the cooking. The vegetables will cook down to very soft consistency by this method.

• *Veggie noodles.* Instead of pasta, try using "noodles" from the low-starch veggie world. Spaghetti squash makes a great substitute for its namesake pasta. To cook, simply cut the squash in half, place it cut side down in a baking dish, add ¼ cup water to the dish, cover tightly, and cook (about 7 to 10 minutes on high in the microwave or about 45 minutes at 350° in the oven). When done, the flesh will easily pull into spaghettilike strands when scraped with the tines of a dinner fork. Dress with olive oil, Parmesan cheese, garlic, or in any low-carb manner you would use to dress pasta. Using a mandoline slicer or vegetable peeler, you can create wide noodlelike strands from zucchini squash. Peel down the length of the squash to make ribbon noodles. Cook them in boiling, salted water, just as you would pasta noodles, until tender (this will take only a couple of minutes). Dress as you would pasta noodles, with cheese sauce, marinara sauce, cream sauce, meats, seafood, etc. As a substitute for very wide noodles, such as lasagna noodles, try using large cabbage or Swiss chard leaves, boiled until tender in salted water. (Many fewer carbs and a reasonable taste approximation.)

• *Potato substitutes.* In many recipes that call for potatoes, you'll find that cooked cauliflower will substitute nicely. For example, you can substitute cauliflower for potatoes in "potato" salad, in mashed "potatoes," and in soups, chowders, or stews. Matchstick julienne of zucchini and yellow squash with onions can make a credible substitute for hash brown "potatoes" for a much lower carb load.

SALADS

• *Meat/poultry/seafood salads.* These are as easy as can be and an entire quick lunch or dinner on one plate. It helps timewise to have washed and stored in the fridge plenty of fresh mixed lettuces and other greens, washed and chopped veggies (broccoli, cauliflower, carrots, celery, radishes, mushrooms, etc.), hard-boiled eggs, and cold meat, fish, or poultry leftovers. Of course, you can always cook them up from scratch, but if you've prepared them in advance you'll be ready to go in no time. Combine 2 cups of greens with ½ cup portions of the low-starch veggies of your choice; chopped or sliced hard-boiled egg, if you like; half a tomato sliced or chopped; and slices or pieces of whatever cold meat, poultry, fish, or seafood you've saved from the day or two before. Sprinkle a bit of crumbled blue cheese or shredded hard cheese on top, and add a few roasted almonds, walnuts, pecans, pine nuts, or sunflower, sesame, or pumpkin seeds for some extra vitamin E and crunch. Top with 1 to 2 tablespoons good vinaigrette dressing and you've got lunch. You can keep the chopped veggies segregated in zip-closure bags or snap-seal plastic or glass containers in the fridge for use as you need them. Again, it doesn't take a lot more time to dice four or five celery stalks or carrots than a single one, or slice a large handful of mushrooms instead of just 2 or 3. Spend a little more time once, and you'll be way ahead of the game.

• *Mixed greens.* Buy several varieties of greens (choose among iceberg, butter, romaine, and red leaf lettuces, also endive, radicchio, spinach, or if it's available in your market, a nice seasonal green mixture). Wash the greens, gently tear into pieces, mix them together, spin dry or wrap in paper toweling to dry in the refrigerator, and store in a greens or lettuce bag or an airtight container. Even a large zip-closure bag lined with a paper towel works well. Then it's easy to grab a couple of handfuls and lightly dress the greens for dinner for just yourself or an entire group. Properly handled, the greens should keep for several days without wilting. They won't, of course, keep after they've been dressed, so dress only what you'll eat at that meal.

• *Fruit salads.* Berries and melons are far and away the best carbohydrate bargains and also happen to be filled with wonderful antioxidant compounds. When you go to the market, grab what looks good and fresh in the berry and melon department and round it out with a bit of what's seasonal—peaches, nectarines, plums, tangerines, grapes, apples, kiwi, etc. Then wash, peel (if appropriate), and chop or slice in a large bowl all the fruits you've bought. Mix well and store covered in the refrigerator. Then, whether you want a side dish with breakfast, an afternoon snack, or dessert after dinner, dip up a ½ cup measure and count in your meal's carb total the average carb load for a ½ cup serving of the fruits you used. For example, we make a tasty, colorful, and low-sugar combination fruit salad using two parts strawberries to one part Valencia orange segments. Two cups fresh sliced strawberries and the sections of a couple of medium Valencia oranges have about 28 total effective carb grams and make six ½ cup servings; therefore, a ½ cup serving has about 4 or 5 grams. Any combination of fruits you like work on any phase of the plan as long as the individual fruits each contain fewer than 7 or 8 grams of effective carbohydrate per ½ cup. That way, the mixture can't possibly contain more than 7 or 8 grams per ½ cup and will probably contain considerably less than that if you use a fair amount of the lower-sugar fruits, like strawberries and raspberries.

SALAD DRESSINGS

Although it's really a simple proposition to make your own dressings, it's not always convenient. If you elect to use commercially prepared dressings (or in some situations have no choice), be aware that most of them—even in relatively nice restaurants—may be made with cheap oils of the partially hydrogenated variety. Don't be afraid to ask the waiter what the dressings contain, what kind of oils were used in their preparation. If there's any doubt about the quality of the ingredients, a simple solution is to ask for olive oil and vinegar to use on your salad. More and more, restaurants make their house vinaigrettes with olive oil, so it may prove less a problem as time goes on. There are also a number of commercially bottled dressings at the stores that use quality oils, no sugar, no artificial ingredients, and so forth. Read the labels carefully, looking for those telltale words *partially hydrogenated,* until you find one that doesn't have them. (Remember that 70 percent of soybean oil is hydrogenated, which may not be stated on the label.) The safest option is to make your own, when you're dining at home anyway, from ingredients you're sure of. Once you get the hang of making your own vinaigrettes, you'll wonder why you ever bought them. To make it quicker and easier, keep a variety of good vinegars on hand (sherry or wine vinegar, herbed vinegar, raspberry vinegar, for example, and perhaps a small bottle of aged balsamic vinegar for just a dash of character), along with garlic, fresh or dried herbs, and good-quality virgin or extra-virgin olive oil. When you're ready to whip it up, in a small bowl or measuring cup combine about ¼ cup of the vinegar or lemon or lime juice (with an added splash of balsamic, if you like), a clove of chopped garlic, a teaspoon or two of a couple of finely chopped fresh herbs (basil, oregano, thyme, dill, rosemary, etc.) or about 1 teaspoon dried herbs, and salt and pepper to taste. Allow the spices to infiltrate the vinegar (or citrus juice) for a few minutes, until just before you're ready to dress your salad. Then slowly drizzle a thin stream of olive oil into the vinegar and spices, whisking like mad (or blending in a small blender) until you've added about ⅓ to ½ cup oil. For best taste, use immediately, but it will store for up to a week in an airtight container in the refrigerator. Shake it well when you reuse it.

SOUPS

Soups really hit the spot in cold weather, and they also expand easily if friends or neighbors unexpectedly drop by at dinnertime. They adapt to an unpredictable eating schedule—ready in just a few minutes if you're pressed for time, able to sit and simmer if necessary—and only get better as leftovers a day or so later, once the flavors have had a chance to combine. To make preparation easy, keep a supply of fresh low-starch veggies, garlic, onions, and canned stewed seasoned tomatoes and broths on hand.

• *Meaty Veggie Soup.* For each serving of this soup, you'll need 1 or 2 cloves garlic, finely chopped; ½ onion, chopped; 1½ to 2 cups chopped mixed low-starch veggies (for example, zucchini, yellow squash, asparagus, broccoli, cauliflower, or carrots); 1 can diced stewed tomatoes (seasoned as you like); and 1 can broth (beef, chicken, vegetable, or mushroom). In addition, you'll want two meal-sized servings of protein—meat, chicken, or seafood— whether it's fresh or leftovers. Heat a couple of tablespoons olive oil in a soup pot or large saucepan and sauté the garlic and onion until limp. If you're cooking the protein fresh in the soup, add small cubes of meat/poultry/seafood now and cook for several minutes, stirring to ensure cooking on all sides and through to the center. Add the fresh veggies and continue to stir to sauté them for a few minutes, until they begin to soften. Add the tomatoes, the broth, and salt and pepper to taste. If you're using leftover meat, poultry, or seafood, add it at this point. Bring soup to a boil, reduce heat, and simmer for a few minutes (up to about an hour) over low heat. For a taste delight, sprinkle a teaspoon or two of finely chopped fresh basil or cilantro onto each bowlful just prior to serving. Double or triple or even quadruple the basic recipe if you've got a large enough pot to accommodate it and store the extra servings in the fridge for lunches or dinners on subsequent days. This is a great way to get a whole meal in a bowl for around 10 effective grams of carb (depending on your veggie choices)!

   • *Tomato-Basil Soup.* Here's another quick and easy—and delicious—soup. It can function as the lunch partner of an entrée salad or any meat entrée (such as leftover chicken breast, steak, ham, burger patties, or shrimp), head to school in the lunch box thermos, or make a splash as the first course of a sit-down dinner. The recipe doubles well, but unless you've got a huge blender, you'll need to make multiple batches to feed a bigger crowd than four. To make two servings of this utterly simple soup, just combine 1 can diced stewed tomatoes (already seasoned with basil and garlic if you like), ½ can vegetable or chicken broth, 2 tablespoons finely chopped fresh basil (or 1 tablespoon dried basil), and 1 or 2 teaspoons of aged balsamic vinegar in the blender and puree until smooth. Pour into a saucepan or soup pot and heat thoroughly. Top each bowlful with a couple of fresh whole basil leaves or with another teaspoon or two of finely chopped fresh basil. It's delicious, colorful, and full of vitamins and phytochemicals important to your health—and has only about 5 or 6 effective carbs per serving.

   • *Garden Gazpacho.* In the warm summer months, what could be better than a chilled soup of fresh garden veggies? Here's a blender version of gazpacho that we often whir up when we don't have time to make a more traditional Andalusian gazpacho. For two servings, combine in the blender 2 fresh ripe medium tomatoes, seeded and quartered; 1 medium cucumber, peeled or not as you prefer; 1 clove fresh garlic, peeled; ½ small yellow bell pepper, stem, seeds, and pith removed; ½ green bell pepper; ¼ red (Spanish) onion, quartered; 1 tablespoon sherry vinegar; 1 tablespoon fresh lime juice (about the juice in ½ lime); 1 teaspoon each of salt and black pepper. Puree in pulse bursts until the veggies are relatively evenly chopped. Each serving will provide about 10 to 12 grams of effective carbohydrate, packed with antioxidant nutrients. Serve it chilled with whatever good protein suits your fancy. We like it with spicy beef or chicken fajita meat or even a lamb burger, with a little guacamole and shredded lettuce, or with grilled salmon or mahi-mahi, or sautéed shrimp and a salad of seasonal mixed greens and vinaigrette.

The idea in cooking is to keep the procedure simple and quick, the food flavorful and fresh, and, as often as you can, the experience of eating a convivial delight. When the order of the day calls for celebration—whether it's a party to mark a family milestone or a more traditional holiday gathering—your new lifestyle should be able to easily accommodate the fun.

15

THE THREE PHASES
OF EATING

MIX-AND-MATCH MEALS FROM
INTERVENTION TO MAINTENANCE

For those of you who don't enjoy the fun of creating your own meal ideas, we've come up with dozens of possibilities for you, whether you're adopting the Hedonist, Dilettante, or Purist approach to your nutritional rehabilitation. To use the mix-and-match system to create a meal, select what you'd like to eat from the Protein Cornerstone Choices lists on the following pages and match it with an entire grouping of foods in the Carbohydrate Accompaniments lists.

Intervention: Getting Started

All people new to the program should begin here, at the Intervention Level, no matter how fit or unfit they may be. Those of you without disorders of blood pressure, blood sugar, or blood lipids or significant amounts of weight to lose will find your stay here a brief one (perhaps only a week or two)—just long enough to adapt to this new way of eating. Once that occurs, you can move quickly through the Transition Level and on to Maintenance. Those readers troubled by any of the many components of the insulin-resistance syndrome will stay at this Intervention Level, eating a diet of adequate protein and good-quality fat and restricting carbohydrate to 7 to 10 ECC grams per meal until these problems are adequately controlled. Then it will be time to move to Transition and Maintenance (the details of which we cover later in the chapter).

Since at least for the first week virtually everyone will begin at Intervention Level, let's look there for an example. For breakfast you might select poached eggs and salmon from the Protein Cornerstone Choices and couple that with a cup of sautéed spinach and a half a fresh tomato, sliced, from the Breakfast Carbohydrate Accompaniments for a delightful and slightly exotic breakfast or brunch. Or when you're rushed, perhaps you'd pick an "on-the-run" meal, such as several hard-boiled eggs and some beef jerky from among the Protein Cornerstone Choices, and couple that with a fresh peach from the Breakfast Carbohydrate Accompaniments. The choices are endless; all you have to do is mix and match them!

Please do take note that the carbohydrate selections for each level are designed to give you *approximately* the prescribed number of grams for that phase. The totals may vary a few grams here or there, but we've tried to select reasonable portions of a wide variety of items and make it all come out even. If you're careful to mix and match and not get into the rut of eating the same thing day after day, these small variances won't matter in the end.

Protein Cornerstone Choices

The following list of protein food should give you plenty of options from which to select when designing your own meals, whether you're in the Intervention, Transition, or Maintenance Level of your correction and whether you opt for the Purist, Dilettante, or Hedonist approach to your rehabilitation. It's an "all for one and one for all" list that should stand in good stead from this moment on. Simply select a food from the protein list at any meal, scale the portion of it to fit your specific requirement (see table 13.3 on page 316), and the cornerstone of the meal is set.

P = Purist, D = Dilettante, H = Hedonist
All protein choices are acceptable for P, D, and H unless otherwise noted.
☺ denotes a special item found in Resources in the appendix.

Eggs any style
Eggs any style + bacon, sausage, fish, or ham
Poached egg + cheese + meat or fish (with cheese: D, H only)
Egg salad (page 361)
Deviled eggs
Scrambled eggs + salmon + cream cheese (with cheese: D, H only)
Crustless Quiche (page 362) with meat, cheese, and/or veggies (with cheese:
   D, H only) (veg will take up all or part of your carb allotment)
Omelet with cheese (D, H only)
Omelet + meat +/− cheese +/− tofu (with cheese: D, H only)
Protein Power Shake (page 362) (includes your carb allotment)
Power Yogurt Cup (page 363) (includes your carb allotment) (D, H only)
Cottage cheese (contains carb) (D, H only)
Tofu, baked or stir-fried (D, H only)
Protein Power Bar ☺ (includes your carb allotment and alone may not be
   sufficient protein for large requirements)
Ham, Canadian bacon, sausage, or slab bacon
Ham, baked, broiled, panfried, smoked
Jerky
Jerky + nuts (nuts have a little carb)
Cold steak
Grilled steak
Roast beef
Steak fajita
Stir-fry beef (no cornstarch)
Chopped beef BBQ (low-sugar sauce only)
Beef kabob
Beef tenderloin
Hamburger steak
Beef brisket

Beef ribs

Kielbasa or Italian sausage

Beef stew (made with only low-starch veggies)

Veal shank, braised (osso buco)

Veal cutlet (nonbreaded)

Pork tenderloin

Pork stir-fry (no cornstarch)

Pork sausage

Turkey hash (no potatoes; substitute cauliflower)

Turkey burger

Cold chicken

Chicken baked, grilled, panfried

Stir-fry chicken (no cornstarch)

Roast chicken

Chicken BBQ (low-sugar sauce only)

Chicken fajita

Chicken salad (page 375)

Meaty Veggie Soup (page 378)

Veggie burger (D, H only)

Fish fillet, baked, grilled, panfried (trout, perch, mahi-mahi, cod, roughy, sea
   bass, catfish)

Tuna steak, grilled, broiled, pan-seared

Salmon, grilled, baked, broiled, poached

Lox (smoked salmon)

Swordfish, grilled, broiled, pan-seared

Shrimp, grilled, broiled, sautéed, boiled

Sardines

Clams or mussels, baked, broiled, sautéed

Oysters, on the half-shell, broiled, baked

Sashimi (salmon, tuna, mackerel, yellowtail, octopus, shrimp, etc.)

Seafood salad (salmon, shrimp, tuna) (page 375)

Calamari, sautéed, baked, grilled, broiled

Lobster, grilled, broiled, sautéed, boiled

Note: See table 13.3, Protein Portions, on page 316 for the amounts of protein sufficient to meet your requirement. Remember, it's fine to combine proteins or to add extra protein to a bar or shake to make it sufficient.

CARBOHYDRATE ACCOMPANIMENTS

INTERVENTION LEVEL

Breakfast

(**P** = Purist, **D** = Dilettante, **H** = Hedonist)
All items are acceptable for P, D, and H unless otherwise noted.
☺ denotes special item found in Resources in the appendix.

½ cup strawberries
1 slice low-carb toast (**H**) with
  butter

---

1 toasted bagel thin (**H**) (slice a
  bagel into 4 thin slices)
butter or cream cheese

½ cup blueberries
½ cup strawberries

---

1 medium peach

½ cup mixed fruit salad (page 376)

---

1 La Tortilla low-carb tortilla ☺ (**H**)
  (use as a breakfast burrito
  wrapper)
1 ounce salsa, hot, medium, or mild

---

1 cup strawberries, blueberries,
  blackberries, or raspberries
1 ounce heavy cream, if desired
  (**D, H**)

½ cup berries (with *Protein Power*
  Shake if made with water
  instead of milk; page 362)

½ serving Paleolithic Punch (page
  366)

---

1 slice low-carb toast or 2 La
  Tortilla tortillas ☺, buttered (**H**)

---

1 fresh tomato, sliced (or halved
  and broiled)
4 asparagus spears topped with a
  little hollandaise sauce (**D, H**
  with sauce)

½ apple, sliced

½ cup melon cubes

---

1 cup steamed or sautéed spinach
½ fresh tomato, sliced
(great topped with poached eggs
  and meat or salmon)

1 broiled portobello mushroom cap
brushed liberally with melted
butter or oil
(great topped with poached egg
with or without meat)

½ cup berries and 1 ounce mixed
nuts/seeds (sunflower and
pumpkin seeds mixed with
almonds make a good combo)
great mixed with 4 ounces yogurt
with protein powder) (D, H)

CARBOHYDRATE ACCOMPANIMENTS

INTERVENTION LEVEL

Lunch and Dinner

(**P** = Purist, **D** = Dilettante, **H** = Hedonist)

All items are acceptable for **P**, **D**, and **H** unless otherwise noted.

☺ denotes special item found in Resources in the appendix.

mixed seasonal greens with
    balsamic vinaigrette
½ cup zucchini
½ cup sliced strawberries

½ cup yellow squash
fresh spinach salad with vinaigrette
    or blue cheese dressing (**D, H**)
½ cup fresh blueberries

---

1 cup broccoli
½ cup red/yellow pepper, sautéed
iceberg lettuce wedge with
    vinaigrette

Chef Salad: 2 cups mixed greens
½ cup each chopped mushrooms,
    broccoli, cauliflower
1 medium tomato, sliced
1 ounce shredded hard cheese
    (**D, H**)
1 hard-boiled egg, topped with 2
    ounces dressing

½ avocado, sliced
½ medium tomato, sliced
2 cups seasonal mixed greens with
    dressing

Caprese Salad: 1 medium tomato,
    sliced (**D, H**)
4 ½-ounce slices fresh mozzarella
    cheese
4 large fresh basil leaves, shredded
olive oil and balsamic vinegar
    dressing

½ cup spaghetti squash
10 asparagus spears
mixed seasonal greens with
    dressing

½ cup sautéed mushrooms
½ roasted red pepper, sliced
iceberg lettuce wedge with dressing

½ cup green beans
½ cup steamed cauliflower,
   buttered
½ fresh sliced tomato, dressed with
   vinaigrette

---

1 cup steamed broccoli (with
   cheese: **D, H**)
½ cup red, yellow, green bell
   pepper, sautéed in olive oil and
   garlic
fresh spinach salad with
   mushrooms, dressed

½ large avocado, dressed on a bed
   of seasonal mixed greens
½ cup mixed fruit salad (page 376)

Caesar Salad, large, no croutons:
1 to 2 cups romaine, torn
1 to 2 tbsp. Caesar Salad dressing
   (no trans fats)
1 to 2 anchovy fillets (optional)
1 medium fresh peach

---

1 cup zucchini ribbon noodles
   (page 374) with garlic, butter,
   and Parmesan (**D, H**)
2 medium tomato halves, broiled
   with butter and sprinkled with
   herbs

---

2 low-carb tortillas ☺ (**H**)
1 cup shredded lettuce
½ medium tomato, chopped
1 ounce shredded Mexican
   cheddar or mozzarella cheese

½ cup Italian sauce (low-carb
   variety)
½ cup spaghetti squash
½ ounce fresh-grated Parmesan
   (**D, H**)
mixed seasonal greens with Italian
   vinaigrette

½ medium pita pocket (**H**)
1 large romaine or butter lettuce
   leaf
1 sliced tomato
1 slice onion
1 tbsp. canola mayonnaise or spicy
   mustard

---

1 slice low-carb bread (**H**)
1 to 2 slices tomato
1 to 2 leaves lettuce
1 to 2 slices onion
1 tbsp. canola mayonnaise +/or
   yellow mustard

---

1 cup stir-fried mixed Chinese
   vegetables (snow peas,
   mushrooms, water chestnuts,
   carrots, bean sprouts, bok
   choy)

---

1 cup of Cabbage Slaw: 2 cups
shredded red and green
cabbage
1 carrot, finely diced
½ cup canola mayonnaise
juice of 1 lemon
1 tbsp. sherry vinegar
2 tsp. Sucralose or saccharine
1 tsp. salt
1 tsp. pepper

1 cup mock potato salad (page
375)

1 cup mashed cauliflower (page
375)
salad of mixed seasonal lettuces
with fresh mushrooms,
peppers, radishes, and avocado
slices, dressed

Greek Salad: 2 cups greens
1 fresh sliced cucumber
1 fresh sliced tomato
1 ounce each black olives and
onion
2 ounces feta cheese

Graduating to Transition

Now that you've accomplished your stated health objectives—or are very close to doing so in the case of weight reduction and fat loss—you're ready to move from the Intervention or corrective level of the plan to one slightly more liberal in carbohydrate. While your protein requirement per meal may remain the same, it may have changed. You should check your new weight against your height on the Minimum Protein Requirement table 13.1 or 13.2 to be sure. With regard to carbohydrates, instead of the 7 to 10 effective grams you've been eating per meal, you'll now be able to enjoy an additional 5 to 8 effective grams per meal; this shift will increase your day's total allotment from a range of 30 to 40 ECC to one of between 55 and 70 ECC grams. What does that add to each meal? Well, the answer depends upon what you want it to add; it could be larger portions of the foods you're already eating—for example, going up from ½ cup berries to 1 cup, or from ½ tomato to a whole one, or from ½ cup squash to a full cup—or it could be adding back in some small portions of things you've been missing, such as rice or pasta. (Of course, that option would apply only to Dilettantes and Hedonists or would mean shifting from the Purist approach to a less stringent one.) At this stage you'll get only about ⅛ cup of these starchy foods if you plan on adding them to one of the Carbohydrate Accompaniments groupings you've been using on the Intervention Level. However, if you've really been hungry for, say, penne, dried beans, or risotto, you could elect to replace an entire meal's carbohydrate allotment with a ⅓-cup portion of one of them, along with your protein and a green salad. Or you could eat the twice-baked *skin* only (scraping as much of the flesh out as possible) of a whole medium potato, dressed with a bit of butter, sour cream, and chives for 10 grams and still have room for salad greens and 1 cup of broccoli or ½ cup of zucchini. The bottom line is that you've now got 15 to 18 ECC grams to spend at each meal, and you can spend them as you like within the limits of your currently chosen plan—that is, your commitment to a Purist, Dilettante, or Hedonist's approach.

For those of you who want some concrete suggestions on how this works in practice, here are some Carbohydrate Accompaniments for Transition Level meals. You'll recognize them from Intervention; take note of how we've augmented them with the extra allotment of carbohydrates. You'll see that in some cases the portion sizes have increased and in others we've added fruit or another vegetable or some starch. And these plans are simply suggestions. You don't have to follow all of them—or, for that matter, any of them—if they're not to your taste. Feel free to use a good carbohydrate counter (such as our new book, *Protein Power LifePlan Gram Counter*) and go to town creating your own delicious Transition Level meals; just be sure to take in an amount of protein sufficient to meet your body's requirement and to keep the total carbohydrate intake per meal between about 15 and 18 ECC grams.

CARBOHYDRATE ACCOMPANIMENTS

TRANSITION LEVEL

Breakfast

(P = Purist, D = Dilettante, H = Hedonist)
All items are acceptable for P, D, and H unless otherwise noted.
☺ denotes special item found in Resources in the appendix.

½ cup strawberries
2 slices low-carb toast (H)
butter

½ toasted bagel (H)
butter or cream cheese

½ cup blueberries
½ cup each strawberries and
    raspberries

1 medium peach
½ cup grapes

1 cup mixed fruit salad (page 376)

1 La Tortilla low-carb tortilla ☺ (H)
    (use as a breakfast burrito
    wrapper)
1 ounce salsa, hot, medium, or mild
⅛ cup rice or pinto beans

1½ cups strawberries, raspberries,
    or blackberries
1 ounce heavy cream, if desired
    (D, H)

1 cup berries with *Protein Power*
    Shake, if made with water
    instead of milk (page 362)

2 servings Paleolithic Punch (page
    366)

2 slices low-carb toast or 2 low-carb
    tortillas ☺, buttered (H)

1 fresh tomato, sliced (or halved
    and broiled)
8 asparagus spears, topped with a
    little hollandaise sauce (with
    sauce: D, H)
½ cup fresh berries

1 apple, sliced

1 cup melon cubes

1 cup steamed or sautéed spinach
½ fresh tomato, sliced (great
    topped with poached eggs and
    meat or salmon)
½ cup fresh strawberries

1 broiled portobello mushroom cap
brushed liberally with melted
butter or oil (great topped with
poached egg with or without
meat)
1 cup sautéed fresh spinach

1 cup berries and 1 ounce mixed
nuts/seeds (sunflower and
pumpkin seeds mixed with
almonds make a good combo)
(great mixed with 4 ounces
yogurt with protein powder)
(**D, H**)

Or add any of the following approximately 5-gram (ECC) carbohydrate allotments to any Intervention Level breakfast to transform it into the Transition Level:

½ cup berries   ½ cup milk   ⅛ cup rice
½ tomato   ½ cup grapes   1 slice low-carb toast
½ kiwi   ½ medium peach   1 low-carb tortilla ☺
½ cup melon   ½ cup cottage cheese   6 asparagus spears

CARBOHYDRATE ACCOMPANIMENTS

TRANSITION LEVEL

Lunch and Dinner

(**p** = Purist, **d** = Dilettante, **h** = Hedonist)
All items are acceptable for **p, d**, and **h** unless otherwise noted.
☺ denotes special item found in Resources in the appendix.

mixed seasonal greens with
    balsamic vinaigrette
1 cup zucchini
½ cup sliced strawberries

---

1 cup yellow squash
fresh spinach salad with vinaigrette
    or blue cheese dressing (**D, H**)
½ cup fresh blueberries

---

1 cup broccoli
½ cup red/yellow pepper, sautéed
iceberg lettuce wedge with
    vinaigrette
1 cup mixed fruit salad (page 376)

Chef Salad: 2 cups mixed greens
½ cup each chopped mushrooms,
    broccoli, cauliflower
1 medium tomato, sliced
1 ounce shredded hard cheese
    (**D, H**)
1 hard-boiled egg, topped with 2
    ounces dressing
½ cup fresh blueberries or
    blackberries

½ avocado, sliced
1 medium tomato, sliced or
    wedged
2 cups seasonal mixed greens with
    dressing

Caprese Salad: 1 medium tomato,
    sliced (**D, H**)
4 ½-oz. slices fresh mozzarella
    cheese
4 large fresh basil leaves, shredded
olive oil and balsamic vinegar
    dressing
1 slice melon with or without
    proscuitto di Parma
½ cup spaghetti squash
10 asparagus spears
mixed seasonal greens with
    dressing

½ cup sautéed mushrooms
1 roasted red pepper, sliced
iceberg lettuce wedge with dressing

½ cup green beans
½ cup steamed cauliflower, buttered
½ fresh tomato, sliced with vinaigrette
½ cup fresh sliced mushrooms
½ fresh avocado, sliced

---

1 cup stir-fried mixed Chinese vegetables (snow peas, mushrooms, water chestnuts, carrots, bean sprouts, bok choy)
½ cup mixed fruit salad (page 376)

---

1 cup of Cabbage Slaw: 2 cups shredded red and green cabbage
1 carrot, finely diced
½ cup canola mayonnaise
juice of 1 lemon
1 tbsp. sherry vinegar
2 tsp. Sucralose or saccharine
1 tsp. salt
1 tsp. pepper

1 cup mock potato salad (page 375)
½ fresh apple, sliced

---

1 cup steamed broccoli (with cheese: D, H)
½ cup red, yellow, green bell pepper, sautéed in olive oil and garlic
fresh spinach salad with mushrooms, dressed
1 Mini Lemon Cheesecake (page 369)

½ large avocado, dressed on a bed of seasonal mixed greens
½ cup mixed fruit salad (page 376)
½ fresh tomato, sliced

Caesar Salad, large, no croutons:
1 to 2 cups romaine, torn
1 to 2 tbsp. Caesar salad dressing (no trans fats)
1 to 2 anchovy fillets (optional)

1 medium fresh peach
5 large fresh strawberries

---

1 cup zucchini ribbon noodles (page 374) with garlic, butter, and Parmesan (D, H)
2 medium tomato halves, broiled with butter and sprinkled with herbs
2 thick onion slices, broiled with olive oil and herbs

---

3 low-carb tortillas ☺ (H)
1 cup shredded lettuce
½ medium tomato, chopped
1 ounce shredded Mexican cheddar or mozzarella cheese (D, H)

½ cup Italian sauce (low-carb variety)
1 cup spaghetti squash
½ ounce fresh-grated Parmesan (D, H)
mixed seasonal greens with Italian vinaigrette

½ medium pita pocket (**H**)
1 large romaine or butter lettuce
    leaf
1 slice tomato
1 slice onion
1 tbsp. canola mayonnaise or spicy
    mustard
½ Valencia orange, sectioned

---

2 slices low-carb bread (**H**)
1 to 2 slices tomato
1 to 2 leaves lettuce
1 to 2 slices onion
1 tbsp. canola mayonnaise and/or
    yellow mustard

---

1 cup mashed cauliflower (page
    375)
salad of mixed seasonal lettuces
    with fresh mushrooms,
    peppers, radishes, and avocado
    slices, dressed
1 Mini Lemon Cheesecake (page
    369) (**D, H**)

Greek Salad: 2 cups greens
1 fresh sliced cucumber
1 fresh sliced tomato
1 ounce each black olives and
    onion
2 ounces feta cheese

Or you can add any of the following approximately 5- to 7-gram (ECC) carbohydrate allotments to any Intervention Level lunch or dinner to transform it
into a Transition Level meal:

½ cup berries
1 cup broccoli
1 cup greens
½ cup okra
½ cup squash
1 glass wine
½ cup melon
1 small peach
1 Mini Lemon
    Cheesecake (page
    369)
2 pieces melba toast
½ artichoke
1 tomato

½ cup leeks
1 cucumber
1 or 2 "lite" beers
½ cup grapes
3 rice crackers
1 pressed rice cake
1 cup cauliflower
1 cup fresh mushrooms
1 cup green beans
1 carrot
3 saltine crackers
½ cup onion
½ fresh apple

½ Valencia orange
1 corn tortilla (small)
½ cup cole slaw (no
    sugar)
¼ cup sweet peas
½ baked potato, *skin
    only*
⅛ cup risotto, pasta, or
    beans
1 low-carb tortilla ☺
5 garlic cloves, roasted
1 slice low-carb bread

(*Note:* Purists would not add any grain items, such as tortillas, bread, crackers, risotto, pasta, or
rice, or any dairy [cheesecake]. Dilettantes would avoid wheat and corn products, such as tortillas,
breads, wheat crackers, or pasta.)

Just Can't Quite Stop Losing

If you continue to lose weight during this period of Transition—and more people than you might imagine do so—you should make a concerted effort to increase your intake of good-quality fats. In other words, eat more of the nutrient- and calorie-dense foods that don't have much of an impact on your insulin, such as nuts, seeds, nut butters, cheeses (unless, of course, you are opting for the Purist ideal), olives, avocados, and the like. Not a particularly tall order, you'd think, for someone to give you license to munch on these kinds of good-quality snacks all day. But it can be harder than you'd think, since they're very filling, too. As our good friend George said of his efforts to maintain his desired weight (that is, to keep it *up,* not get it *down*) after succeeding in reclaiming his health with Protein Power nutrition: "If there's something you can get from eating roasted almonds, then I've got it!" Every day, he eats a cup or more of almonds that he roasts himself with a little butter and salt—and each cup contains more than 1,300 calories! Despite that, he remains leaner, healthier, and more energetic than he's been in years.

If your weight continues to drop despite an increase in your intake of good fats, it's time to slide up to the Maintenance Level of carbohydrate intake and begin living the plan for the long haul. Let's see what that adjustment in your intake would bring in the way of added food.

Learning to Maintain—Most of the Time

Congratulations! If you're ready to make the shift from Transition Level to Maintenance, that means that you've achieved the health goals you set for yourself at the start of your nutritional and lifestyle rehabilitation. If you have lowered your triglycerides, raised your HDL ("good" cholesterol), improved your blood-lipid ratios, lowered your blood pressure, stabilized your blood sugar readings, or trimmed your waistline—or, as is typically the case, all of the above—you're ready to graduate from Transition to Maintenance and begin to enjoy the wellness you were born to have. For some of you, the road from Intervention to Maintenance may have taken only a month or six weeks; if you fall into that category, count yourself both lucky and smart for not letting your health problems get too far ahead of you before taking steps to halt them. Make a vow to yourself right now never to let them creep back into your life by forsaking what you now know to be the right way for you to eat.

Other people aren't so lucky. For those with more serious medical problems or a significant number of pounds to lose, the rehabilitative process may take a year or even more. But so what! Even if it does take a year to accomplish, what's that weighed against the reward of spending the rest of your life healthy, strong, and full of enough energy to really enjoy it? But the longer it takes to reclaim your health, the more serious you should be about defending your claim. Those of you who suffered serious insulin-related problems at the outset of this journey must never, never forget that you inherited the tendency for your insulin metabolism to become unhinged in the face of a diet too high in carbohydrates. And that tendency never goes away. Although you've now taken back control of your metabolism and can maintain that control as long as you wish, all it would take for the specter of insulin resistance and hyperinsulinemia to arise once more would be for you to fool yourself into believing that some sort of magic has occurred and you can eat anything you want at any time. Unless we missed something, nobody bopped you on the head with a magic wand and decreed you lean and healthy. No magic *"poof!"* caused your triglycerides to fall from the stratosphere back into the normal range or your blood pressure and blood sugar to drop. Eating right did. Your own hard work got you to this healthy place. Your knowledge of how foods affect your body and your application of that knowledge got you there. Returning to the kind of diet that eons of development and refinement designed got you here. And remembering those things will keep you here.

RATCHET UP YOUR CARBS—VERY CAREFULLY

Now that you're ready to head into a Maintenance Level carbohydrate intake, you're probably wondering exactly what that will mean in terms of the additional foods available to you. In terms of your protein choices and fat choices, things remain the same. Check your weight against table 13.1 or 13.2 to see what your minimum protein serving size should be at your new weight but remember that with protein, that's always a minimum; if your appetite desires more, you can have more without disrupting your metabolic harmony.

As far as your intake of carbohydrate foods is concerned, just as with your shift to the Transition Level, moving to Maintenance could mean larger portions of the things you've already been eating—and for those adhering to a strict Purist philosophy, that will indeed most often be the case—or it could mean a reintroduction of slightly larger portions of some of the sweeter, starchier, higher-carbohydrate foods that you've for the most part done without during your rehabilitation. But take great care as you do this business of increasing starchy or sugary things; these kinds of foods have incredible potential to unhinge your insulin metabolism if you overdo them, particularly early on in your move to your Maintenance carbohydrate level. We recommend—based on our personally having taken care of thousands of people with this problem—that you increase your carbohydrate intake slowly, deliberately, and according to the prearranged plan that we've outlined in table 13.6, Carbohydrate Intake Guidelines.

No doubt you're wondering how many carbs you'll be allowed in Maintenance per meal or per day. Although we'd love to give you that number, unfortunately, we don't know it. Everyone differs in what he or she will tolerate in the carbohydrate department while still maintaining the health benefits and lean body that going through this nutritional rehabilitation has wrought. A number of factors come into play in determining where things will settle, among them how disordered your metabolism was to begin with, your current state of insulin sensitivity, the number of overall calories you consume each day, and your level of physical activity. Let's look at each of these and see how they figure in.

You'll remember from chapter 2, "The Insulin Connection," the classic research study of Claire Hollenbeck and Gerald Reavan's team that showed that 75 percent of even "apparently normal" people overproduce insulin to some degree when they consume carbohydrates. But the degree to which they do so varies; out of one hundred people, about twenty-five can tolerate a load of carbohydrate without raising their insulin levels much (we call them the Metabolically Gifted and Talented), about twenty-five will experience an insulin rise of a modest amount, about twenty-five will see their insulin level rise considerably, and for the last twenty-five, insulin levels will go screaming upward to levels as high as individuals with type II diabetes. So, depending upon where you began this journey—that is, which of these groups you'd have fallen into if you'd been among the subjects in this classic medical study—you may be more or less sensitive to the reintroduction of increasing amounts of carbohydrate into your diet. Or, in simple terms, some people will tolerate more carbohydrate than others will.

And your caloric intake and output also exert an impact on how many carbohydrates you'll tolerate while remaining in control metabolically. The more physically active you become—that is, the more calories you burn each day—the more calories and carbohydrate you'll likely be able to tolerate in Maintenance. The reverse of this statement is also true: the less active you are, the fewer carbohydrate grams you'll tolerate. Remember this relationship, the balance between carbohydrates and activity. For example, what would happen if you were accustomed to being physically active and you became injured—sprained an ankle, broke a leg, or tore a muscle? Your normal level of calorie output from exercise would, of course, abruptly decline, and when it did, you would have to just as abruptly drop your carbohydrate intake (to Transition Level or, depending upon the extent of your incapacitation, even Intervention Level) or you would gain weight and begin to lose your grip on metabolic control. Once you recovered and were able to resume your previous level of exercise, you'd be able to return to your higher carbohydrate intake. How high?

Again, we wish we could tell you with certainty the number of grams you'll tolerate, but we can't. No one number will fit all, and finding your precise balance point will be a matter of trial and error. As you progress from Transition to Maintenance, in the first week, you'll add about 5 ECC grams of carbohydrate to each meal, giving you an additional 15 or so grams a day. Hold at this level for a week or so to see if you'll remain stable. If you do, creep up another 5 grams per meal the next week or add a 5- to 10-gram snack and hold again. See how you feel at that level of intake. If all seems okay, creep up another 5 grams per meal again each week until you reach the point that you begin to see some cracks in your metabolic control—for example, you begin to retain a little fluid (tight rings, tight shoes, puffy eyes in the morning), see your weight inch up a bit, or your lab values (particularly triglycerides) rise slightly. When you see these signs, back down to the last intake at which you were stable and felt good. And although we don't know precisely where your control point will be, years of experience helping our patients find their way to Maintenance has shown us that the vast majority of people will tolerate a number of carbohydrate grams each day that is approximately equal to the minimum number of grams of protein their body requires. For example, if you calculate your minimum protein requirement at 27 grams per meal, you'll probably be able to tolerate 27 grams of carbohydrate per meal in Maintenance. (Take note that we specified carbohydrate grams equal to your *calculated minimum protein requirement*—not equal to the amount of protein you eat in a given meal. You may eat more grams of protein than your minimum requirement if you like, but your carb limit can't expand accordingly!)

Although this rule of thumb won't hold true in all cases, most people can tolerate this 1:1 ratio without much ado; very physically active or very insulin-sensitive people may perhaps tolerate as much as one-third more carbohydrate grams than their calculated minimum number of protein grams. And there will also be the less tolerant few who won't be able to tolerate a carbohydrate intake much beyond their Transition Level day in and day out without unhinging their control slightly. As you're seeking your Maintenance number of carbohydrate grams, keep these rough figures in mind to help guide your stepwise increases. When you reach the point that your carbohydrate grams per meal equal your minimum protein requirement, stop to assess your metabolic stability, your weight, blood pressure, and sense of well-being. Perhaps even have some blood tests (insulin, blood sugar, triglycerides, cholesterol readings) repeated to help you and your physician make the determination of whether or not you'll be able to go higher on carbs on a day-to-day basis.

Once you've got your number, try to stick to it most of the time and you'll find maintaining your lean, healthy body isn't as tough as you've been told.

To modify your Transition meals to begin the first week of Maintenance, you'll simply add increments of about 5 ECC to each meal. Here's how the total carbohydrate allotment in the first week of Maintenance might look:

CARBOHYDRATE ACCOMPANIMENTS

MAINTENANCE LEVEL WEEK 1

Breakfast

P = Purist, D = Dilettante, H = Hedonist)
All items are acceptable for P, D, and H unless otherwise noted.
☺ denotes special item found in Resources in the appendix.

1 cup strawberries
2 slices low-carb toast (H)
butter

½ toasted bagel (H)
butter or cream cheese
½ tomato, sliced

---

1 cup blueberries
½ cup each strawberries and
    raspberries

---

1 medium peach
1 cup grapes

1½ cup mixed fruit salad
(page 376)

1½ servings Paleolithic Punch
    (page 366)

---

2 slices low-carb toast or
2 low-carb tortillas ☺, buttered (H)
1 medium peach

---

1 fresh tomato, sliced (or halved
    and broiled)
8 asparagus spears, topped with a
    little hollandaise sauce (with
    sauce: D, H)
1 cup fresh berries

---

1 apple, sliced
2 ounces roasted almonds

1½ cup melon cubes

---

1 cup steamed or sautéed spinach
1 fresh tomato, sliced (great topped
    with poached eggs and meat or
    salmon)
1 cup fresh strawberries

---

1 La Tortilla low-carb tortilla ☺ (H)
    (use as a breakfast burrito
    wrapper)
1 ounce salsa, hot, medium, or mild
¼ cup rice or pinto beans (D, H)

2 cups strawberries, raspberries, or blackberries

1 ounce heavy cream, if desired. (**D, H**)

---

1 cup berries with *Protein Power* Shake made with 8 ounces milk

---

1 broiled portobello mushroom cap brushed liberally with melted butter or oil (great topped with poached egg meat) with or without 1 cup sautéed fresh spinach

½ tomato, broiled with herbs and olive oil

---

1 cup berries and 2 ounces mixed nuts/seeds (sunflower and pumpkin seeds mixed with almonds make a good combo) great mixed with 8 ounces yogurt with protein powder) (**D, H**)

Or add any of the following approximately 5-gram (ECC) carbohydrate allotments to any Transition Level breakfast to transform it into the Maintenance Level Week 1:

½ cup berries	½ cup milk	⅛ cup rice
½ tomato	½ cup grapes	1 slice low-carb toast
½ kiwi	½ medium peach	1 low-carb tortilla
½ cup melon	½ cup cottage cheese	6 asparagus spears

Or occasionally replace your entire breakfast allotment of carbohydrates with any of these treats, each of which will cost you about 20 to 25 ECC grams:

2 slices raisin bread (**H**)

⅔ cup oatmeal, butter, sweetener (**D, H**)

½ cup rice, butter, artificial sweetener (**D, H**)

1 small (7″) waffle, ½ cup berries (**H**)

½ English muffin, butter, 2 tsp. jam (**H**)

1 small oat bran muffin (**H**)

½ cup oatmeal, ½ cup berries (**D, H**)

1 small crescent roll (**H**)

1 small flour tortilla (**H**)

CARBOHYDRATE ACCOMPANIMENTS

MAINTENANCE LEVEL WEEK 1

Lunch and Dinner

(**P** = Purist, **D** = Dilettante, **H** = Hedonist)
All items are acceptable for **P**, **D**, and **H** unless otherwise noted.
☺ denotes special item found in Resources in the appendix.

mixed seasonal greens with ½ fresh
   tomato and balsamic
   vinaigrette
1 cup zucchini
½ cup sliced strawberries

---

1 cup yellow squash
fresh spinach salad with vinaigrette
   or blue cheese dressing (**D**, **H**)
1 cup fresh blueberries

---

1 cup broccoli
1 cup red/yellow pepper, sautéed
iceberg lettuce wedge with
   vinaigrette
1 cup mixed fruit salad (page 376)

Chef Salad: 2 cups mixed greens
½ cup each chopped mushrooms,
   broccoli, cauliflower
1 medium tomato, sliced
1 ounce shredded hard cheese
   (**D**, **H**)
1 hard-boiled egg, topped with 2
   ounces dressing
1 cup fresh blueberries or
   blackberries

½ avocado, sliced
1 medium tomato, sliced or
   wedged
2 cups seasonal mixed greens with
   dressing
½ cup each broccoli, cauliflower
2 ounces roasted sunflower seeds

Caprese Salad: 1 medium tomato,
   sliced (**D**, **H**)
4 ½-ounce slices fresh mozzarella
   cheese
4 large fresh basil leaves, shredded
olive oil and balsamic vinegar
   dressing
2 to 3 slices melon with or without
   proscuitto di Parma
½ cup spaghetti squash
10 asparagus spears
mixed seasonal greens with
   dressing

1 cup steamed broccoli (with cheese: **D, H**)

1 cup red, yellow, green bell pepper, sautéed in olive oil and garlic

fresh spinach salad with mushrooms, dressed

1 Mini Lemon Cheesecake (page 369) (**D, H**)

½ large avocado, dressed on a bed of seasonal mixed greens

½ cup mixed fruit salad (page 376)

1 fresh tomato, sliced or wedged

Caesar Salad, large, no croutons:

1 to 2 cups romaine, torn

1 to 2 tbsp. Caesar salad dressing (no trans fats)

1 to 2 anchovy fillets (optional)

1 medium fresh peach

5 large fresh strawberries

2 ounces roasted almonds

1½ cup zucchini ribbon noodles (page 374) with garlic, butter, and Parmesan (**D, H**)

2 medium tomato halves, broiled with butter and sprinkled with herbs

2 thick onion slices, broiled with olive oil and herbs

---

3 low-carb tortillas ☺ (**H**)

1 cup shredded lettuce

½ medium tomato, chopped

1 ounce shredded Mexican cheddar or mozzarella cheese (**D, H**)

½ cup Italian sauce (low-carb variety)

1 cup spaghetti squash

½ ounce fresh-grated Parmesan (**D, H**)

mixed seasonal greens with Italian vinaigrette

½ cup sautéed mushrooms

1 roasted red pepper, sliced

iceberg lettuce wedge with dressing

½ cup green beans

½ cup steamed cauliflower, buttered

1 fresh tomato, sliced with vinaigrette

½ cup fresh sliced mushrooms

½ fresh avocado, sliced

1½ cups stir-fried mixed Chinese vegetables (snow peas, mushrooms, water chestnuts, carrots, bean sprouts, bok choy)

½ cup mixed fruit salad (page 376)

½ cup pasta, olive oil, garlic or cream sauce (**H**)

salad greens with vinaigrette

1½ cup mixed zucchini, mushroom, peppers, onion, and tomatoes (for soup)

1 cup of Cabbage Slaw: 2 cups shredded red and green cabbage
1 carrot, finely diced
½ cup canola mayonnaise
juice of 1 lemon
1 tbsp. sherry vinegar
2 tsp. Sucralose or saccharine
1 tsp. salt
1 tsp. pepper

1 cup mock potato salad (page 375)
1 fresh apple, sliced

½ cup butter beans (D,H)
green salad with ½ cup mushrooms
½ fresh tomato, with vinaigrette

½ cup Great Northern or kidney beans
green salad with vinaigrette
½ cup canned, stewed tomatoes

½ medium pita pocket (H)
1 large romaine or butter lettuce leaf
1 slice tomato
1 slice onion
1 tbsp. canola mayonnaise or spicy mustard
½ Valencia orange, sectioned

---

2 slices low-carb bread (H)
1 to 2 tomato slices
1 to 2 leaves lettuce
1 to 2 slices onion
1 tbsp. canola mayonnaise and/or yellow mustard
½ fresh apple, sliced

---

1 cup mashed cauliflower (page 375)
salad of mixed seasonal lettuces with 1 cup fresh mushrooms, peppers, radishes and ½ avocado sliced, dressed
1 Mini Lemon Cheesecake (page 369) (D, H)

---

1 "lite" burger bun (H) with 1 lettuce leaf, 1 slice tomato, mayonnaise, mustard, pickles

---

Greek Salad: 2 cups greens
1 fresh sliced cucumber
1 fresh sliced tomato
1 ounce each black olives and onion
2 ounces feta cheese

1 fresh Valencia orange, sectioned

½ cup buttered corn (H)
green salad with ½ fresh tomato, dressed with vinaigrette

½ cup black-eyed peas
½ cup turnip greens
2 green onions

And remember, you can add any of the following approximately 5- to 7-gram (ECC) carbohydrate allotments to any Transition Level lunch or dinner to transform it into a Maintenance Level Week 1 meal. These also serve as ideas for adding the 5-gram meal increments each week as you progress to your final Maintenance Level intake.

½ cup berries	1 tomato	½ fresh apple
1 cup broccoli	½ cup leeks	½ Valencia orange
1 cup greens	1 cucumber	1 corn tortilla (small)
½ cup okra	1 or 2 "lite" beers	½ cup cole slaw (no
½ cup squash	½ cup grapes	sugar)
1 glass wine	3 rice crackers	¼ cup sweet peas
½ cup melon	1 pressed rice cake	½ baked potato, *skin*
1 small peach	1 cup cauliflower	only
1 Mini Lemon	1 cup fresh mushrooms	⅛ cup risotto, pasta, or
Cheesecake (page	1 cup green beans	beans
369)	1 carrot	1 low-carb tortilla ☺
2 pieces melba toast	3 saltine crackers	5 garlic cloves, roasted
½ artichoke	½ cup onion	1 slice low-carb bread

(Note: Purists would not add any dairy items (cheesecake) or grain items, such as tortillas, bread, crackers, risotto, pasta, or rice. Dilettantes would avoid wheat and corn products, such as tortillas, breads, wheat crackers, or pasta.)

Stumbling Upon the Honey Tree

Does maintaining a certain limit on carb intake mean that you can never have a "starch and sugar blowout" again? Does it mean that you'll never again taste a Triple Fudge Brownie Delight, Deep-Dish Blackberry Cobbler à la Mode, or Warm Bread Pudding with Bourbon Sauce? Nope. It doesn't in the least. Even our ancient ancestors stumbled into a honey tree once in a while, and from the published accounts of such occurrences in contemporary hunter-gatherer tribes, when they did, it was party time! Super Bowl Sunday! Christmas morning! If they'd had fireworks, they would have filled the air with trailing sparkles of gold and blue and red! Apparently, among hunter-gatherers, news of a honey find spreads as quickly as rave reviews of a hot new restaurant, and in short order the eager group assembles, with young and old alike eating the honey until they're all, quite literally, drunk on it. To be true to your Paleolithic heritage, you should occasionally do likewise. Treat yourself to something sinfully rich and totally luscious every now and then. Not every night, certainly, perhaps not

408   *The Protein Power LifePlan*

even every week or month, but once in a while, as we do, pretend you've stumbled into a honey tree and eat your fill in celebration of such a rare and delightful find. Make your celebration of the honey tree as joyous—and guilt-free—as it would have been to your ancient ancestors. Have a big helping of the "pleasure nutri-ent" for a special occasion—your birthday, anniversary, or a spe-cial or traditional holiday. Once in a while, it's good for you to do it.

That's not to say that a "honey drunk" comes without conse-quence; there's no escaping your own biochemistry. A sudden shower of sugar (or starch) into your bloodstream will occasion a whopping rise in insulin almost immediately. And with it, you'll retain some fluid—the next morning your eyes will be puffy, your rings tight, your waistbands and socks will leave "tread marks." Buckle down the next day or two, returning even to an Interven-tion Level of carb intake, and you'll quickly restore balance to your insulin metabolism again.

And that's how you'll wend your way through the coming years. Just as we've done now for a decade and a half ourselves, strive to maintain a controlled and tolerable carbohydrate intake most of the time, saving visits to the honey tree for special occa-sions (so-called because they occur *occasionally*) and recovering from the party afterward. It's such a simple plan, but by adhering to it you'll be able to enjoy the remainder of your life healthier, fitter, leaner, and sound in mind and spirit.

APPENDIX

MICRONUTRIENT ROUNDUP

NUTRIENT	MULTIVITAMIN FOR BASIC HEALTH	FOR DISEASE-SPECIFIC RECOMMENDATIONS INCREASE THE SUPPLEMENTATION OF "BASIC" TO THESE TOTAL AMOUNTS.*							
		DIABETES	HEART DISEASE	CHOLESTEROL	TRIGLYCERIDES	OBESITY	DISEASES OF THE EYE	AUTOIMMUNE DISORDERS	VEGETARIANS
Vitamin A (as beta carotene)	25,000 IU								
Vitamin C	200 IU	500						1000	
Vitamin D_3 (optional)	400 IU								
Vitamin E (mixed)	400 IU	800	800	800	800		800		
Vitamin K_1	100 mcg								
Thiamine	50 mg								
Riboflavin	15 mg								
Niacin	30 mg								
Niacinamide	130 mg								
Vitamin B_6 (as Pyridoxal-5'-Phosphate)	15 mg		30						
Folate	800 mcg		1200						
Vitamin B_{12}	500 mcg		1000						1000
Biotin (optional)	400 mcg								
Pantothenic Acid	400 mg								

Supplement				
Calcium (optional)	300 mg			
Magnesium*	400 mg	600	600	
Chromium	200 mcg	1000	500	
(as Niacin bound or Picolinate)				
Selenium	100 mcg			
Zinc	15 mg			
Copper	1.5 mg			
Manganese	2.0 mg			
Molybdenum	100 mcg			
Boron	3 mg			
Potassium	≥99 mg	396	396	396
Alpha-Lipoic Acid	200 mg	600	600	
Bilberry				
L-Carnitine†	2 g	4 g	4 g	
CoQ10	100 mg	300	200	
Vanadyl Sulfate†	5–10 mg			
L-Glutamine†	20–40 g			
Methionine†	2 g			
Taurine†	2 g			

*If two or more categories apply, take the highest *single* dose. Do not add doses together.
†Take before meals 3 times per day every other month.

In addition to what you'll find here, be sure to periodically check our web site, www.eatprotein.com, where we list new products as we find them.

FOOD PRODUCTS

SWEETENERS

Sucralose (Splenda)
Web: www.synergydiet.com/splendaproducts.asp
This web site sells much more than Splenda. We make no recommendations about their other products, as we've not examined them.

Isomalt
A mostly nonabsorbable sweetener that holds up to cooking. Distributed by:
Palatinit of America, Inc.
101 Gibraltar Dr.
Suite 2B
Morris Plains, NJ 07950
(for technical information)
Phone: (800) 476-6258 or (201) 326-9508

GRAIN THINGS

Whole-wheat fat-free tortillas with an ECC of 3–7. They freeze very well.
La Tortilla Factory
3635 Standish Ave.
Santa Rose, CA 95407
Phone: (800) 446-1516

Thin, crunchy crackers made of brown rice and salt, under 2 grams ECC each:
Hol-Grain Brown Rice Crackers
Conrad Rice Mill, Inc.

307 Ann St.
New Iberia, LA 70560

Organic bread products, with no preservatives and no added fat. Not
very low carb, but high quality:
Alvarado St. Bakery
Rohnert Park, CA 94928

NATURAL BEEF PRODUCTS

Cates Family Farm
5992 CTH T
Spring Green, WI 53588
Phone: (608) 588-2836

Coleman Natural Products
5140 Race Court Unit 4
Denver, CO 80216
Phone: (800) 442-8666

Denver Buffalo Company
1120 Lincoln St.
Suite 905
Denver, CO 80203-9790
Phone: (800) BUY-BUFF or (800) 289-2833

WILD GAME

Game Sales International
2456 E. 13th St.
Loveland, CO 80537
Phone: (800) 729-2090

Game Exchange/Polarica
105 Quint St.
San Francisco, CA 94124
(800) 426-3872
    or

73 Hudson St.
New York, NY 10013
Phone: (800) 426-3487

MEAL REPLACEMENT BARS, SHAKES

Protein Power Bars and *Protein Power* Shakes
Great-tasting high-protein bars in four flavors with 30 grams protein and 7 to 10 ECC; shakes with 22 grams protein and 3 ECC per serving. A product of ProGenesis Corp., Brentwood, CA, distributed by Nutritional Wisdom. Phone: (888) 325-4606.

> Ultimate Protein System Bars and Shakes
> A product of Country Life
> Hauppauge, NY 11788
> Available at many retail grocery and health food centers.

> Unipro Perfect Protein Shakes
> A Product of Unipro Performance Nutrition
> San Clemente, CA 92673
> Phone: (800) 621-6070
> Available at many retail grocery and health food centers.

BEVERAGES

> TAZO Teas
> PO Box 66
> Portland, OR 97207
> (for catalog) Phone: (800) 299-9445
> Available at many retail groceries and health food stores.

PICKLED VEGETABLES

Gourmet pickles, fancy relishes, and garnishments.

The Pickle Sisters
7509 Cantrell Rd.
Little Rock, AR 72207
Phone and fax: (501) 664-0811
Be sure to ask about their *Protein Power LifePlan* Instant Hors d'oeuvres and their "Boomslang Venom" olive oil vinaigrette.

VEGETABLE WASH

> Healthy Harvest Fruit and Vegetable Rinse
> PO Box 861

Madison, CT 06442
Phone: (203) 245-2033

BRAIN FOOD

FOREIGN LANGUAGE SOFTWARE

Learn to Speak Series
The Learning Company
One Athenaeum St.
Cambridge, MA 02142
Phone: (617) 494-1200
Web: www.learningco.com

[Language] Now Series
Transparent Language Products
22 Proctor Hill Rd.
PO Box 575
Hollis, NH 03049-0575
Phone: (603) 465-2230
E-mail: info@transparent.com
Web: www.transparent.com

Tell Me More Series
Auralog
3333 E. Camelback Rd.
Suite 250
Phoenix, AZ 85018
Web: www.auralog.com

Self-Study Series
Syracuse Language
5790 Widewaters Pkwy.
Syracuse, NY 13214-2845
Phone: (800) 797-5264
E-mail: customerservice@syrlang.com
Web: www.syrlang.com

HOME AND IN-RESIDENCE SUMMER STUDY COURSES

St. John's College
Summer Classics Program

1160 Camino Cruz Blanca
Santa Fe, NM 87501
Phone: (505) 984-6104
Fax: (505) 984-6003
E-mail: classics@mail.sjcsf.edu
Web: www.sjcsf.edu

College of Santa Fe
Elderhostel
1600 St. Michael's Dr.
Santa Fe, NM 87505

Washington and Lee University
Office of Special Programs
Lexington, VA 24450
Phone: (540) 463-8723
Fax: (540) 463-8478
E-mail: rfure@WLU.edu

Ten Blue Windows
Poetry and Creative Writing Workshops
2566 Camino Chueco
Santa Fe, NM 87505
Phone: (505) 471-5575

LECTURES ON TAPE

The Teaching Company
Great Lecturer Series
7405 Alban Station Court
Suite A107
Springfield, VA 22150-2318
Phone: (800) 832-2412
Fax: (703) 912-7756

MEDITATION AND RELAXATION

A guided course in how-to (4 cassette tapes and a manual).
Learn to Meditate
Patricia Carrington, Ph.D.

Pace Educational Systems, Inc.
61 Kingsley Rd.
Kendall Park, NJ 08824
Phone: (800) 297-9897
Fax: (732) 297-0778
Available in many bookstores.

Meditation Made Easy
Lorin Roche, Ph.D.
HarperSanFrancisco, 1998
Book and cassette set available at many bookstores or through the
    publisher.

MUSIC

Mozart for Your Mind (Philips Classic Productions, 1995) (a division of
PolyGram Records, Inc., New York).

Music for the Mozart Effect, Vols. I, II, and III
Spring Hill Music
PO Box 800
Boulder, CO 80306
Phone: (303) 938-1188
Fax: (303) 938-1191

The Mozart Effect: Music for Children, Vols. I and II
Atlantic Recording Corporation
1290 Avenue of the Americas
New York, NY 10020
Web: www.childrensgroup.com

SUGGESTED AND RELATED READING

Because of space limitations, we are unable to include the lengthy bibliography of research data upon which we base our program and the
material contained in *The Protein Power LifePlan*. You'll find the complete bibliography on the Internet at our web site www.eatprotein.com,
or you may send a large (10 × 13) self-addressed and stamped ($3.00
postage) envelope to Drs. Eades/CCMM, PMB 504, 6525 Gunpark
Drive 370, Boulder, Colorado, 80301-3346, and we'll send you a copy.

COOKBOOKS

Aidells, Bruce. *The Complete Meat Cookbook* (Houghton Mifflin, 1998). A wonderful guidebook for those who love meat. Many recipes are not in sync with our philosophy, so you'll have to pick and choose those not heavily laced with starchy accompaniments.

Bittman, Mark. *How to Cook Everything* (Macmillan, 1998) and *Living Low-Carb* (Little, Brown, 2000). One of the best basic cookbooks we've ever seen. If you wonder how to cook almost anything, this book will tell you how! Again, not all recipes are *Protein Power LifePlan*–friendly, but use it as a guide for learning to cook.

Fran McCullough. *The Low-Carb Cookbook* (Hyperion, 1997). An excellent resource for anyone following this plan, giving carb counts for most recipes. Beware, however, the use of recipes containing aspartame!

IMPROVING BRAIN FUNCTION AND VISION

Crook, T. H., and B. Adderly. *The Memory Cure* (Pocket Books, 1999). Filled with information about the research on and benefits of supplemental phosphatidylserine.

Jourdain, Robert. *Music, The Brain, and Ecstacy—How Music Captures Our Imagination* (Avon, 1998). An in-depth examination of the structure of music, exploring the origins of sound, tone, melody, harmony, rhythm, and the interaction of the human brain with these components. A fascinating work.

Rosenbauer, Wolfgang. *Better Vision Naturally* (Sterling, 1998) (English translation from German). An incisive, short book, containing simple daily and weekly exercises to increase eye strength and improve circulation and vision.

Schmidt, M. A. *Smart Fats* (Frog, 1997).

Winter, Arthur, M.D., and Ruth Winter, M.S., *Brain Workout* (St. Martin's, 1997). A wonderful book on execising your brain for maximum performance of memory, sensory perception, and intelligence. Includes dozens of suggested exercise techniques preserve, restore, and improve your brain's potential.

EXERCISE

Chu, Donald A. *Explosive Power and Strength* (Human Kinetics, 1996). For more information call (800) 747-4457 or visit www.humankinetics. com on the Web.

Chu, Donald A. *Jumping into Plyometrics* (Human Kinetics, 1998).

NUTRITION

Our partner, Dr. Ron Rosedale, is hard at work on a book, titled *Capturing the Fire of Life,* detailing his own Purist version of nutrition, diabetes, and health. It should be available within the year, so check our web site (eatprotein.com) for details about its release when they become known, or write to Dr. Rosedale at our clinic in Boulder (see address below).

PHYSICIAN INFORMATION*

We will send information about our program and the specific tests we use to any physician who requests it. We will also be happy to consult by phone with any physician who desires assistance in treating a complex patient with our regimen. Please contact our office, the Colorado Center for Metabolic Medicine, at the address below.

NEWSLETTERS, CRUISES, OTHER INFORMATION

For information about the newsletter we're planning, *Protein Power Cruises,* or other questions, write to us at:
Drs. Eades
6525 Gunpark Dr. 370
PMB 504
Boulder, CO 80301
Please direct your inquiry for proper delivery, either Attn: Newsletter or Attn: Information.

Or check our web site:
eatprotein.com

---

*Due to ambiguities in the medical and legal systems, we regret that we cannot make diagnoses by phone or mail or answer individual specific medical questions on patients we have not personally cared for except through their physician. We can, however, respond to general questions that relate to our program and how to use it.

½ cup green beans
½ cup steamed squash,
    buttered (1 tbsp.)
½ fresh sliced tomato
    vinaigrette

1 cup steamed broccoli with
    cheese sauce
½ cup red, yellow, green bell
    pepper, sautéed in olive oil and
    garlic
fresh spinach salad with
    mushrooms, dressed

½ large avocado, sliced, with
    ¼ of seasonal mixed berries
½ cup mixed fruit salad

Caesar Salad, large, no croutons
1 to 2 cups romaine lettuce
1 to 2 tbsp. Caesar dressing (look for
    no trans fats)
1 to 2 anchovy fillets (optional)
1 medium fresh peach

1 cup zucchini ribbon pasta
    (page 374) with olive oil
    and Parmesan
2 medium tomato halves, broiled
    with butter and
    herbs

INDEX

Page numbers of illustrations and charts appear in italics.

CARBOHYDRATE

Lunch

Portion   Discussion

ll items are acceptable for
denotes special item found in

mixed seasonal greens with tossed
    tomato and balsamic
    vinaigrette
cup zucchini
cup sliced strawberries

cup yellow squash

    or blue cheese dressing (p. 3
cup fresh blueberries

cup broccoli
cup red/yellow peppers, jarre
iceberg lettuce wedge with
    vinaigrette
cup mixed fruit salad (page 35

her Salad: 2 cups mixed greens
cup each chopped mushrooms,
    broccoli, cauliflower
medium tomato, sliced
ounce shredded hard cheese
    (p. 3)
hard-boiled egg, topped with 2
    ounces dressing
cup fresh blueberries or
    blackberries